Viral Keratitis

Bhavana Sharma
Radhika Tandon • Jeewan Singh Titiyal
Editors

Viral Keratitis

Springer

Editors
Bhavana Sharma
Department Of Ophthalmology
All India Institute of Medical Sciences
Bhopal, Madhya Pradesh, India

Radhika Tandon
Dr RP Centre for Ophthalmic Sciences
All India Institute of Medical Sciences
New Delhi, Delhi, India

Jeewan Singh Titiyal
Dr RP Centre for Ophthalmic Sciences
All India Institute of Medical Sciences
New Delhi, Delhi, India

ISBN 978-981-95-3147-9 ISBN 978-981-95-3148-6 (eBook)
https://doi.org/10.1007/978-981-95-3148-6

This Springer imprint is published by the registered company Springer Nature Singapore Pte Ltd.
The registered company address is: 152 Beach Road, #21-01/04 Gateway East, Singapore 189721, Singapore

Dedicated to my parents.

For the unwavering support, and boundless belief that has shaped every aspect of my life and made this endeavor possible.

I owe them everything.

Foreword

> There are in fact two things, science and opinion; the former begets knowledge, the latter ignorance.
> Hippocrates (460 BC–377 BC), from: *The Canon Law* sect. 4, in *Hippocrates*, trans. W. H. S. Jones (1923), Vol. 2, 265.

Medical textbooks serve as critical sources of information to our medical students, residents-in-training, and physicians in all phases of their careers. The best texts remain treasured items for lifetimes on the bookshelves of every physician. In the field of Ophthalmology, those of us with copies of *System of Ophthalmology*, by Sir Stewart Duke-Elder (CV Mosby Company), still find invaluable insights and perspectives that would otherwise be erased by history, with literature references from past centuries not discoverable online.

Medical texts enable a deeper dive into topics than can be accomplished in a simple review article—a book's chapters permit a focused approach into each distinct facet of the subject matter. The multitude of perspectives offered by different authors within the same book creates a depth and range not possible in a single review article. And in the era of digital, online medical education in a forever multi-tasked world, a textbook offers a deeper meditation on a topic than hit-and-run internet searches with the resultant, brief and often incorrect, artificially generated summaries can match.

Here cometh a new and scholarly tome, *Viral Keratitis*, superbly edited by Professors Bhavana Sharma, Radhika Tandon, and Jeewan Singh Titiyal. This work fills a critical unmet need in the ophthalmic literature by addressing the full spectrum of issues and concerns faced by practitioners when treating patients with corneal infections caused by viruses. With a particularly in-depth focus on the three most commonly encountered viral etiologies of keratitis in humans, namely, herpes simplex virus, varicella zoster virus, and adenovirus, the reader will quickly discern the commonalities and differences in how the cornea responds clinically to these three disparate pathogens. This leads inevitably to a deeper consideration of the fundamentals of corneal pathophysiology and immunology. As George Waring and Merlyn Rodrigues so eloquently illuminated in their classic article, "Patterns of pathologic response in the cornea" (*Surv Ophthalmol* 1987;31:262–6), the cornea can respond to insult in only a limited number of ways. Overlap in clinical findings among different etiologies of viral keratitis can lead to confusion in diagnosis, then to errors in management, and finally to missed opportunities to preserve and/or restore vision. Discussions of the subtleties in clinical presentation and natural history of these three most common viral infections of the cornea, as found in this new text, along with chapters on less common entities, will enable a higher level of clinical practice by corneal specialists and generalists alike. This new text by Sharma, Tandon, and Titiyal will therefore fill a gap unmet by currently available books, or by the internet.

The All-India Institute of Medical Sciences (AIIMS) was established in 1965 through an Act of the Parliament of India, and is the largest government hospital in the country. Its Dr. Rajendra Prasad Centre for Ophthalmic Sciences, named for the first President of India and known as "RP Centre," was established in 1967 and is now the leading center in India for training young ophthalmologists. Over one-half million patients are seen at RP Centre every year, and their ophthalmologists have the privilege of seeing, and the attendant responsibility of caring for, the entire spectrum of corneal disorders, including both common and rare viral causes of keratitis. This book will well serve every ophthalmologist seeking to better understand viral etiologies of corneal disease, their manifestations, and their diagnosis and treatments. With this new book, Professors Sharma, Tandon, and Titiyal all leaders at AIIMS and respected worldwide for their expertise and knowledge, have met the oft-repeated maxim at the RP Center: "Tamso Ma Jyotirgamaya" (from darkness to light).

Enjoy!

Respectfully offered on April 11, 2025.

James Chodosh

Professor and Chair, Ophthalmology
and Visual Sciences, Professor
Neurosciences, Professor
Molecular Genetics and Microbiology
University of New Mexico School of Medicine
Albuquerque, NM, USA

Edith Ives Cogan Professor of Ophthalmology
Emeritus, Harvard Medical School
Albuquerque, NM, USA

Preface

It gives me great pleasure to be part of this book on Viral Keratitis, a condition that remains both common and challenging in everyday ophthalmic practice. Through this work, we have aimed to bring together clear, practical, and up-to-date information to help eye care professionals manage these cases more effectively.

The book features contributions from experienced clinicians and researchers across leading ophthalmic institutes in India. It covers the complete spectrum of viral keratitis—from Herpes Simplex and Herpes Zoster to Adenoviral infections. It begins with essential background topics such as risk factors, antiviral agents, post-viral dry eye, and key clinical trials that have shaped current practice. We have also included practical and emerging areas such as neurotrophic keratitis and surgical decision-making in complex cases. The focus throughout has been to make the content useful not only for academic learning but also for everyday clinical decision-making.

What makes this book especially useful is its structured and easy-to-follow format. Each topic flows logically—from how a condition develops, to how it presents, and finally, how it should be managed. To aid learning, chapters include diagrams, flowcharts, and clinical photographs. These features are particularly helpful for residents and young ophthalmologists beginning to manage such cases.

It has been a pleasure to collaborate once again with Dr. Bhavana Sharma, with whom I previously co-edited a book on Corneal Emergencies, and with Prof. Radhika Tandon. I extend my sincere thanks to all contributing authors for writing their chapters with such clarity and commitment. I would also like to thank Springer Publications and their team for their support in bringing this book to completion.

I hope this book serves as a handy and trusted guide for anyone involved in the care of patients with viral keratitis.

New Delhi, India　　　　Jeewan Singh Titiyal

Preface

Viral keratitis is one among the most important causes of corneal morbidity worldwide, affecting individuals across all age groups and geographies. Its clinical complexity, recurrent nature, and potential for vision-threatening complications emphasizes the critical need for timely diagnosis, effective management, and ongoing research. As advancements in virology, immunology, and therapeutics continue to shape our understanding, the management of viral keratitis has evolved into a multidisciplinary endeavor.

This textbook was conceived to serve as a comprehensive and practical resource for ophthalmologists, residents, fellows, and researchers. It brings together the expertise of renowned clinicians to provide in-depth experiential knowledge of the pathogenesis, clinical presentations, diagnostic modalities, and current as well as emerging treatment options for various forms of viral keratitis. Particular emphasis has been placed on herpes simplex virus (HSV) and varicella-zoster virus (VZV) keratitis, given their prevalence and clinical importance, while also addressing less common but equally important viral etiologies, including adenovirus, cytomegalovirus, and emerging pathogens.

Each chapter has been carefully structured to integrate current evidence with practical clinical insights, highlighting both foundational knowledge and cutting-edge developments. Flow diagrams, comparative tables, and illustrative photographs have been included to enhance learning and clinical application.

We hope that this textbook will not only deepen the reader's understanding of viral keratitis but also contribute to improved patient care through evidence-based, thoughtful, and compassionate practice.

We are grateful to all contributors for their dedication, and to the readers—both current and future—whose commitment to excellence in ophthalmic care inspires this work.

New Delhi, India　　　　Radhika Tandon

Preface

Viral keratitis with its diverse clinical presentations, challenging course and potential for sight-threatening complications, necessitates a comprehensive and up-to-date resource for clinicians, researchers, and students alike. This book endeavors to fill a critical gap in the existing literature by providing the first dedicated, in-depth knowledge on all aspects of viral keratitis. Spanning over 28 meticulously crafted chapters in five sections, this volume aims to provide a holistic understanding of viral keratitis, catering to a broad audience, the students, clinical fellows, researchers, and general ophthalmologists who will benefit from the in-depth analysis of current knowledge and identification of areas for informed guided decision.

The strength of this book is further amplified by the invaluable contributions of leading experts in the field of cornea who have shared their knowledge and experience as co-authors. Their insights and perspectives have been instrumental in ensuring the accuracy, relevance, and clinical utility of the information presented herein.

It is the culmination of several decades of experience in clinical care, academics, and a dedicated focus on corneal diseases. As editors, we bring a robust background in both clinical practice and academic research, having actively participated in the diagnosis and management of viral keratitis. This deep-seated understanding of the challenges and intricacies of viral keratitis has been the driving force behind this comprehensive undertaking.

It is our sincere hope that the book will serve as an indispensable resource, fostering a deeper understanding of viral keratitis and contributing to improved patient care and outcomes.

Bhopal, India Bhavana Sharma

Preface

Viral keratitis remains one of the most prevalent and potentially sight-threatening ocular conditions worldwide. It constitutes a significant proportion of avoidable corneal blindness and necessitates timely diagnosis and intervention to prevent irreversible visual impairment. Given its clinical importance and the complexity of its management, a comprehensive understanding of viral corneal diseases is essential for ophthalmologists at all levels of practice.

This book is a comprehensive compilation of the various viral corneal disease encountered by ophthalmologists in their day-to-day practice. The content is supplemented by illustrative tables, diagnostic flowcharts, and high-quality clinical images, designed to enhance comprehension and facilitate practical application. Additionally, key learning points are highlighted at the end of each chapter to aid in quick reference and revision.

It was my privilege to work as associate editor in this book with some of the most esteemed corneal experts, which enriched my understanding of viral corneal diseases and their practical management in everyday clinical settings. I would like to express my sincere gratitude to Professor Bhavana Sharma for her invaluable guidance and support throughout this remarkable learning platform.

Bhopal, India　　　　Priyanka

Acknowledgments

The creation of this book has been fueled by a shared passion for advancing knowledge within the academic sphere. The time devoted to this project reflects not just a professional commitment but a personal dedication to providing a much-needed resource for the ophthalmic community.

I am profoundly grateful to Professor James Chodosh for lending his esteemed expertise and insightful perspective in writing the foreword to this book. His significant contributions to the field of corneal infections and his profound understanding of viral keratitis have added immense value and prestige to this work. Professor Chodosh's endorsement and thoughtful introduction will undoubtedly enhance the book's reach and impact within the academic and clinical communities. His willingness to share his time and wisdom is deeply appreciated.

This endeavor is the result of collective effort, guidance, and support of my respected co-editors Prof. J. S. Titiyal and Prof. Radhika Tandon who have been a constant source of inspiration for ophthalmic fraternity. Without their unwavering support, guidance, and critical review this book would not have seen the light of the day.

My sincere gratitude to all coauthors who are distinguished experts in the field of cornea for contributing their invaluable knowledge and time. The insightful chapters have been instrumental in shaping the comprehensive nature of this work and has been crucial in ensuring the quality and coherence of this book.

My Appreciation goes to the associate editor Dr. Priyanka for her meticulous support in bringing out this volume. The support of my senior residents, Dr. Nikhila C. Jain, Dr. Parul Mittal, and Dr. Brindha Periasamy, has been instrumental in thoughtful curation of the chapters.

I am deeply indebted to my family for their unwavering support and patience, throughout the demanding process of writing and editing this book. To my daughters, whose constant encouragement has been a motivation for me to make them proud. To my husband and siblings, whose belief in the power of education has been a guiding force in all my academic pursuits.

My sincere appreciation to the publisher Springer Nature for their professionalism, and commitment to bringing this project to fruition. Their expertise in publishing has been essential in shaping this book into its final form.

To all who have contributed, directly or indirectly, to this endeavor, I offer my heartfelt thanks.

I do hope this book serves as a valuable resource for the ophthalmic community and contributes to the advancement of knowledge in the field of viral keratitis.

Professor and Head of Ophthalmology
All India Institute of Medical Sciences Bhopal
Bhopal, India

Bhavana Sharma

Contents

About the Editors

Bhavana Sharma is Professor and Head of Ophthalmology and Dean Examinations at prestigious All India institute of Medical Sciences Bhopal. She is an ophthalmologist clinician-scientist working mainly in the field of Cataract, Cornea, and Ocular surface diseases. With over 100 peer-reviewed publications and over 200 conference presentations she leads the way in academics and research. She is credited with two reference text book on "Corneal Emergencies" and "Viral Keratitis" in addition to chapters in various textbooks. She has worked as the principal Investigator for various projects, including multicentric collaborative research projects funded by esteemed government and other funding agencies such as DST, ICMR, and MOHFW. She has been accorded several awards including best papers of cornea, cataract, and trauma and coveted best of best paper award. She has been awarded by national societies for significant contribution toward academics which includes achievement award by All India Ophthalmic Society and honor award of IJO in addition to national resource teacher gold plaque, Gurusamman and Shushrut Samman by forum of Ophthalmic teachers of India. She has been conferred with Hon. Fellowship of all India Collegium of Ophthalmology in cornea for her illustrious career and contribution toward Corneal transplantation. She is in the editorial board member of various peer-reviewed ophthalmic journals. She serves as reviewer to most national and international ophthalmology journals including *JAMA*; *Eye and Vision*; *APJO*; *International Ophthalmology*; *Clinical Ophthalmology*; *Cornea*; *PLOS One*; *IJO*, etc. She is frequently invited as guest faculty in conferences and CMEs in addition to conducting Instruction courses. She has served as Vice president, Treasurer, and General Secretary of Divisional Ophthalmic Societies in addition to chair of various institutional and government committees including academic and research committees. She has had active involvement in supporting institutions in developing transplant programs and enhancing eye banking facilities. She has been involved in establishing the Centre for Low Vision Rehabilitation at AIIMS Bhopal in addition to developing various specialty and surgical services at AIIMS Bhopal.

Radhika Tandon is a renowned ophthalmologist and academician, currently serving as Chief and Professor at Dr. Rajendra Prasad Centre for Ophthalmic Sciences, All India Institute of Medical Sciences (AIIMS), New Delhi. With over 30 years of experience in clinical ophthalmology, medical education, and ophthalmic research, she is widely recognized for her expertise in corneal diseases, ocular surface disorders, and regenerative therapies. A trailblazer in the field of limbal stem cell transplantation, she played a pivotal role in developing stem cell-based treatments for ocular surface reconstruction, significantly advancing care for patients with corneal blindness. She has led several multidisciplinary extramural and intramural projects in collaboration with leading institutions such as IIT Delhi and under the aegis of national funding agencies like the Department of Biotechnology (DBT), Department of Health Research (DHR), and Indian Council for Medical Research (ICMR).

She has an extensive academic portfolio with over 350 peer-reviewed publications in high-impact international and national journals. Her scholarly work also includes 25+ book chapters in authoritative ophthalmology textbooks and reference works, contributing significantly to the academic and clinical discourse in her field. In recognition of her expertise, she has held several prominent positions, including Chairperson of the National Eye Bank at AIIMS and member of various expert committees constituted by the national agencies.

An inspiring educator and mentor, she has guided numerous postgraduate and doctoral students, many of whom now occupy key positions in academia and clinical practice. Her academic leadership and commitment to excellence have earned her several national accolades and invitations to speak at major international conferences.

Beyond her research and teaching, she is actively involved in public health outreach and national policy initiatives in eye care. Her dedication to innovation, evidence-based medicine, and patient-centric care continues to transform lives and inspire the next generation of clinician-scientists in India and beyond.

Jeewan Singh Titiyal is a distinguished ophthalmologist who has made significant contributions to the field of ophthalmology in India and internationally. He is the former Chief of the Dr. RP Centre for Ophthalmic Sciences and Dean (Research) at the All India Institute of Medical Sciences (AIIMS), New Delhi. He completed his MBBS at AIIMS, New Delhi, followed by Junior and Senior Residency specializing in Ophthalmology with a focus on Cornea, Cataract, and Refractive Surgery. He was honored with a Doctor of Science (DSc) (Honoris Causa) by the Hemwati Nandan Bahuguna Uttarakhand Medical Education University, Dehradun, and was awarded the FRCOphth (Hon.) by the Royal College of Ophthalmologists, London, UK.

He has made significant academic and research contributions, with over 380 publications, more than 9000 citations, and 7 books, along with over 60 chapters. He is among the top-cited researchers in ophthalmology in India from 2021 to 2024, according to the Stanford University list of the top 2% most cited scientists in the world. He made history as the first Indian to perform live surgery at the American Society of Cataract & Refractive Surgeons (ASCRS) in the USA. His expertise has led him to deliver over 2000 lectures, and he has been an invited faculty member at more than 200 international and national conferences, including over 100 live surgical demonstrations. He has received more than 30 Best Paper, Best Poster, and Best Video Awards at various international and national forums. He has also contributed two patents to the field.

His outstanding achievements have earned him numerous national and international honors. He was awarded the Padma Shri by the President of India in 2014. He has also received the Distinguished Service Award from the Asia-Pacific Academy of Ophthalmology, the Senior Achievement Award from the American Academy of Ophthalmology, and the APACRS Certified Educator (ACE) Award. In addition, he was honored with the P. Siva Reddy International Award and the R.P. Dhanda Award for his contributions to eye banking and corneal transplantation, and was bestowed with the Guru Dronacharya Award by Vision 2020 Right to Sight, India.

He has trained more than 2000 students, teachers, and leaders in the field of ophthalmology. He played a pivotal role in formulating ophthalmic guidelines for the COVID-19 pandemic and post-pandemic era, and he has collaborated with the Ministry of Health & Family Welfare, ICMR, and WHO on various national surveys related to blindness. He has also worked on providing comprehensive healthcare services and building capacity in remote tribal areas of Jharkhand, Uttarakhand, Ladakh, and the Andaman & Nicobar Islands.

In addition to his academic and clinical work, he has held significant leadership roles in national ophthalmic societies. He is current President (elect) of the All India Ophthalmological Society (AIOS).

1 Introduction

Bhavana Sharma

Viral keratitis is an infectious disease of the cornea caused by viral agents. Among the various types of keratitis, viral keratitis stands out as a significant concern due to its potential to cause recurrent episodes, ongoing inflammation and resultant visual impairment. Several viruses have been implicated, with, Adeno virus, Herpes simplex virus (HSV), and Varicella-zoster virus (VZV) being the most common agents. These viruses often lie dormant in the body after initial infection, mainly in the trigeminal ganglion, and can reactivate later, leading to keratitis.

This chapter aims to provide an overview of viral keratitis, covering its etiology, pathogenesis, clinical manifestations, diagnosis, treatment, preventive measures, and recent advances.

1.1 Etiology

Common etiological agents implicated in the causation of viral keratitis include the following:

1.1.1 Herpes Simplex Virus (HSV)

HSV keratitis stands as one of the most common and challenging forms of viral keratitis, affecting the cornea and potentially leading to significant visual impairment. HSV is a double-stranded DNA virus belonging to the Herpesviridae family and it exists in two distinct serotypes: HSV-1 and HSV-2. While HSV-1 is the predominant cause of HSV keratitis, HSV-2 is primarily associated with genital herpes and can occasionally lead to ocular involvement through autoinoculation or direct viral spread [1, 2].

1.1.2 Varicella-Zoster Virus (VZV)

VZV belongs to the herpesvirus family and is responsible for causing chickenpox during primary infection and shingles (herpes zoster) upon reactivation. VZV can cause ocular complications, when the virus affects the ophthalmic branch of the trigeminal nerve. Ocular involvement typically occurs during the reactivation of latent VZV residing in the sensory ganglia, leading to Herpes Zoster Ophthalmicus (HZO) [3, 4].

1.1.3 Adenovirus Keratitis

Adenoviruses, belonging to the Adenoviridae family, are common pathogens responsible for various respiratory and ocular infections. Adenovirus keratitis typically arises from the serotypes of adenovirus that can infect the eye, primarily types 3, 4, 8, 19, and 37. These viruses are highly contagious and often spread through

B. Sharma (✉)
Department of Ophthalmology, AIIMS Bhopal, Bhopal, Madhya Pradesh, India

B. Sharma et al. (eds.), *Viral Keratitis*, https://doi.org/10.1007/978-981-95-3148-6_1

direct contact with ocular or respiratory secretions of infected individuals. Transmission commonly occurs in settings such as swimming pools, ophthalmic clinics, or crowded environments where close contact is frequent.

1.1.4 Other Viruses

While HSV, VZV, and adenovirus are common viruses, several rare viruses have also been reported to cause this condition:

1. Rubeola (Measles) Virus: Measles is a highly contagious viral infection caused by the rubeola virus. While keratitis is not a common complication of measles, it can be seen in severe cases.
2. Epstein-Barr Virus (EBV): EBV, a member of the herpesvirus family, has been associated with infectious mononucleosis and can rarely cause keratitis. EBV keratitis typically presents as a unilateral stromal keratitis with diffuse corneal opacification [5].
3. Cytomegalovirus (CMV): CMV infection, is usually associated with retinitis in immunocompromised individuals; however it can also cause keratitis. CMV keratitis may present as unilateral or bilateral stromal keratitis with characteristic multifocal coin-shaped lesions in endothelium [6].
4. Human T-cell Lymphotropic Virus Type 1 (HTLV-1): HTLV-1 is a retrovirus associated with adult T-cell leukaemia/lymphoma and HTLV-1-associated myelopathy/tropical spastic paraparesis. HTLV-1-associated keratitis has been reported, often in individuals with concomitant HTLV-1 uveitis [7].
5. West Nile Virus (WNV): West Nile virus is primarily transmitted to humans through the bite of infected mosquitoes. While West Nile fever and neuroinvasive disease are the most common clinical manifestations, ocular involvement, including keratitis, has been reported in rare cases [8].
6. Coxsackievirus: Coxsackievirus, a member of the Enterovirus genus, is primarily associated with hand-foot-and-mouth disease and other systemic illnesses. However, rare cases of coxsackievirus-associated keratitis have been reported.

1.2 Incidence

The global incidence of HSV keratitis is estimated to be around 1.5 million, with 40,000 new cases of severe monocular visual impairment or blindness annually. Studies have estimated the prevalence of HSV keratitis to range from approximately 5 to 20 cases per 100,000 population per year [9, 10]. The prevalence tends to be higher in temperate climates where HSV-1 is endemic. VZV keratitis is less common than HSV keratitis; however, it still contributes to a notable proportion of viral keratitis cases. The prevalence of VZV keratitis may vary depending on the incidence of herpes zoster in the population. HZO accounts for 10–20% of all herpes zoster cases.

1.3 Structure of Viruses Causing Viral Keratitis

Most viruses share common structural features. A general overview of the structure of viruses is as follows:

1. *Capsid*: The capsid is the protein shell that encloses the viral genetic material (DNA or RNA). It provides protection to the viral genome and helps in the transmission of the virus. The capsid can have various shapes, such as icosahedral, helical, or complex.
2. *Viral Genome*: The viral genome can be either DNA or RNA, single-stranded or double-stranded, depending on the virus type. The genome carries the genetic information necessary for virus replication and assembly. In the case of RNA viruses, some may have positive-sense RNA (which can be directly translated into proteins) or negative-sense RNA (which must be transcribed into a complementary strand before protein synthesis).

3. *Surface Proteins*: Viruses have surface proteins, including viral glycoproteins, that play crucial roles in viral attachment, entry, and host cell recognition. These proteins interact with specific receptors on the surface of host cells, facilitating virus entry into the cell.
6. *Complications*: Viral keratitis can lead to various complications, including neovascularization, opacities, scars, facets, and non-healing ulcers. Viral ulcers generally do not perforate owing to simultaneous angiogenesis of the involved area with stromal necrotising keratitis being an exception.

1.4 Pathogenesis of Viral Keratitis

1. *Primary infection*: Viral particles can enter the eye through various routes such as direct contact with contaminated fingers, contact lenses, or through droplets from coughing or sneezing. Once in the eye, the virus attaches to the surface of corneal epithelial cells. It may enter the cells through receptor-mediated endocytosis or by fusing directly with the cell membrane.
2. *Active viral replication*: The virus replicates within the corneal epithelial cells and keratocytes, leading to the destruction of these cells. The replication process triggers an immune response, causing inflammation in the affected area.
3. *Spread and Secondary Infection*: As the infection progresses, the virus can spread to neighbouring corneal cells, leading to widespread inflammation and tissue damage. Secondary bacterial infection may also occur due to compromised corneal integrity.
4. *Inflammatory Response*: The immune system responds to the viral infection by releasing inflammatory mediators such as cytokines and chemokines. This inflammatory response contributes to the symptoms of keratitis, including pain, redness, and swelling.
5. *Reactivation/Recurrent Infections*: In cases of HSV keratitis, the virus can establish latency within sensory nerves of the face, including the trigeminal nerve. Periodic reactivation of the virus can lead to recurrent episodes of keratitis, often triggered by factors such as stress, sunlight exposure, or immunosuppression.

1.5 Clinical Manifestations

Viral keratitis is often underdiagnosed owing to its varied clinical presentation. It can mimic bacterial keratitis, mycotic keratitis, acanthamoeba keratitis, or ocular surface disorders due to overlapping signs and symptoms. Thus non-responding keratitis should be revaluated for viral affection with high index of suspicion. The common manifestations include the following:

- Epithelial Keratitis: Presenting as Dendritic or Geographic Ulcers.
- Non-necrotizing Stromal Keratitis.
- Necrotizing Stromal Keratitis.
- Endothelial Keratitis.
- Neurotrophic Keratitis.
- Metaherpetic Ulcers.
- Uveitis: Scleritis: Episcleritis: Retinitis: Optic Neuritis.
- Oculomotor Palsies: Postherpetic Neuralgia (PHN).

1.6 Management

Management of HSV keratitis aims to control viral replication, alleviate symptoms, and prevent complications. Treatment modalities include [11, 12] the following:

1. *Topical Antiviral Therapy*: Topical antiviral agents such as Acyclovir 3%, Ganciclovir 15%, or Trifluridine 1% are commonly prescribed to inhibit viral replication and promote healing.

2. *Oral Antiviral Medications*: In cases of severe or recurrent HSV keratitis, oral antiviral medications such as Acyclovir, Valacyclovir, or Famciclovir may be warranted for systemic control of the infection.
3. *Topical Corticosteroids*: Short-term use of topical corticosteroids may be considered to reduce ocular inflammation and prevent scarring; however, their use requires cautious monitoring to avoid exacerbating viral replication.
4. *Debridement*: In cases of dendritic keratitis or persistent epithelial defects, therapeutic corneal debridement may be performed to remove necrotic tissue and promote epithelial healing.

1.7 Future Directions

Research into viral keratitis continues to evolve, with ongoing efforts to improve diagnosis, treatment, and prevention strategies, namely:

1. *Antiviral Therapies*: There is ongoing research for exploration of new antiviral agents, such as small molecule inhibitors and gene editing technologies, aimed at disrupting viral replication and reducing corneal inflammation [13].
2. *Topical Therapies*: Optimized dosing regimens and delivery systems to enhance the penetration of antiviral agents into the cornea and improve treatment outcomes [14].
3. *Biologic Therapies*: Biologic agents, such as monoclonal antibodies and cytokine inhibitors, are under investigation as potential adjunctive treatments for viral keratitis. These agents target specific immune pathways involved in the pathogenesis of corneal inflammation, offering targeted therapy with potentially fewer side effects than traditional immunosuppressive agents [14].
4. Vaccines: Research into the development of vaccines against HSV and other viruses implicated in viral keratitis is ongoing. Vaccination strategies aim to prevent primary infection or reactivation of latent virus, thereby reducing the incidence and severity of viral keratitis and its associated complications.

1.8 Conclusion

Viral keratitis represents a substantial burden of ocular health, leading to significant morbidity and potential vision loss if not promptly diagnosed and treated. Efforts to improve diagnostic capabilities, enhance access to healthcare services, implement preventive measures, and effective treatments are essential for mitigating the impact of viral keratitis on individuals and communities worldwide.

References

1. Liesegang TJ. Herpes simplex virus epidemiology and ocular importance. Cornea. 2001;20(1):1–13. https://doi.org/10.1097/00003226-200101000-00001.
2. Farooq AV, Shukla D. Herpes simplex epithelial and stromal keratitis: an epidemiologic update. Surv Ophthalmol. 2012;57(5):448–62. https://doi.org/10.1016/j.survophthal.2012.02.002.
3. Kalogeropoulos CD, Bassukas ID, Moschos MM, Tabbara KF. Eye and periocular skin involvement in herpes zoster infection. Med Hypothesis Discov Innov Ophthalmol. 2015;4(4):142–56.
4. Liesegang TJ. Herpes zoster virus infection. Curr Opin Ophthalmol. 2004;15(6):531–6. https://doi.org/10.1097/01.icu.0000143686.68103.46.
5. Matoba AY. Ocular disease associated with Epstein-Barr virus infection. Surv Ophthalmol. 1990;35(2):145–50. https://doi.org/10.1016/0039-6257(90)90069-8.
6. Koizumi N, Inatomi T, Suzuki T, for the Japan corneal Endotheliitis Study Group, et al. Japan corneal Endotheliitis Study Group. Clinical features and management of cytomegalovirus corneal endotheliitis: analysis of 106 cases from the Japan corneal endotheliitis study. Br J Ophthalmol. 2015;99(1):54–8. https://doi.org/10.1136/bjophthalmol-2013-304625. Epub 2014 Jul 29
7. Nakao K, Ohba N. Clinical features of HTLV-I associated uveitis. Br J Ophthalmol. 1993;77(5):274–9. https://doi.org/10.1136/bjo.77.5.274.
8. Rousseau A, Haigh O, Ksiaa I, Khairallah M, Labetoulle M. Ocular manifestations of West Nile

virus. Vaccines (Basel). 2020;8(4):641. https://doi.org/10.3390/vaccines8040641.

9. McCormick I, James C, Welton NJ, Mayaud P, Turner KME, Gottlieb SL, Foster A, Looker KJ. Incidence of herpes simplex virus keratitis and other ocular disease: global review and estimates. Ophthalmic Epidemiol. 2022;29(4):353–62. https://doi.org/10.1080/09286586.2021.1962919.
10. James C, Harfouche M, Welton NJ, et al. Herpes simplex virus: global infection prevalence and incidence estimates, 2016. Bull World Health Organ. 2020;98(5):315–29. https://doi.org/10.2471/BLT.19.237149.
11. Chodosh J, Ung L. Adoption of innovation in herpes simplex virus keratitis. Cornea. 2020;39 Suppl 1(1):S7–S18. https://doi.org/10.1097/ICO.0000000000002425.
12. Wilhelmus KR. Antiviral treatment and other therapeutic interventions for herpes simplex virus epithelial keratitis. Cochrane Database Syst Rev. 2015;1(1):CD002898. https://doi.org/10.1002/14651858.CD002898.pub5.
13. Kim TH, Lee SW. Therapeutic application of genome editing technologies in viral diseases. Int J Mol Sci. 2022;23(10):5399. https://doi.org/10.3390/ijms23105399.
14. Žigrayová D, Mikušová V, Mikuš P. Advances in antiviral delivery systems and chitosan-based polymeric and Nanoparticulate antivirals and antiviral carriers. Viruses. 2023;15(3):647. https://doi.org/10.3390/v15030647.

Risk Factors

2

Priyanka, Harsha Saxena, Parul Mittal, and Bhavana Sharma

Abstract

Viral keratitis remains a significant concern due to its potential to cause recurrent episodes, ongoing inflammation, and resultant visual impairment. Virulence and pathogenicity play crucial roles in determining the severity and outcomes of viral keratitis. Compromised immune status, direct transmission, contact lens wear, particularly extended or overnight wear, environmental factors, occupational, climate, trauma, associated comorbidities, etc., are various risk factors for viral keratitis. Family history and hereditary patterns also play a significant role in the susceptibility to various health conditions, including viral keratitis. Hand hygiene, eye protection, contact lens care, etc., are various preventive measures to reduce the risk factors for viral keratitis. Health education initiatives play a key role in promoting awareness about viral keratitis, emphasizing preventive measures, and encouraging early intervention.

Keywords

Viral Keratitis · Immune status · Factors · Preventive measures

2.1 Introduction

Viral keratitis remains a fairly common entity, yet it often remains underdiagnosed owing to varied clinical course. Common viral pathogens include Herpes Simplex Virus (HSV), Varicella Zoster Virus (VZV), and Adenovirus. These viruses have been extensively studied for their impact on the cornea and their role in causing keratitis [1–3]. Understanding the virology and pathogenesis is essential for precise diagnosis, tailored treatment strategies, and optimal clinical outcomes for patients affected by this sight-threatening condition. Knowledge about the risk factors is important not only for overall management but also for allowing healthcare providers to identify individuals who are more susceptible to viral keratitis. By understanding the risk factors, healthcare professionals can develop targeted prevention strategies to reduce the incidence and severity [4]. Furthermore, awareness of risk factors can influence treatment decisions and help tailor therapy to address the specific viral etiology and associated factors contributing to keratitis.

Priyanka · P. Mittal · B. Sharma (✉)
AIIMS Bhopal, Bhopal, Madhya Pradesh, India

H. Saxena
Vision First Eye Hospital, Neo Hospital, Noida, India

B. Sharma et al. (eds.), *Viral Keratitis*, https://doi.org/10.1007/978-981-95-3148-6_2

2.2 Risk Factors

2.2.1 Virus-Related Risk Factors

2.2.1.1 Risk Factors Related to Specific Virus

(a) Herpes Simplex Virus (HSV)

HSV-1: Herpes simplex virus type 1 is typically associated with oral herpes infections.

HSV-2: Herpes simplex virus type 2 is primarily known for causing genital herpes, which is usually transmitted through sexual contact. While less common, HSV-2 can also be a cause of ocular herpes infections, particularly in cases of neonatal herpes or through autoinoculation from genital lesions.

Impact of Previous HSV Infection on the Development of Viral Keratitis:

Reactivation of latent virus from trigeminal ganglia or other nerve ganglia can lead to recurrent episodes of ocular herpes [5]. Previous HSV infection can predispose individuals to more severe forms of herpetic keratitis, including stromal inflammation, corneal scarring, and vision-threatening complications like corneal neovascularization or corneal perforation [6].

(b) Varicella-Zoster Virus (VZV)

Individuals with compromised immune function, such as those undergoing immunosuppressive therapy or with conditions like HIV/AIDS, are at an increased risk of VZV reactivation and subsequent development of VZV-related keratitis (Table 2.1). Older individuals, particularly those over 50 years of age, have a higher risk of developing Herpes Zoster and associated ocular complications, including VZV keratitis. Patients with a history of herpes zoster in the ophthalmic division of the trigeminal nerve are at a heightened risk of developing VZV keratitis due to the proximity of eye.

(c) Adenovirus

Adenoviruses are a common family of viruses known to cause a variety of clinical manifestations, including respiratory infections, gastrointestinal illnesses, and ocular diseases. Adenoviral keratitis is a form of viral eye infection that can lead to significant ocular morbidity. Transmission of infection occurs through the following modes (Table 2.1):

Direct Contact: Transmission of adenoviruses leading to keratoconjunctivitis often occurs through direct contact with infected respiratory secretions or ocular secretions. Close personal contact or exposure to contaminated surfaces can facilitate viral transmission.

Ocular-Trauma: Adenoviral keratitis can also occur following ocular trauma, such as foreign body injuries or contact lens-related trauma, where the virus gains access to the cornea through compromised epithelial barriers, leading to infection and inflammation.

Crowded Environments: Individuals in settings with high population density, such as schools, daycare facilities, and hostels are at an increased risk of adenoviral infections due to the ease of viral transmission in crowded environments.

Poor Hygiene Practices: Lack of proper hand hygiene, sharing of personal items, and inadequate disinfection of surfaces can contribute to the spread of adenoviruses and increase the likelihood of developing adenoviral keratitis.

Contact Lens Wear: Contact lens wearers, especially those who do not adhere to proper hygiene practices or lens care protocols, are at a higher risk of adenoviral keratitis. Prolonged contact lens wear can create microtrauma on the corneal surface, providing a portal of entry for adenoviral infection.

Table 2.1 Showing pathophysiological mechanisms of involvement

S. no	Virus	Mechanism	Risk factors
1	Herpes simplex virus (HSV)	Direct viral invasion of corneal epithelial cells causing inflammation and cell death.	Close contact with infected individuals Stress UV light exposure Contact lens wear Viral pathogenicity. Genetic predisposition Immunosuppression (e.g systemic steroid, HIV, organ transplant)
2	Varicella-zoster virus (VZV)	Reactivation of latent virus in the trigeminal ganglion leading to keratitis	Older age Immunosuppression (e.g. cancer, HIV) Physical/psychological stress UV light exposure Viral pathogenicity. Exposure to infected individuals
3	Adenovirus	Direct viral infection causing epithelial cell destruction and inflammation, following an upper respiratory tract infection or conjunctivitis	Recent upper respiratory infection Exposure to infected individuals-fomites Contact lens wear Poor hygiene Crowded living conditions Healthcare-associated exposure Virulence School children
4	Cytomegalovirus (CMV)	Direct viral invasion and replication in corneal endothelial cells, often in immunocompromised patients	Immunosuppression (e.g., AIDS, organ transplant) Increasing age Co-infection with other viruses Viral latency and reactivation Viral pathogenicity Close contact with infected bodily fluids Healthcare workers Caregivers
5	Epstein-Barr virus (EBV)	Associated with keratitis through immune-mediated mechanisms rather than direct invasion, often associated with systemic EBV infection.	Immunosuppression Co-infection with other viruses Stress Previous EBV infection UV light exposure Viral latency and reactivation potential Pathogenicity of the virus Poor nutrition Close contact with infected individuals

(d) Other Viral Infections

Zika Virus: Emerging evidence suggests that Zika virus can cause ocular manifestations, including keratitis, in infected individuals. The virus is primarily transmitted through mosquito bites and has been linked to cases of viral keratitis with varying degrees of severity [7].

MERS-CoV (Middle East Respiratory Syndrome Coronavirus): Although primarily known for respiratory illnesses, MERS-CoV has been associated with ocular complications, including keratitis. Infection with MERS-CoV can lead to systemic manifestations that may impact ocular health and increase the risk of keratitis [8].

2.2.1.2 Virulence and Pathogenicity

(i) Strain variations and mutations

Virulence and pathogenicity play crucial roles in determining the severity and outcomes of viral keratitis. Understanding how strain variations and mutations in viral pathogens affect virulence and pathogenicity can provide insights into disease progression and treatment response. Different strains of a virus may possess varying abilities to infect corneal tissue, replicate within host cells, evade the immune response, and cause tissue damage. Studies have shown that specific HSV-1 strains may be more virulent in causing severe forms of herpetic keratitis, leading to prolonged inflammation, scarring, and vision loss in affected individuals.

Mutations in viral genomes can result in altered virulence factors, increased pathogenicity, or changes in viral behavior within the host. These mutations may arise spontaneously or under selective pressures, such as antiviral treatments, immune responses, or environmental conditions. In the context of viral keratitis, mutations in key viral genes, such as those encoding viral surface proteins or enzymes involved in replication, can impact the ability of the virus to infect corneal cells, evade immune detection, or establish persistent infections [9, 10].

(ii) Viral load and replication efficiency

Viral load and replication efficiency are important factors that influence the severity, progression, and clinical outcomes of viral keratitis. The quantification of viral load, which represents the amount of viral genetic material present in ocular tissues or fluids, provides valuable insights into the dynamics of viral replication and the host-pathogen interaction in keratitis.

High viral loads in the cornea or surrounding tissues may correlate with more severe ocular symptoms, extensive tissue damage, and a greater risk of complications in viral keratitis patients. The replication efficiency of viral pathogens in corneal cells determines their ability to establish productive infections, spread within the ocular tissue, and evade host immune responses. Viruses with high replication efficiency may cause rapid progression of keratitis, leading to extensive tissue damage, inflammation, and visual impairment.

2.2.1.3 Latency and Reactivation

(i) Mechanisms of viral latency

Following primary infection, certain viruses associated with keratitis, such as herpes simplex virus (HSV), and varicella-zoster virus (VZV), have the ability to establish latency in sensory ganglia, including the trigeminal ganglion for ocular herpes infections. During latency, the viral genome persists in a transcriptionally silent state within the neuronal nuclei, evading immune surveillance and antiviral treatments. Viral latency is maintained through various immune evasion mechanisms, including the suppression of viral gene expression, the inhibition of apoptosis in latently infected neurons, and the modulation of host immune responses to minimize viral antigen presentation. During latency, viral genomes may express latency-associated transcripts (LATs), which play a role in maintaining the latent state, promoting neuronal survival, and facilitating reactivation in response to external stimuli or host factors [11, 12].

(ii) Triggers for reactivation

Reactivation of latent viruses like herpes simplex virus (HSV) and varicella-zoster virus (VZV) can lead to recurrent episodes of viral keratitis. Various factors, including stress, ultraviolet (UV) exposure, trauma, and immunosuppression, can serve as triggers for viral reactivation in the cornea.

Psychological stress and physical stressors can weaken the immune system and disrupt the delicate balance that maintains viral latency. Stress-induced changes in cortisol levels and immune function may contribute to the reactivation of latent viruses in the cornea.

Prolonged exposure to ultraviolet radiation from sunlight can trigger viral reactivation in individuals with latent herpes viruses. UV radiation-induced damage to corneal epithelial cells and local immune suppression may create an environment conducive to viral replication. Physical trauma to the eye, such as corneal abrasions, surgeries, or contact lens wear, can disrupt the corneal epithelium and provide entry points for viral particles to reactivate and infect corneal cells. Trauma-induced inflammation and tissue damage may trigger viral shedding and recurrence of keratitis.

2.2.2 Host Factors

- *Genetic Predisposition*

  Understanding the genetic predisposition to the development of keratitis can provide valuable insights into individual variability in disease susceptibility and severity.

  HLA Genes: Human leukocyte antigen (HLA) genes, particularly HLA class I and II alleles, have been implicated in modulating the immune response and susceptibility to viral infections. Certain HLA genotypes have been associated with an increased risk of herpes simplex keratitis and other viral keratitis subtypes [13].

  Interferon Genes: Variations in genes encoding interferons, key components of the antiviral immune response, have been linked to altered susceptibility to viral infections, including those leading to keratitis. Polymorphisms in interferon genes may influence the host's ability to mount an effective antiviral defense [14, 15].

  Toll-Like Receptor (TLR) Genes: TLRs play a crucial role in recognizing viral pathogens and initiating the innate immune response. Genetic variations in TLR genes have been associated with altered susceptibility to viral infections, including viral keratitis [16].

  Family history and hereditary patterns play a significant role in the susceptibility to various health conditions, including viral keratitis. Studies have reported instances of familial clustering of viral keratitis, suggesting a potential genetic predisposition to the condition within certain families. Family history assessment is essential in identifying individuals at higher risk of developing keratitis and may facilitate early intervention and monitoring [17, 18].

  Genetic factors impacting corneal health, such as structural integrity, immune response, and inflammatory regulation, can influence susceptibility to viral keratitis. Examination of hereditary patterns in corneal diseases provides valuable insights into the complex interplay between genetic predisposition and environmental factors in keratitis development. Family history evaluation for viral keratitis can guide genetic counseling and screening efforts aimed at identifying at-risk individuals and families.
- *Immune Status*

  – Immunocompromised states

  Immunocompromised states, such as HIV/AIDS and organ transplant recipients, pose a significant risk factor for viral keratitis. The compromised immune function in these individuals can lead to an increased susceptibility to viral infections, including those affecting the cornea.

  Patients with HIV/AIDS are more prone to developing viral keratitis due to progressive decline in immune function associated with the disease. The impaired immune response in HIV-infected individuals can result in reactivation of latent viral infections, such as herpes simplex virus and varicella-zoster virus, leading to keratitis [19].

Organ transplant recipients are often immunosuppressed, making them susceptible to viral infections, including viral keratitis. Immunosuppressive medications reduce the body's ability to fight off viral pathogens, increasing the risk of developing keratitis post-transplantation [20]. Immunocompromised individuals with viral keratitis may face challenges in treatment response and disease recurrence due to their compromised immune status. Close monitoring and specialized management strategies, including antiviral therapy and modification of immunosuppressive regimens, are essential in this population to prevent vision-threatening complications [21].

– Immunosuppressive therapies

Immunosuppressive therapies, such as corticosteroids and chemotherapy, are known to increase the risk of viral keratitis by compromising the immune system's ability to effectively respond to viral infections. Prolonged or high-dose corticosteroid therapy can suppress the immune response and predispose individuals to viral keratitis. Corticosteroids can inhibit the inflammatory response needed to control viral replication in the cornea, potentially leading to reactivation of latent viral infections or increased susceptibility to new viral infections [22].

Patients undergoing chemotherapy often experience immunosuppression, which can predispose them to viral infections, including viral keratitis. The weakened immune system in chemotherapy recipients may compromise the cornea's ability to defend against viral pathogens, increasing the risk of keratitis development [23]. Close monitoring, early intervention, and potential modification of immunosuppressive regimens are essential to minimize the risk of viral keratitis-related complications in patients receiving such treatments [24].

- *Age and Gender*

Age-related susceptibility patterns play a significant role in the development and progression of viral keratitis. Children and infants may be at increased risk of viral keratitis due to immature immune systems and higher likelihood of direct contact with viral pathogens. Additionally, behaviors such as rubbing the eyes and poor hygiene practices are common in pediatric populations, further predisposing them to viral infections. Young adults may also be susceptible to viral keratitis, particularly due to lifestyle factors, such as contact lens wear, increased outdoor activities, and participation in contact sports, which can increase the risk of exposure to viral pathogens. Middle-aged adults may experience a shift in susceptibility patterns as age-related changes in the immune system occur. Factors such as stress, underlying health conditions, and environmental exposures may contribute to the increased risk of viral keratitis in this age group. The elderly are more susceptible to viral keratitis due to age-related decline in immune function (immunosenescence), presence of comorbidities, and higher rates of ocular surface disorders. These factors can increase the vulnerability of the elderly to viral infections.

– Gender differences in prevalence and severity

Studies have shown varying prevalence rates of viral keratitis between genders, with some suggesting a higher incidence in males while others report no significant gender-based differences. Hormonal, anatomical, and behavioral factors may contribute to potential variations in viral keratitis prevalence between males and females.

Hormonal fluctuations, particularly estrogen levels in females, have been suggested to influence the immune response and susceptibility to infectious diseases, including viral keratitis. Variances in behavior, such as hygiene practices, contact lens usage, and occupational or recreational activities, may contribute to gender disparities in viral keratitis prevalence and severity.

2.2.3 Environmental Factors

- *Geographical Distribution*

An understanding of the regional prevalence and endemic zones of viral keratitis can provide valuable insights into the geographic distribution of the condition and the impact of environmental and genetic factors on its occurrence. In the United States, viral keratitis, particularly caused by Herpes Simplex Virus (HSV), is a significant cause of infectious corneal disease. Studies have reported varying regional prevalence rates, with higher incidence seen in areas with a higher population density and greater exposure to potential risk factors.

The Asia-Pacific region, including countries like India, China, and Japan, has been noted to have a relatively high prevalence of viral keratitis, attributed to factors such as overcrowding, poor hygiene practices, and increased exposure to infectious agents. Varicella Zoster Virus (VZV) keratitis is also prevalent in this region.

Data on viral keratitis prevalence in Africa is limited; however, studies have indicated a notable burden of the condition, especially in areas with limited access to healthcare services and poor sanitation. Adenovirus keratitis outbreaks have been reported in some African countries. Europe has reported varying prevalence rates of viral keratitis across different countries. Studies have highlighted the impact of climate factors, population demographics, and healthcare infrastructure on the distribution of viral keratitis cases in Europe [25].

Specific endemic zones for viral keratitis, such as tropical regions with high humidity and poor sanitation, have been identified. These areas may experience a higher incidence of viral keratitis due to increased viral shedding, vector presence, and suboptimal access to ophthalmic care.

- *Climatic Influence on Viral Activity and Transmission*

Climate plays a significant role in influencing viral activity and transmission, including viruses associated with ocular diseases such as viral keratitis. Temperature can affect the survival and replication of viruses. Warmer temperatures may enhance viral replication rates in certain viruses, potentially increasing the risk of transmission. In the context of viral keratitis, temperature variations can impact the survival of infectious viral particles on environmental surfaces and affect transmission dynamic [26].

Humidity levels can influence the stability of viruses in the environment. Low humidity levels can desiccate viral particles, potentially reducing their viability, while high humidity may promote viral survival and transmission. Waterborne viruses can survive in moist environments and pose a risk for transmission through contact with contaminated surfaces or aerosols. Changes in precipitation patterns due to climate variability can influence the spread of viruses causing ocular infections. Seasonal changes, such as temperature fluctuations and shifts in humidity levels, can impact viral activity and transmission patterns. Viral keratitis outbreaks may exhibit seasonal variability, with increased cases during certain times of the year that correlate with climatic conditions favoring viral transmission.

Climate change can have profound effects on viral transmission dynamics by altering temperature, precipitation patterns, and ecological conditions. Changes in climate variables may expand the geographic range of viruses, impact vector populations, and influence the incidence of viral diseases, including ocular infections like viral keratitis.

- *Socioeconomic Status*

Access to healthcare and sanitation plays a crucial role in preventing, diagnosing, and managing viral keratitis and other ocular conditions. Poor sanitation practices, such as inadequate hand hygiene, improper contact lens care, and environmental contamination, can contribute to the transmission of viruses that cause keratitis. Rural population may face challenges in accessing specialized eye care services for the diagnosis and management of viral keratitis. Limited availability of eye care professionals, long travel distances, and socioeconomic barriers can hinder rural residents from receiving timely treatment. Strategies to improve telemedicine services and mobile eye clinics can enhance access to care in rural areas.

Health education initiatives play a key role in promoting awareness about viral keratitis, emphasizing preventive measures, and encouraging early intervention. International collaboration, resource allocation, and policy interventions aimed at improving healthcare infrastructure and ensuring basic sanitation facilities can contribute to disease prevention and control.

- *Overcrowded Living Conditions*

Crowded living conditions can facilitate the transmission of viruses responsible for keratitis, such as Herpes Simplex Virus (HSV) and varicella-zoster virus (VZV). Close contact among individuals in crowded settings increases the likelihood of viral shedding and subsequent infection. High population density can exacerbate the risk of outbreaks of viral keratitis.

In overcrowded environments, maintaining proper hygiene practices can be challenging, leading to an increased risk of viral transmission. Poor sanitation, lack of access to clean water, and inadequate waste disposal can contribute to the spread of infectious agents.

Urban areas with high population density and inadequate living conditions may be particularly vulnerable to outbreaks of viral keratitis. Factors such as shared living spaces, limited access to healthcare facilities, and poor sanitation can contribute to the transmission of viruses. Urban planning strategies that promote better housing, sanitation, and healthcare infrastructure are essential for mitigating the impact of viral infections.

Settings such as childcare facilities and schools, characterized by close contact and shared amenities, can serve as hotspots for viral transmission, including viruses causing keratitis. Proper hygiene protocols, regular disinfection of surfaces, and prompt identification of symptomatic individuals are essential in preventing outbreaks of viral keratitis in childcare and educational settings.

- *Occupational Exposure*

Healthcare workers and laboratory personnel play a crucial role in the prevention, diagnosis, and management of viral keratitis and other infectious diseases. These frontline professionals are at an increased risk of exposure to infectious agents, including viruses that cause keratitis, during the course of their work. Healthcare workers and laboratory personnel need to adhere to strict infection control practices to prevent the transmission of viral keratitis and other eye infections in healthcare settings. This includes measures such as hand hygiene, proper use of personal protective equipment (PPE), disinfection of equipment, and safe handling of infectious materials to minimize the risk of exposure.

2.2.4 Behavioral Factors

- *Personal Hygiene*
  - Hand hygiene practices

  Proper hand hygiene can effectively reduce the spread of pathogens from contaminated surfaces to the eyes, thereby lowering the risk of developing infections. Thoroughly washing the hands for at least 20 s, including the back of the hands, between the fingers, and under the nails, is crucial for effective hand hygiene.

  Alcohol-based hand sanitizers with at least 60% alcohol content can be used as an alternative for disinfecting the hands. Hands should be washed or sanitized at key times, including before and after contact with the eyes, before handling contact lenses, and after touching potentially contaminated surfaces.
  - Sleep patterns and stress levels

  Disrupted sleep patterns, such as insufficient sleep, poor sleep quality, or irregular sleeping hours, can contribute to elevated stress levels. Chronic sleep disturbances can interfere with the body's ability to manage stress effectively, leading to increased susceptibility to stress-related health issues, including anxiety, depression, and cardiovascular problems.

Adequate and restful sleep plays a crucial role in regulating stress hormones, such as cortisol, and promoting overall well-being. Prolonged exposure to high stress levels and disrupted sleep patterns is associated with a range of adverse health outcomes, including compromised immune function and consequent susceptibility to infections.

- *Medical History and Comorbidities*
  - Previous Episodes of Viral Keratitis as a Risk Factor for Recurrence:

  Individuals who have experienced viral keratitis caused by viruses such as Herpes Simplex Virus (HSV) or Varicella Zoster Virus (VZV) are at an increased risk of recurrence due to viral reactivation. These viruses can remain latent in the trigeminal ganglion and reactivate during times of stress or immunosuppression. In some cases, the inflammatory response triggered by a previous episode of viral keratitis may persist, creating an environment conducive to viral replication and recurrent infections [27].

  If a previous episode of viral keratitis was not adequately treated or if there was poor adherence to treatment regimens, the infection may not have been completely resolved, increasing the likelihood of recurrence. Some viral strains may have a higher propensity for recurrence due to their specific virulence factors or ability to evade the host immune response.
- *Systemic Diseases*

  Systemic diseases like diabetes mellitus, other metabolic syndromes, and autoimmune diseases (e.g., rheumatoid arthritis, lupus) remain an important predisposition both for primary infection and disease reactivation.

2.2.5 Conclusion

Transmission through fomites/direct contact/aerosols, environmental factors, immunosuppression, and emerging virus strains are major risk factors for viral keratitis. Factors such as contact lens wear, crowded environments, and poor hygiene practices also increase susceptibility to viral infections of the cornea. By identifying and addressing these risk factors, public health interventions can be more effectively targeted to prevent viral keratitis transmission within communities.

Preventive measures play a crucial role in mitigating the risk of viral keratitis. This includes promoting good hygiene practices, proper contact lens care, and avoiding close contact with individuals exhibiting viral symptoms. Immunizations for preventable viral infections like varicella can aid in reducing the incidence of viral keratitis. Effective management strategies involve early diagnosis, prompt initiation of antiviral therapy, and tailored treatment approaches based on the specific viral pathogen involved.

Key Points

1. Viral keratitis often remains underdiagnosed owing to varied clinical course.
2. Compromised immune system, previous eye injuries, extended contact lens wear, poor hygiene, associated comorbidities, and environmental/genetic factors are important risk factors for viral keratitis.
3. Recognizing and addressing these factors can influence treatment decisions and targeted prevention strategies to reduce the incidence and severity.
4. This will help tailor therapy to address the specific viral etiology and associated factors contributing to them.

References

1. Tsatsos M, MacGregor C, Athanasiadis I, Moschos MM, Hossain P, Anderson D. Herpes simplex virus keratitis: an update of the pathogenesis and current treatment with oral and topical antiviral agents. Clin Experiment Ophthalmol. 2016;44(9):824–37.
2. Litt J, Cunningham AL, Arnalich-Montiel F, Parikh R. Herpes zoster Ophthalmicus: presentation, complications, treatment, and prevention. Infect Dis Ther. 2024;13(7):1439–59.
3. González-López JJ, Morcillo-Laiz R, Muñoz-Negrete FJ. Adenoviral keratoconjunctivitis: an update. Arch Soc Esp Oftalmol. 2013;88(3):108–15.
4. Green M, Apel A, Stapleton F. Risk factors and causative organisms in microbial keratitis. Cornea. 2008;27(1):22–7.

5. Theil D, Derfuss T, Paripovic I, Herberger S, Meinl E, Schueler O, et al. Latent herpesvirus infection in human trigeminal ganglia causes chronic immune response. Am J Pathol. 2003;163(6):2179–84.
6. Giménez F, Suryawanshi A, Rouse BT. Pathogenesis of herpes stromal keratitis--a focus on corneal neovascularization. Prog Retin Eye Res. 2013;33:1–9.
7. Ventura CV, Ventura LO. Ophthalmologic manifestations associated with Zika virus infection. Pediatrics. 2018;141(Suppl 2):S161–6.
8. Abdul-Kadir MA, Lim LT. Human coronaviruses: ophthalmic manifestations. BMJ Open Ophthalmol. 2020;5(1):e000630.
9. Moshirfar M, Kelkar N, Peterson T, Bradshaw J, Parker L, Ronquillo YC, et al. The impact of antiviral resistance on herpetic keratitis. Eye Contact Lens. 2023;49(3):127–34.
10. Petrillo F, Petrillo A, Sasso FP, Schettino A, Maione A, Galdiero M. Viral infection and antiviral treatments in ocular pathologies. Microorganisms. 2022;10(11):2224.
11. Grinde B. Herpesviruses: latency and reactivation – viral strategies and host response. J Oral Microbiol. 2013;25(5):10. https://doi.org/10.3402/jom.v5i0.22766.
12. Goldstein RS, Kinchington PR. Varicella zoster virus neuronal latency and reactivation modeled in vitro. Curr Top Microbiol Immunol. 2023;438:103–34.
13. Samandary S, Kridane-Miledi H, Sandoval JS, et al. Associations of HLA-A, HLA-B and HLA-C alleles frequency with prevalence of herpes simplex virus infections and diseases across global populations: implication for the development of an universal CD8+ T-cell epitope-based vaccine. Hum Immunol. 2014;75(8):715–29.
14. Bourdon M, Manet C, Montagutelli X. Host genetic susceptibility to viral infections: the role of type I interferon induction. Genes Immun. 2020;21(6–8):365–79.
15. Ren J, Antony F, Rouse BT, Suryawanshi A. Role of innate interferon responses at the ocular surface in herpes simplex virus-1-induced herpetic stromal keratitis. Pathogens. 2023;12(3):437.
16. Jin X, Qin Q, Chen W, Qu J. Expression of toll-like receptors in the healthy and herpes simplex virus-infected cornea. Cornea. 2007;26(7):847–52.
17. Chan YK, Dick AD, Hall SM, Langmann T, Scribner CL, Mansfield BC, et al. Inflammation in viral vector-mediated ocular gene therapy: a review and report from a workshop hosted by the Foundation Fighting Blindness, 9/2020. Transl Vis Sci Technol. 2021;10(4):3.
18. Azher TN, Yin XT, Tajfirouz D, Huang AJ, Stuart PM. Herpes simplex keratitis: challenges in diagnosis and clinical management. Clin Ophthalmol. 2017;11:185–91.
19. Olusanya BA, Oshun PO. Management of herpes zoster ophthalmicus in people with HIV infection. Cochrane Database Syst Rev. 2018;2018(1):CD008770.
20. Lee DH, Zuckerman RA, AST Infectious Diseases Community of Practice. Herpes simplex virus infections in solid organ transplantation: guidelines from the American Society of Transplantation Infectious Diseases Community of Practice. Clin Transpl. 2019;33(9):e13526.
21. Binkley R. Herpetic keratitis, patience is a virtue: HSK in immunocompromised patient. OCP. 2021;27:5–14.
22. Sharma B, Soni D, Mohan RR, Sarkar D, Gupta R, Chauhan K, et al. Corticosteroids in the management of infectious keratitis: a concise review. J Ocul Pharmacol Ther. 2021;37(8):452–63.
23. Koganti R, Yadavalli T, Shukla D. Current and emerging therapies for ocular herpes simplex virus Type-1 infections. Microorganisms. 2019;7(10):429.
24. Sarikonda G, von Herrath MG. Immunosuppressive mechanisms during viral infectious diseases. In: Suppression and regulation of immune responses, vol. 677. Humana Press; 2010. p. 431–47.
25. Zhang Y, Xu X, Wei Z, Cao K, Zhang Z, Liang Q. The global epidemiology and clinical diagnosis of *Acanthamoeba* keratitis. J Infect Public Health. 2023;16(6):841–52.
26. Lowen AC, Steel J. Roles of humidity and temperature in shaping influenza seasonality. J Virol. 2014;88(14):7692–5.
27. Cook WJ, Kramer MF, Walker RM, Burwell TJ, Holman HA, Coen DM, et al. Persistent expression of chemokine and chemokine receptor RNAs at primary and latent sites of herpes simplex virus 1 infection. Virol J. 2004;1:5. https://doi.org/10.1186/1743-422X-1-5. PMID: 15507126; PMCID: PMC524517.

Antiviral Agents and Pharmacotherapeutics

3

Shivani Joshi, Noopur Gupta, Neiwete Lomi, M. Vanathi, and Radhika Tandon

Abstract

From idoxuridine to valganciclovir, there have been a number of antiviral agents discovered and further studied for the treatment of viral keratitis. As clinicians, it is necessary to understand the different mechanisms of action of various drugs. The pharmacotherapeutics of these drugs determine which drug is best suited for each aetiology. Viral keratitis is an umbrella term used to describe infections caused by Herpes simplex virus (HSV), Varicella zoster virus (VZV), Adenovirus, Cytomegalovirus (CMV), Epstein Barr virus (EBV) and others. Viral keratitis has a wide range of presentations from dendritic to stromal to endothelitis. After determining the type of presentation, choice of antiviral agents along with other pharmacological agents like steroids is ascertained to achieve the best possible outcome and improve the quality of life of patients with viral keratitis.

Keywords

Antiviral drugs · Viral Keratitis · Herpes Simplex · Varicella Zoster

S. Joshi · N. Gupta (✉) · N. Lomi · M. Vanathi · R. Tandon
R. P. Centre, AIIMS New Delhi, New Delhi, India

3.1 Introduction

After William Prosoff's discovery of Idoxuridine as an anti-cancer drug in 1959, Herbert Kaufman introduced it as an antiviral medication for herpes simplex keratitis in 1962 [1, 2].

Due to its corneal toxicity and inability to penetrate corneal epithelium, acyclovir emerged as a highly effective drug for viral keratitis throughout the spectrum of its presentations. Trifluridine, valaciclovir, ganciclovir, valganciclovir and famciclovir are some of the other antiviral agents that are currently in use for viral keratitis. This chapter aims to describe the pharmacotherapeutics of these agents and current advances in the field of management of viral keratitis.

3.2 Manifestations of Viral Keratitis

Amongst the different viruses which have been reported to cause keratitis, the herpes simplex virus (HSV) is the dominant cause. Other agents of viral keratitis include the cytomegalovirus (CMV), the varicella-zoster virus (VZV), Epstein-Barr virus (EBV) and adenovirus.

3.2.1 Herpes Simplex Virus (HSV)

There are two types of HSV—HSV 1 and HSV 2. Most ocular infections are due to HSV 1. The

B. Sharma et al. (eds.), *Viral Keratitis*, https://doi.org/10.1007/978-981-95-3148-6_3

global incidence of herpes keratitis is reported to be 1.5 million cases [3]. In a primary HSV -1 infection, ocular involvement is 8% with recurrence rates reported as 9.6% after 1 year, 22.9% after 2 years, 40% after 5 years and 67% after 10 years [4, 5].

The pathomechanism of reactivation of HSV 1 is not yet well understood but it is agreed that some stress factor induces the reactivation of the virus that resides in the trigeminal ganglion and travels via ophthalmic nerves in retrograde fashion to cause recurrent keratitis. Herpes simplex keratitis has been classified as epithelial, stromal, endothelial and neurotrophic based on the depth or pattern of involvement [6]. Epithelial keratitis is the most common manifestation which could range from granular spots, punctate lesions to branching dendritic lesions and geographical ulcers. The swollen borders of these dendrites are the sign of intraepithelial cell infiltration by the active virus. Characterized by diminished corneal sensation, diagnosis is usually on clinical basis, although viral Polymerase Chain reaction (PCR) is a confirmatory tool. Stromal keratitis can be disciform, necrotizing and immune type. Disciform keratitis consists of circular, focal stromal oedema with keratic precipitates and Descemet membrane folds. Necrotizing keratitis is caused by the active virus with dense white stromal infiltrates and corneal oedema with an increased risk of stromal melting. Immune keratitis is due to antigen–antibody complex deposition. Endothelitis can be disciform, linear, sectoral or diffuse, associated with endothelial dysfunction, keratic precipitates and corneal oedema, Descemet membrane folds and anterior chamber inflammation. Neurotrophic or meta-herpetic keratitis is due to the damage to corneal nerves by the virus which can lead to persistent epithelial defects.

3.2.2 Varicella Zoster Virus (VZV)

Herpes zoster ophthalmicus is a sight-threatening condition presenting as a vesicular rash along the distribution of the ophthalmic branch of trigeminal nerve along with epithelial infection as pseudoidentities or punctate keratitis. These dendrites are smaller and lack the terminal bulb like that of herpes simplex. Larger ulcers with stromal infiltration lead to corneal opacity after healing of ulcer. Nummular lesions in superficial stroma and sclerokeratitis may also be seen with VZV.

3.2.3 Cytomegalovirus (CMV)

Transmission rate of CMV from a mother with primary infection is 30–40% [7]. 40% of the infants with CMV infections develop auditory, ocular and neurological diseases. CMV has emerged as an etiological agent for viral endothelitis because of the large number of positive PCR results from aqueous samples. 24.1% of viral keratitis with corneal oedema were positive for CMV DNA as reported by Kandori et al. [8]. CMV has viral-tropism for CD34 + myeloid progenitor cells as well as for pulmonary, corneal endothelium, retinal and salivary tissue. CMV endothelitis presents as coin-shaped keratic precipitates, corneal oedema and anterior chamber inflammation. CMV epithelial and stromal keratitis have been reported in Acquired Immunodeficiency Syndrome (AIDS) patients.

3.2.4 Ebstein Barr Virus (EBV)

EBV keratitis is rare and seen as dendritic lesions of epithelium or as infiltrates in deeper stroma. In more severe cases, it can lead to corneal necrosis [5].

3.2.5 Adenovirus

Adenovirus infection presents as keratoconjunctivitis with multifocal nummular corneal infiltrates in most cases, along with chemosis, hyperaemia, tarsal and epibulbar follicles [9].

3.3 Clinical Trials in Viral Keratitis

Various clinical trials have been done for herpes simplex as described below (Tables 3.1 and 3.2).

Table 3.1 Herpetic Eye Disease Study (1992–1996)

Title	Purpose	Method	No. of patients	Follow-up	Conclusion
HEDS—I SKN	To evaluate efficacy of topical steroids in HSV stromal keratitis	Topical 1% prednisolone phosphate drops 8 times/day tapered over 10 weeks in addition to trifluridine	106	16 weeks	Faster resolution of stromal keratitis and fewer treatment failures
HEDS—I SKS	To evaluate efficacy of oral acyclovir (400 mg 5 times/day) in addition to topical steroids and antiviral	Oral acyclovir was given 5 times/day for 10 weeks in addition to topical prednisolone phosphate as described in SKN	104	16 weeks	No apparent benefit in adding oral acyclovir
HEDS—I IRT	To evaluate efficacy of adding oral acyclovir in treatment of HSV iridocyclitis	Oral acyclovir (400 mg 5 times/day) was given for 10 weeks in addition to topical prednisolone phosphate and trifluridine	50	16 weeks	Although not statistically significant, results showed benefit of adding oral acyclovir to treatment of HSV iridocyclitis

Table 3.2 Herpetic Eye Disease Study II (1992–1996)

Title	Purpose	Method	No. of patients	Follow-up	Conclusion
HEDS—II EKT	To evaluate the benefit of oral acyclovir in epithelial keratitis to prevent recurrence	Oral acyclovir (400 mg 5times/day) was given for 21 days in addition to topical trifluridine	287	One year	There was no benefit in addition of oral acyclovir in preventing development of stromal keratitis or iritis
HEDS—II APT	To evaluate the long-term benefit of oral acyclovir treatment in prevention of recurrences	Oral acyclovir (400 mg twice a day) was given for 1 year in patients with recent history of HSV keratitis but no active disease	703	One year	Oral acyclovir reduced the probability by 41% that any form of herpetic eye disease would return in patients who had infection in the previous year and 50% reduction in the rate of return of a more severe form of disease.
HEDS—II RFS	To evaluate the effect of psychological, environmental or biological factors on recurrences of HSV eye disease	All subjects filled out questionnaires weekly for 1 year to track acute and chronic stressors		One year	Psychological stress does not appear to be a trigger of recurrences of HSV keratitis

3.3.1 Zoster Eye Disease Study (ZEDS)

The primary aim of ZEDS was to determine whether suppressive antiviral treatment with oral valacyclovir for 12 months delays the occurrence of specific forms of HZO keratitis and iritis. As a secondary objective, the ZEDS investigators assessed whether the study drug reduces the incidence or severity of postherpetic neuralgia. Although the primary outcome did not show a benefit of suppressive valacyclovir treatment, secondary study outcomes demonstrated treatment superiority at the 18-month endpoint and a reduced number of multiple episodes of keratitis or iritis at both 12 and 18 months. These results support consideration of 1 year of suppressive valacyclovir treatment for HZO [10].

3.4 Classification of Antiviral Agents

As discussed above, human herpesvirus (HHV) genome is responsible for most of the viral keratitis. The herpesvirus genome consists of a non-

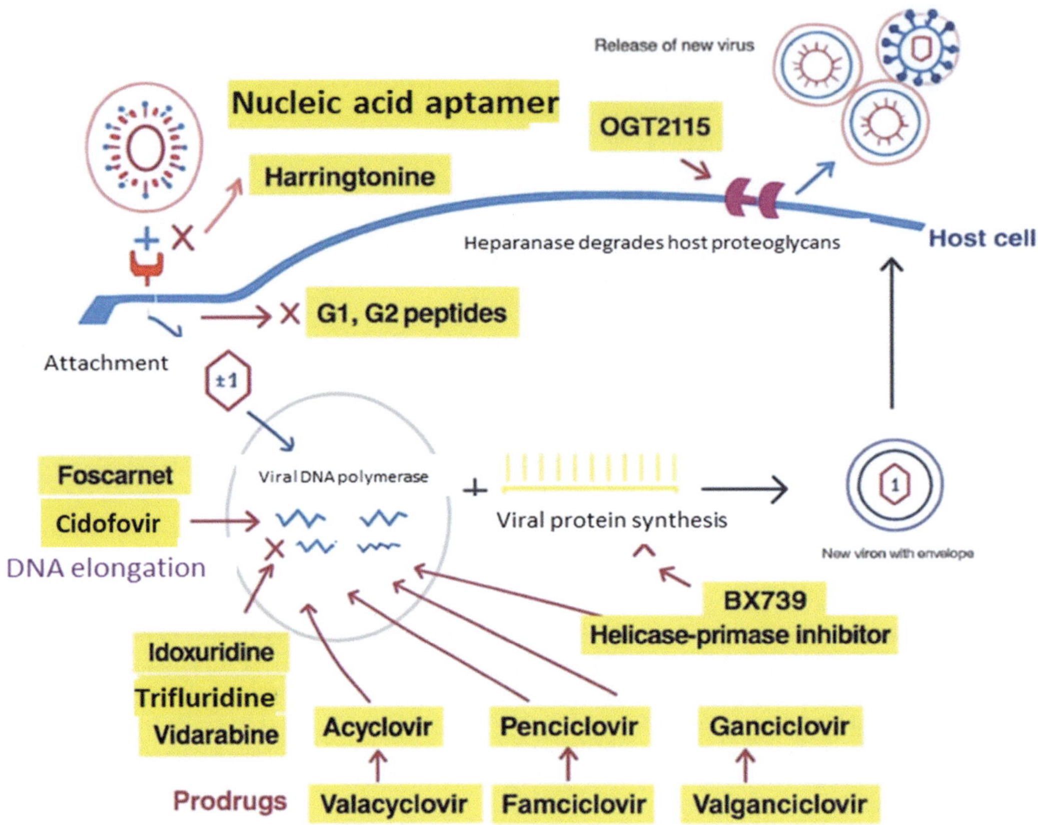

Fig. 3.1 Antiviral agents according to their mechanism of action

Table 3.3 Classification of antiviral agents

Nucleoside analogue	Nucleotide analogue	Pyrophosphate analogue	Newer drugs
Idoxuridine	Cidofovir	Foscarnet	BX759
Trifluridine			Nucleic acid aptamers
Vidarabine			Cationic peptide therapies
Acyclovir			CRISPR/cas 9 system
Ganciclovir			OGT 2115
Prodrugs			Antibodies
Famciclovir			
Valcyclovir, valganciclovir			

segmented, linear, double-stranded DNA (dsDNA) molecule. The virion consists of an icosahedral nucleocapsid surrounded by a lipid envelope. The replication cycle of herpes virus takes place in the host nucleus. The currently available antivirals act on specific stages in the life cycle of the virus (Fig. 3.1).

The antiviral agents can be classified as follows (Table 3.3).

3.5 Pharmacotherapeutics

3.5.1 Idoxuridine (IDU)

Structure—thymidine analogue.

Mechanism of action—The drug incorporates as thymidine in viral DNA, resulting in impaired transcription and translation, thereby producing defective viral progeny. Idoxuridine triphosphate inhibits DNA polymerase and dTMP synthetase, disrupting their function.

Clinical use—0.1% IDU was the first antiviral introduced in 1962 commercially. It is useful only for HSV epithelial keratitis. As it does not penetrate through intact cornea, it is ineffective in herpetic iritis and stromal keratitis. It is usually given for a maximum of two weeks to avoid corneal toxicity.

Adverse effects—Contact dermatitis, punctate epithelial keratopathy, follicular conjunctivitis, lacrimal punctal stenosis and occlusion, and lid margin keratinization when used topically. It is teratogenic, mutagenic and potentially carcinogenic, therefore IDU is not used systemically.

Resistance—HSV resistance to IDU occurs due to modification of the thymidine kinase (TK) gene. Viral strains resistant to this drug have been isolated from patients with keratitis treated with idoxuridine.

3.5.2 Trifluridine

Structure—Fluorinated pyrimidine nucleoside.

Mechanism of action—Trifluridine is similar to IDU and competitively inhibits incorporation of thymidine triphosphate into viral DNA resulting in non-functional DNA.

Clinical use—1% trifluridine has similar efficacy as of 0.1% IDU.

Adverse effects—Prolonged use of trifluridine causes irritation, delayed epithelial healing, conjunctival keratinization and scarring. Discontinuation of the drug often reverses these adverse effects. Trifluridine is limited to topical use because of its cytotoxicity, teratogenicity, mutagenicity and carcinogenicity.

3.5.3 Vidarabine

Structure—Purine arabanosyl nucleoside.

Mechanism of action—Vidarabine is virustatic. It inhibits viral DNA synthesis by inhibiting terminal deoxynucleotidyl transferase and DNA polymerase. Topically applied vidarabine crosses the cornea in minor amounts in corneas with intact epithelium. If given intravenously, vidarabine is rapidly deaminated by adenosine deaminase to the less effective Ara-HX form or other non-effective metabolites. To enhance the antiviral efficacy of vidarabine therapy, potent inhibitors of adenosine deaminase are administered with the drug.

Clinical use—Topical vidarabine 3% ointment has been found to be effective in herpetic keratitis and keratouveitis in both animal models and in humans. Systemic administration is reserved for HSV or drug-resistant VZV in life-threatening situations due to its systemic toxicity.

Adverse effects—Vidarabine is minimally toxic when applied topically. Systemic administration requires large amount of intravenous fluid administration because of the compound's relative insolubility, in turn causing stress on cardiovascular and renal system.

Resistance—Vidarabine-resistant viruses with changes in the DNA polymerase gene have been isolated [11].

3.5.4 Acyclovir

Structure—Acyclovir is a purine nucleoside, a guanosine analogue which is characterized by the absence of carbon atoms at 2′and 3′ positions.

Mechanism of action—Acyclovir acts by viral DNA chain termination and rapid inactivation of viral DNA polymerase. Acyclovir is phosphorylated (activated) to acyclovir monophosphate specifically by herpesvirus-encoded thymidine kinase. This is absent in non-infected cells, making acyclovir very selective and hence less toxic. Acyclovir monophosphate is further phosphorylated to acyclovir diphosphate and triphosphate by viral and cellular enzymes. Acyclovir triphosphate (ACVTP) competes for deoxyguanosine triphosphate (dGTP), the natural substrate for virus-specific DNA polymerase and is incorporated irreversibly onto the growing viral DNA chains, thus causing chain termination. Acyclovir exhibits effective action on HSV-1 and HSV-2, VZV, EBV and, to a lesser extent, CMV. This drug has been reported to be 160 times more effective than vidarabine and 10 times more effective than idoxuridine [12]. Acyclovir has been shown to suppress latent virus reactivation in trigeminal ganglion, but it does not eliminate latency within the ganglion.

Clinical Use—Acyclovir is formulated as a 3% ointment with polyethylene glycol (PEG) due to its lipophilic nature. It is indicated in herpetic epithelial keratitis five times a day for 1–3 weeks. Oral acyclovir is also indicated in both HSV and VZV keratitis. For HSV stromal keratitis and endothelitis, iridocyclitis, oral acyclovir 400 mg five times a day for the initial 2–3 weeks followed by a maintenance dose of 400 mg twice a day is given. For Herpes Zoster Ophthalmicus, the inhibitory doses for VZV are much higher so oral Acyclovir 800 mg five times a day is advised. According to the HEDS trial oral acyclovir prevents recurrence of any form of ocular HSV by 41% when given at a dose of 400 mg twice a day [13].

Adverse Effects—When applied topically for a long duration, acyclovir is seen to be epitheliotoxic. Systemically, nephrotoxicity is the main adverse effect of the drug. It is related to the route of elimination of the drug, being caused by the accumulation of non-soluble drug crystals in the renal tubules. With long-term usage of oral acyclovir for the purpose of prophylaxis of recurrence, we must monitor serum electrolytes, blood urea and creatinine. Renal toxicity is evidenced by an increase in serum creatinine, the appearance of urine sediment or signs of acute renal failure. Hydration of all patients should be monitored and patients with renal insufficiency should have reduced doses and prolongation of the intervals between dosing to minimize this risk. Rare central nervous system toxicity, delirium tremens and coma have been reported. Other common side effects are gastrointestinal distress and headache. There is no evidence that acyclovir is a carcinogen or teratogen, and at therapeutic doses for ocular disease, there is no reported adverse effect on the hematopoietic or immune system.

3.5.5 Ganciclovir

Structure—This drug is an acyclic pyrimidine nucleoside of deoxyguanosine. Ganciclovir is structurally similar to acyclovir but because of the additional hydroxyl group (-OH) there is an expanded drug activity. Besides HSV, it also inhibits the replication of CMV.

Mechanism of action—Ganciclovir causes viral DNA chain termination and inhibits viral DNA polymerase. The incorporation of the drug triphosphates destabilizes the viral DNA strands and leads to the suppression of DNA elongation.

Clinical use—Because of the additional hydroxyl group, ganciclovir is 25 times more potent than acyclovir against CMV. It is the drug of choice for CMV keratitis. Ganciclovir was marketed as FDA-approved 0.15% gel in 2009. It has higher potency than acyclovir against HSV therefore a lower concentration of 0.15% is effective. Oral bioavailability is poor with only 5–10% drug being absorbed when given orally but has been administered at 1000 mg thrice a day for 8 weeks for prevention and treatment of recurrent HSV stromal keratitis and endothelitis [14].

Adverse effects—Conjunctival hyperaemia, punctate keratopathy and ocular irritation have been reported with topical ganciclovir. Systemic ganciclovir has been associated with granulocytopenia, thrombocytopenia, anaemia, azoospermia, and a rise in serum creatinine.

3.5.6 Valacyclovir

Structure—L -Valine ester of acyclovir.

Mechanism of action—On ingestion, this drug is immediately changed to acyclovir by the enzyme valacyclovir hydrolase in the digestive tract. The oral bioavailability is several times that of acyclovir. The antiviral mechanism is the same as that of acyclovir.

Clinical use—Oral valacyclovir 500 mg twice daily for 7–10 days can be used for HSV infections and 1 g thrice daily for 7–10 days for HZO.

Adverse effects—Valacyclovir is nephrotoxic and kidney function tests are to be monitored.

3.5.7 Famciclovir

Structure—Acyclic guanine derivative.

Mechanism of action—Famciclovir is a prodrug for penciclovir. It has an action similar to acyclovir by inhibiting viral DNA polymerase.

Clinical use—Famciclovir has a better oral bioavailability as compared to acyclovir. This drug is used in the dosage of 500 mg thrice daily for 7 days for acute HSV and HZO infections.

Adverse effects—This drug is nephrotoxic. Dose adjustment is required when given in concurrence with other nephrotoxic medication.

3.5.8 Valganciclovir

Structure—L-valine ester salt of Ganciclovir.

Mechanism of action—Valganciclovir has significantly higher oral bioavailability (60%) than ganciclovir (9%). After oral administration, it is rapidly converted to ganciclovir by intestinal and hepatic esterases. The mechanism of action is the same as that of ganciclovir.

Clinical use—Valganciclovir is used in the treatment of CMV retinitis. It has been reported to be successful in herpes simplex keratitis not responding to conventional antiviral treatment [15]. Valganciclovir is given at an induction dose of 900 mg twice daily for 10 days followed by 900 mg once daily as a prophylactic dose.

Adverse effects—Bone marrow suppression, nephrotoxicity.

3.5.9 Cidofovir

Structure—Cytosine nucleotide analogue.

Mechanism of action—Cidofovir is a competitive inhibitor of viral DNA polymerases and therefore inhibits viral DNA elongation.

Clinical use—The drug is mainly used for CMV infections resistant to ganciclovir and foscarnet. Because of its poor oral bioavailability, it is usually given intravenously with probenecid to prevent nephrotoxicity. Although more commonly used for CMV retinitis, animal studies have found that 0.2–0.5% topical cidofovir was as effective as trifluridine in treating HSV epithelial keratitis [16]. Topical cidofovir has also been suggested for usage in acyclovir-resistant herpes keratitis [17].

Adverse effects—This drug is nephrotoxic and requires systemic monitoring when administered.

3.5.10 Foscarnet

Structure—Non-nucleoside analogue to pyrophosphate.

Mechanism of action—Foscarnet selectively inhibits the pyrophosphate binding site on viral DNA polymerase and finally prevents the incorporation of nucleotides into the growing DNA strand. Acyclovir is a guanosine analogue that requires phosphorylation by the viral thymidine kinase (TK) prior to conversion to its active form. Foscarnet does not utilize thymidine kinase for its action, therefore does not develop resistance due to this gene.

Clinical usage—Foscarnet is administered intravenously for ganciclovir-resistant CMV retinitis, but topical formulation of 1.2% -1.4% has shown to be useful in acyclovir-resistant herpes keratitis [17]. In 1998, Fabricius et al. studied various concentrations of topical foscarnet in 10 patients with HSV keratitis and found that corneal toxicity developed in patients using 1.9% foscarnet, but the medication was well tolerated by those using 1.2% and 1.4% foscarnet [18].

Adverse effects—When administered intravenously, foscarnet can cause nephrotoxicity. Topical administration of 1.9% has shown cornea toxicity.

3.5.11 Newer Drugs

3.5.11.1 BX759

This drug inhibits various kinases in the virus causing inhibition of AKT signalling pathway phosphorylation which impedes viral protein synthesis and results in slowing of viral activity within cells. The precise mechanism by which BX795 acts on AKT and the long-term effects of BX795 treatment still must be elucidated [19].

3.5.11.2 Helicase

Primase inhibitors—Oral BAY 57–1293, a Helicase-primase inhibitor has been studied and found to be a substitute for eye drops as an effective treatment for herpetic keratitis and might be useful in treating stromal keratitis and iritis, as well as preventing recurrences of ocular herpes in animal models [20].

3.5.11.3 Aganirsen

This drug works as an antisense oligonucleotide, inhibiting insulin receptor substrate-1 expression. Aganirsen eye drops have been found to reduce corneal neovascularization during healing of viral keratitis [21].

3.5.11.4 Harringtonine

This drug is a natural alkaloid. It has shown to be effective in HSV- 1 infections by suppressing the herpes virus entry mediator expression, thus preventing viral entry of HSV-1 into the host cell [22].

3.5.11.5 Nucleic Acid Aptamers

They are short oligonucleotides with the ability to bind to a wide variety of molecular targets. Two RNA aptamers, designated aptamer-1 and aptamer-5 were able to bind to the HSV-1 protein gD with high specificity and thus inhibit the viral protein interaction with its receptor. The lack of toxicity reported with these aptamers and their ability to inhibit HSV-1 and HSV-2 infections with great specificities and low concentrations make aptamers an attractive treatment option to be further studied [23].

3.5.11.6 Cationic Peptide Therapies

G1 and G2 peptide therapies have shown to inhibit viral entry into cells of HSV-1. Peptide derived from HIV TAT-cd protein if given early at a concentration at 1 mg/ml has shown to decrease viral keratitis [5].

3.5.11.7 CRISPR-Cas9

Currently, CRISPR- Cas9 systems can reduce HSV-1 replication significantly in both infected cells and cells experiencing a reactivation of HSV-1 from quiescence. Future in vitro and in vivo studies are needed to examine the effects of CRISPR-Cas9 on HSV-1 infections and optimize the system to eradicate latent viral particles [24].

3.5.11.8 OGT 2115

Heparanase is an enzyme which is capable of cleaving heparan sulphate. It is important for HSV-1 release from infected corneal cells. OGT 2115 has been characterized as an inhibitor of heparanase enzymatic activity. It hinders viral egress from corneal cells [25].

3.5.11.9 Antibodies

Krawczyk et al. developed a humanized monoclonal antibody, designated mAb hu2c, against the viral glycoprotein gB. MAb hu2c proved to be effective in neutralizing wild-type and drug-resistant strains of HSV-1, blocking the spread of the virus between cells. Animal studies have shown that it is useful to decrease the viral load even for ocular infections [26, 27].

3.5.12 Newer Drug Delivery Models—Lipid-Based Nanocarriers and Polymeric-Based Nanocarriers

3.5.12.1 Lipid-Based Nanocarriers

Lipid-based nanocarriers—includes liposomes and niosomes, solid lipid nanoparticles (SLNs) and nanostructured lipid carriers (NLCs) and nanoemulsions. Liposomes consist of single or multiple phospholipid bilayers arranged in a vesicular shape, surrounding an inner aqueous core. They improve the ocular bioavailability of drugs by their interaction with the corneal surface. Chetoni et al. found that acyclovir liposomes (LIPO-ACVs) have a 11-fold greater bioavailability in aqueous humour of rabbits in comparison with the currently available ointment [28]. Niosomes are synthesized using non-ionic surfactants instead of phospholipids and they possess better stability and longer shelf-life as compared to liposomes. Akhter et al. evaluated the ocular retention and intraocular delivery of ganciclovir entrapped in niosomes, which were pre-coated with chitosan and found that chitosan coating increased ocular retention due to its interaction with the negatively charged components on the corneal surface of rabbits [29].

3.5.12.2 Polymeric-Based Nanocarriers

These include nanomicelles, polymeric nanoparticles and nanosuspensions. Nanomicelles are colloidal drug delivery systems made up of amphiphilic surfactant units that increases the solubility of hydrophobic drugs in aqueous solution by encapsulating them in the lipophilic core. Acyclovir polymeric micelles have been developed and the effects studied on bovine cornea and sclera and showed better penetration through the sclera than in the cornea [30]. Polymeric nanoparticles in the form of acyclovir with poly (lactic-co-glycolic acid) ACV—PLGA have been studied and found that these nanoparticles are relatively safe and non-toxic in animal studies [31].

3.6 Vaccines

Heiligenhaus et al. described immunization with a synthetic peptide of glycoprotein D (gD) of HSV-l in a murine model of herpes stromal keratitis in 1995. Their results suggest that immunization with gD (5–23) stimulates both humoral and cellular immune mechanisms which protect against HSV-l keratitis [32]. In 1998, Nesburn et al. reported efficacy of periocular recombinant glycoprotein D from HSV-1 (gD1) as a vaccine in rabbit models [33]. Pivetti-Pezzi et al. reported a reduction in the number and duration of relapses in herpes simplex virus 1-related keratitis/keratouveitis after giving a vaccine with heat shock-inactivated herpes simplex virus type 1 [34]. in 2021, Nabi et al. reported protection against HSV keratitis in mice models after giving live attenuated vaccine (VC2) [35]. Various other subunit, live attenuated and DNA/RNA vaccine trials are underway, but none have been approved yet for usage [36].

Centers for Disease Control and Prevention (CDC) recommends that all adults 50 years of age and older and people 19 years of age and older who are or will become immunocompromised receive the recombinant zoster vaccine, adjuvanted (Shingrix; GSK). The most common side effects of vaccination are local injection-site reactions or mild systemic reactions, but rarely, ophthalmologic reactivation of HZ has been reported [37, 38].

3.7 Conclusion

Viral keratitis, primarily caused by herpes simplex virus, presents significant clinical challenges due to its diverse manifestations and potential for recurrence. Agents such as acyclovi, and ganciclovir form the quintessential components in the armamentarium against the virus with ongoing clinical trials exploring the efficacy and safety of newer modalities. These modalities, including lipid-based and polymeric nanocarriers, aim to enhance therapeutic outcomes by improving ocular bioavailability. Further, vaccines to preventing herpes keratitis have shown significant promise for clinical use, although no vaccines are currently approved for clinical use.

Key Points

1. Viral keratitis can present as various manifestations. These must be recognized, and treatment has to be targeted to the particular manifestation.

2. Currently available topical and oral antivirals are effective in the management of viral keratitis.
3. HEDS trial has given recommendations on the use of oral acyclovir.
4. Mechanism of action and adverse effects of each drug should be well understood while advising these drugs.
5. Oral administration of antiviral agents requires systemic monitoring.
6. Newer drugs and modes of drug delivery are under study to better target viral activity.

References

1. Prusoff WH. Synthesis and biological activities of iododeoxyuridine, an analog of thymidine. Biochim Biophys Acta. 1959;32(1):295–6.
2. Kaufman H, Martola EL, Dohlman C. Use of 5-iodo-2′-deoxyuridine (IDU) in treatment of herpes simplex keratitis. Arch Ophthalmol Chic Ill 1960. 1962;(68):235–9.
3. Reynaud C, Rousseau A, Kaswin G, M'garrech M, Barreau E, Labetoulle M. Persistent impairment of quality of life in patients with herpes simplex keratitis. Ophthalmology. 2017;124(2):160–9.
4. Farooq AV, Shukla D. Herpes simplex epithelial and stromal keratitis: an epidemiologic update. Surv Ophthalmol. 2012;57(5):448–62.
5. Koganti R, Yadavalli T, Naqvi RA, Shukla D, Naqvi AR. Pathobiology and treatment of viral keratitis. Exp Eye Res. 2021;205:108483.
6. Holland EJ, Schwartz GS. Classification of herpes simplex virus keratitis. Cornea. 1999;18(2):144–54.
7. Stagno S, Pass RF, Cloud G, Britt WJ, Henderson RE, Walton PD, et al. Primary cytomegalovirus infection in pregnancy. Incidence, transmission to fetus, and clinical outcome. JAMA. 1986;256(14):1904–8.
8. Kandori M, Inoue T, Takamatsu F, Kojima Y, Hori Y, Maeda N, et al. Prevalence and features of keratitis with quantitative polymerase chain reaction positive for cytomegalovirus. Ophthalmology. 2010;117(2):216–22.
9. Bialasiewicz A. Adenoviral Keratoconjunctivitis. Sultan Qaboos Univ Med J. 2007;7(1):15–23.
10. Cohen EJ, Troxel AB, Liu M, Hochman JS, Baratz KH, Mian SI, et al. ZEDS Trial Research Group. Low-Dose Valacyclovir in Herpes Zoster Ophthalmicus: The Zoster Eye Disease Randomized Clinical Trial. JAMA Ophthalmol. 2025;143(4):269–76. https://doi.org/10.1001/jamaophthalmol.2024.6114. PMID: 40048183; PMCID: PMC11886868.
11. Paintsil E, Cheng YC. Antiviral agents. In: Schaechter M, editor. Encyclopedia of microbiology; 2009. p. 223–57. https://doi.org/10.1016/B978-012373944-5.00178-4.
12. Grieco MH. Therapy of viral infections. Bull N Y Acad Med. 1982;58(8):711–20.
13. Wilhelmus KR, Gee L, Hauck WW, Kurinij N, Dawson CR, Jones DB, et al. Herpetic eye disease study: a controlled trial of topical corticosteroids for herpes simplex stromal keratitis. Ophthalmology. 1994;101(12):1883–96.
14. Wang X, Wang L, Wu N, Ma X, Xu J. Clinical efficacy of Oral ganciclovir for prophylaxis and treatment of recurrent herpes simplex keratitis. Chin Med J. 2015;128(1):46–50.
15. Koseoglu ND, Strauss BR, Hamrah P. Successful Management of Herpes Simplex Keratitis with Oral Valganciclovir in patients unresponsive or allergic to conventional antiviral therapy. Cornea. 2019;38(6):663–7.
16. Kaufman HE, Varnell ED, Thompson HW. Cidofovir and experimental herpetic stromal disease. Arch Ophthalmol. 1999;117(7):925–8.
17. De Clerck I, Walgrave V, Snoeck R, Andrei G, Blanckaert J, Mulliez E, et al. Putting drug resistant epithelial herpes keratitis in the spotlight: a case series. Am J Ophthalmol Case Rep. 2022;25:101268.
18. Fabricius EM. Foscarnet eyedrops in recurrence prophylaxis of herpes simplex virus keratitis. Acta Ophthalmol Scand. 1998;76(6):754–7.
19. Shukla D, Jaishankar D. Targeting Akt phosphorylation by a small molecule inhibitor generates an effective strategy to curb corneal herpes simplex virus type-1 infection. Invest Ophthalmol Vis Sci. 2018;59(9):4931.
20. Kaufman HE, Varnell ED, Gebhardt BM, et al., et al. Efficacy of a helicase-primase inhibitor in animal models of ocular herpes simplex virus type 1 infection. J Ocul Pharmacol Ther Off J Assoc Ocul Pharmacol Ther. 2008;24(1):34–42.
21. Cursiefen C, Viaud E, Bock F, Geudelin B, Ferry A, Kadlecová P, et al. Aganirsen antisense oligonucleotide eye drops inhibit keratitis-induced corneal neovascularization and reduce need for transplantation: the I-CAN study. Ophthalmology. 2014;121(9):1683–92.
22. Liu Y, You Q, Zhang F, Chen D, Huang Z, Wu Z. Harringtonine inhibits herpes simplex virus type 1 infection by reducing herpes virus entry mediator expression. Front Microbiol. 2021;12:722748.
23. Yadavalli T, Agelidis A, Jaishankar D, Mangano K, Thakkar N, Penmetcha K, et al. Targeting herpes simplex Virus-1 gD by a DNA Aptamer can be an effective new strategy to curb viral infection. Mol Ther Nucleic Acids. 2017;9:365–78.
24. Yin D, Ling S, Wang D, Dai Y, Jiang H, Zhou X, et al. Targeting herpes simplex virus with CRISPR–Cas9 cures herpetic stromal keratitis in mice. Nat Biotechnol. 2021;39(5):567–77.
25. Suryawanshi RK, Patil CD, Agelidis A, et al. Pathophysiology of reinfection by exogenous HSV-1 is driven by heparanase dysfunction. Sci Adv.

2023;9(17):eadf3977. https://doi.org/10.1126/sciadv.adf3977.
26. Koganti R, Yadavalli T, Shukla D. Current and emerging therapies for ocular herpes simplex virus Type-1 infections. Microorganisms. 2019;7(10):429.
27. Labib BA, Chigbu DI. Clinical management of herpes simplex virus keratitis. Diagnostics. 2022;12(10):2368.
28. Chetoni P, Rossi S, Burgalassi S, Monti D, Mariotti S, Saettone MF. Comparison of liposome-encapsulated acyclovir with acyclovir ointment: ocular pharmacokinetics in rabbits. J Ocul Pharmacol Ther. 2004;20(2):169–77. https://doi.org/10.1089/108076804773710849.
29. Akhter S, Ramazani F, Ahmad MZ, Ahmad FJ, Rahman Z, Bhatnagar A, et al. Ocular pharmacoscintigraphic and aqueous humoral drug availability of ganciclovir-loaded mucoadhesive nanoparticles in rabbits. Eur J Nanomedicine. 2013;5(3):159–67.
30. Li Z, Liu M, Ke L, et al. Flexible polymeric nanosized micelles for ophthalmic drug delivery: research progress in the last three years. Nanoscale Adv. 2021;3(18):5240–54. https://doi.org/10.1039/d1na00596k.
31. Pandey M, Choudhury H, Abdul-Aziz A, Bhattamisra SK, Gorain B, Su JST, et al. Advancement on sustained antiviral ocular drug delivery for herpes simplex virus keratitis: recent update on potential investigation. Pharmaceutics. 2021;13(1):1.
32. Heiligenhaus A, Wells PA, Foster CS. Immunisation against HSV-1 keratitis with a synthetic gD peptide. Eye Lond Engl. 1995;9(Pt 1):89–95.
33. Nesburn AB, Burke RL, Ghiasi H, Slanina SM, Wechsler SL. A therapeutic vaccine that reduces recurrent herpes simplex virus type 1 corneal disease. Invest Ophthalmol Vis Sci. 1998;39(7):1163–70.
34. Pivetti-Pezzi P, Accorinti M, Colabelli-Gisoldi RA, Pirraglia MP, Sirianni MC. Herpes simplex virus vaccine in recurrent herpetic ocular infection. Cornea. 1999;18(1):47–51.
35. Nabi R, Lewin AC, Collantes TM, Chouljenko VN, Kousoulas KG. Intramuscular vaccination with the HSV-1(VC2) live-attenuated vaccine strain confers protection against viral ocular Immunopathogenesis associated with γδT cell Intracorneal infiltration. Front Immunol. 2021;12:789454. https://doi.org/10.3389/fimmu.2021.789454.
36. Krishnan R, Stuart PM. Developments in vaccination for herpes simplex virus. Front Microbiol. 2021;12:798927. https://doi.org/10.3389/fmicb.2021.798927.
37. Jabbour S, Shekhawat NS, Chen A, Woreta FA. Presumed herpes zoster Ophthalmicus reactivation following recombinant zoster vaccination. Cornea. 2021;40(2):248.
38. Lehmann A, Matoba A. Reactivation of herpes zoster stromal keratitis after HZ/su Adjuvanted herpes zoster subunit vaccine. Ophthalmology. 2018;125(11):1682.

Clinical Trials in Viral Keratitis

4

Pranita Sahay, Kanchita Pandey,
Prafulla Maharana, and Brindha Periasamy

Abstract

Herpes simplex and Herpes zoster viruses are the common causes of viral keratitis with variable clinical presentation. The treatment options for viral keratitis primarily include antivirals and steroids. Researchers have done various studies to understand the rationale of these two drugs tailored to the clinical presentation of viral keratitis. This chapter provides a detailed description of the landmark trial, herpetic eye disease study (HEDS), and an overview of the Zoster Eye Disease Study (ZEDS).

Keywords

HEDS · ZEDS · Clinical trials · Viral keratitis

4.1 Introduction

The clinical spectrum of viral keratitis includes epithelial keratitis (dendritic/geographic), stromal keratitis (immune/necrotizing), and viral kerato-uveitis, with varying visual outcomes [1, 2]. Each entity has a different management approach with topical or systemic antivirals and steroids [1]. Before the HEDS trial, the role of topical corticosteroids in the treatment of herpes simplex virus (HSV) stromal keratitis remained uncertain. Additionally, it was unclear whether the addition of an oral antiviral to a treatment regimen that included topical corticosteroids and antivirals would offer any additional benefit. HEDS I trial was aimed to address these gaps. HEDS II trial addressed the role of oral acyclovir in preventing the progression and recurrence of HSV keratitis.

4.2 Herpetic Eye Disease Study (HEDS)

The Herpetic Eye Disease Study (HEDS) is a landmark series of clinical trials that significantly influenced the treatment guidelines for HSV keratitis. It explored topical corticosteroids in combination with antiviral agents (topical and systemic) for various stages of HSV anterior segment disease. The study was initiated in 1989 and the guidelines proposed by HEDS is still considered a gold standard in the management of viral keratitis.

4.2.1 Design

HEDS was a prospective, randomized, double-masked, placebo-controlled, and multicentric clinical trial that was conducted in two phases, each with three trials as described in Table 4.1.

P. Sahay · K. Pandey · P. Maharana (✉)
R. P. Centre, AIIMS Delhi, Delhi, India

B. Periasamy
AIIMS Bhopal, Bhopal, Madhya Pradesh, India

B. Sharma et al. (eds.), *Viral Keratitis*, https://doi.org/10.1007/978-981-95-3148-6_4

Table 4.1 Phases of HEDS

HEDS I (1989 to 1992)	HEDS II (1992 to 1994)
3 therapeutic trials	2 preventive trials 1 cohort trial (epidemiological study)

4.2.2 Purpose

HEDS was designed around a set of questions that the trials intended to explain and offer a protocol for treating HSV anterior segment disease.

1. Are topical steroids effective in HSV stromal keratitis along with topical trifluridine?
2. Should oral acyclovir be added to topical steroids and trifluridine regimen in HSV stromal keratitis?
3. Does oral acyclovir aid in better resolution of HSV iritis in patients already using topical steroids and trifluridine?
4. Does early treatment of HSV epithelial keratitis with oral acyclovir prevent progression to stromal keratitis and iridocyclitis?
5. Is low-dose oral acyclovir prophylaxis helpful in preventing HSV recurrence?
6. What are the triggers/predictors of HSV recurrence?

4.2.3 Herpetic Eye Disease Study 1 (HEDS I)

HEDS I was conducted from May 1989 to 1992. The first phase of the trial answered first three questions of HEDS in three parts and assessed the efficacy of oral acyclovir and topical steroids for treating HSV stromal keratitis and iritis.

1. HSV Stromal Keratitis not on Steroid (HEDS-SKN).
2. HSV Stromal Keratitis on Steroids (HEDS-SKS).
3. HSV Iridocyclitis Receiving Topical steroids (HEDS-IRT).

4.2.3.1 HEDS—SKN Trial

(a) *Study question:* Are topical steroids effective in HSV stromal keratitis along with topical trifluridine?

(b) *Protocol:* Trial recruited 106 patients with active HSV stromal keratitis and randomized into two arms. The simplified form of study protocol is shown in the Flowdiagram 4.1. Patients were evaluated weekly for 10 weeks, every other week until week 16, and again at 6 months.

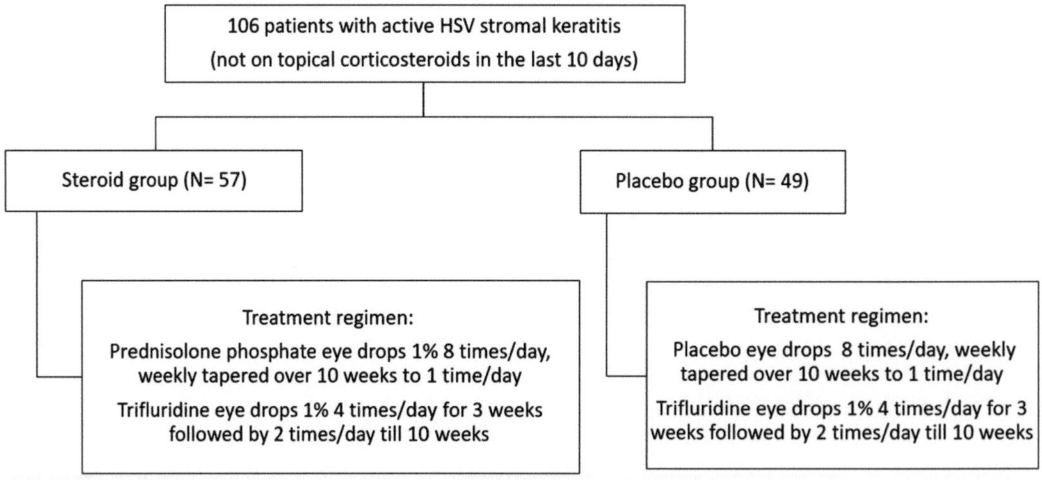

Flowdiagram 4.1 Showing simplified protocol of HEDS -SKN trial

(c) *Results:* Steroid group participants had clinical resolution in 26 days, which was faster than the placebo group (72 days). Treatment failure was more in placebo group which was 73% at 10 weeks and 76% at 16 weeks when compared to steroid group. There was no difference between the groups in terms of final visual outcome and recurrence of HSV. The results are summarized in Table 4.2.

(d) *Inference:* Topical prednisolone phosphate 1% in HSV stromal keratitis helps in faster clinical resolution, reduction in disease progression, and fewer treatment failures. Also, a delay in the prescription of topical steroids does not affect the final visual outcome [3].

Table 4.2 Results of HEDS—SKN trial

Study outcomes	Steroid group	Placebo group
Median time from randomization to clinical resolution	26 days	72 days
Treatment failure (persistence/ progression of stromal keratitis)		
At 10 weeks	26%	73%
At 16 weeks	49%	76%
Final visual outcome	No difference	
HSV recurrence	No difference	

4.2.3.2 HEDS-SKS Trial

(a) *Study question:* Should oral acyclovir be added to topical steroids and trifluridine regimen in HSV stromal keratitis?

(b) *Protocol:* They recruited 104 patients with active HSV stromal keratitis and randomized into two arms. The simplified form of study protocol is shown in Flowdiagram 4.2.

(c) *Results*: Similar results were noted between the groups in terms of treatment success (Acyclovir group—18% Vs. Placebo group—19%) and failure (Acyclovir group—75% Vs. Placebo group—74%). The final visual outcome was better in the acyclovir group; however, the difference was statistically insignificant. The results are summarized in Table 4.3.

(d) *Inference:* Addition of oral acyclovir to topical steroids and trifluridine regimen in HSV stromal keratitis has no apparent benefit in terms of visual outcome and resolution time. Double antiviral therapy (oral + topical) has no compounding effect in HSV stromal keratitis [4].

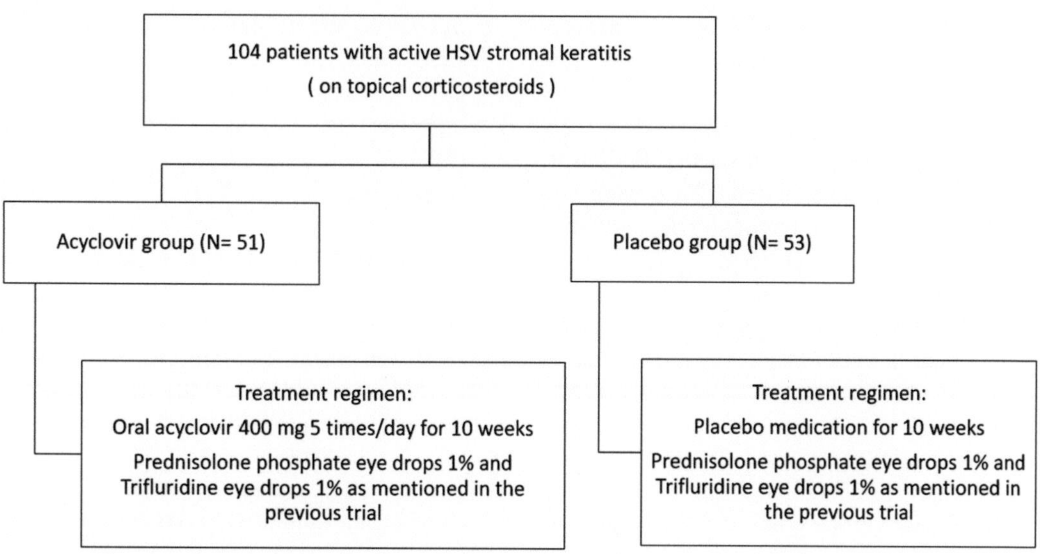

Flowdiagram 4.2 Showing simplified protocol of HEDS -SKS trial

Table 4.3 Results of HEDS—SKS trial

Study outcomes	Acyclovir group	Placebo group
Treatment success	18%	19%
Treatment failure	75%	74%
Visual outcome		
Improvement	58%	39%
No improvement	36%	49%
Worsening	6%	13%

Table 4.4 Results of HEDS—IRT trial

Study outcomes	Acyclovir group	Placebo group
Treatment success	41%	32%
Treatment failure	50%	68%

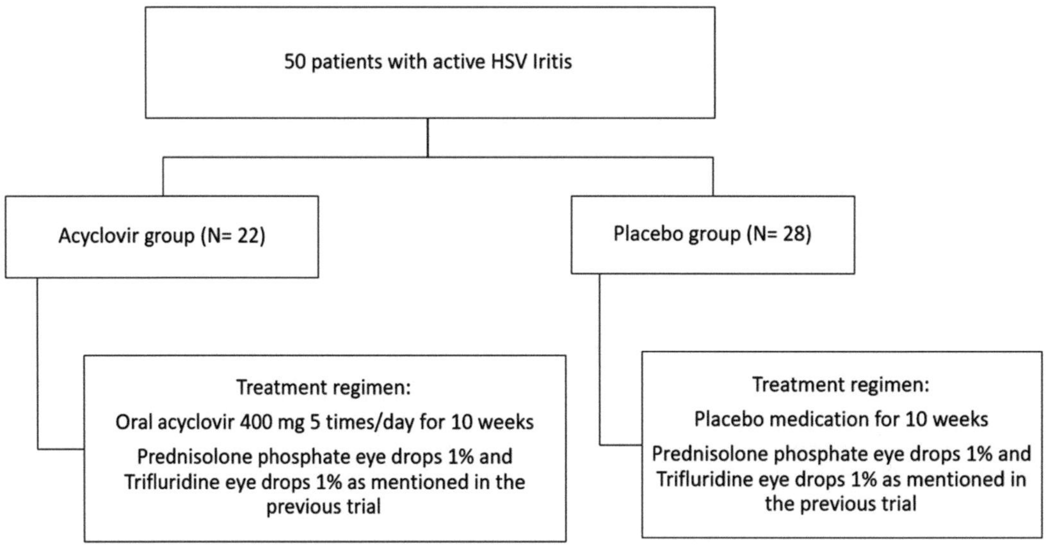

Flowdiagram 4.3 Showing simplified protocol of HEDS -IRT trial

4.2.3.3 HEDS-IRT Trial

(a) *Study question:* Does oral acyclovir aid in better resolution of HSV iritis in patients already using topical steroids and trifluridine?

(b) *Protocol:* The sample size planned was 104 but only 50 patients with active HSV iritis were enrolled over 4 years. They were randomized into two groups. The simplified form of study protocol is shown in Flowdiagram 4.3. Patients were followed weekly for 10 weeks, then every 2 weeks for the next 6 weeks of post-treatment, and at 26 weeks. The trial was stopped because of the small sample size and statistically conclusive results were not formulated.

(c) *Results:* Treatment success was similar between acyclovir group (41%) and placebo group (32%). However, placebo group had higher treatment failure of 68% when compared to acyclovir group which was 50%. The results are summarized in Table 4.4.

(d) *Inference:* Adding oral acyclovir to topical steroids and trifluridine regimen in HSV iritis may be beneficial (noted after 3 weeks of treatment). But this needs further validation [5].

4.2.4 Herpetic Eye Disease Study II (HEDS II)

HEDS II was conducted from October 1992 to 1994. This second phase of the trial answered next three questions of HEDS in 3 parts.

1. HSV Epithelial Keratitis Trial (HEDS-EKT).
2. Acyclovir Prevention Trial (HEDS-APT).
3. Recurrence Factor Study (HEDS-RFS).

4.2.4.1 HEDS-EKT Trial

(a) *Study question:* Does early treatment of HSV epithelial keratitis with oral acyclovir prevent progression to stromal keratitis and iridocyclitis?

(b) *Protocol:* They recruited 287 patients with active HSV epithelial keratitis and randomized into two arms. The simplified form of study protocol is shown in Flowdiagram 4.4. Patients were followed up for 1 year with 8 visits.

(c) *Results:* In both groups, the rate of progression of HSV epithelial keratitis to stromal keratitis or iritis was similar (Acyclovir group—11% vs Placebo group—12%) but, there was no difference in recurrence of HSV epithelial keratitis. The risk of developing stromal keratitis or iritis was higher in patients with previous episodes of HSV stromal keratitis or iritis (23%) than in patients without such a history (9%).

(d) *Inference:* Adding oral acyclovir in HSV epithelial keratitis does not prevent the progression to stromal keratitis and iridocyclitis. The risk of developing stromal keratitis or iritis was higher in patients with a prior history of HSV eye disease. In addition, history of stromal keratitis/iritis variant of HSV eye disease had a higher risk when compared to epithelial keratitis in the development of recurrences [6].

4.2.4.2 HEDS-APT Trial

(a) *A study question:* Is low-dose oral acyclovir prophylaxis helpful in preventing HSV recurrence?

(b) *Protocol:* They recruited 703 patients with a history of HSV eye disease within the last 1 year but have been inactive, and not on any treatment, in the last 1 month. They were randomized into two groups. The simplified form of study protocol is shown in Flowdiagram 4.5. Patients were followed up during 1 year of treatment with 5 visits and 6 months of post-treatment period with 3 visits. Episodes of recurrence during the trial were treated with the standard regimen as indicated, but patients continued to receive the oral acyclovir or placebo for the entire 1 year.

(c) *Results:* The recurrence rate of HSV eye disease was 19% and 32% in acyclovir group and placebo group, respectively. There was 50% reduction in HSV stromal keratitis recurrence in acyclovir group. This effect was seen only in patients with history of HSV stromal keratitis. Study also showed that oral acyclovir prophylaxis reduced the incidence of epithelial keratitis from 11% to 9% and that of stromal keratitis from 13% to 8%. Multiple recurrences were noted in 4% in acyclovir group and 9% in placebo group.

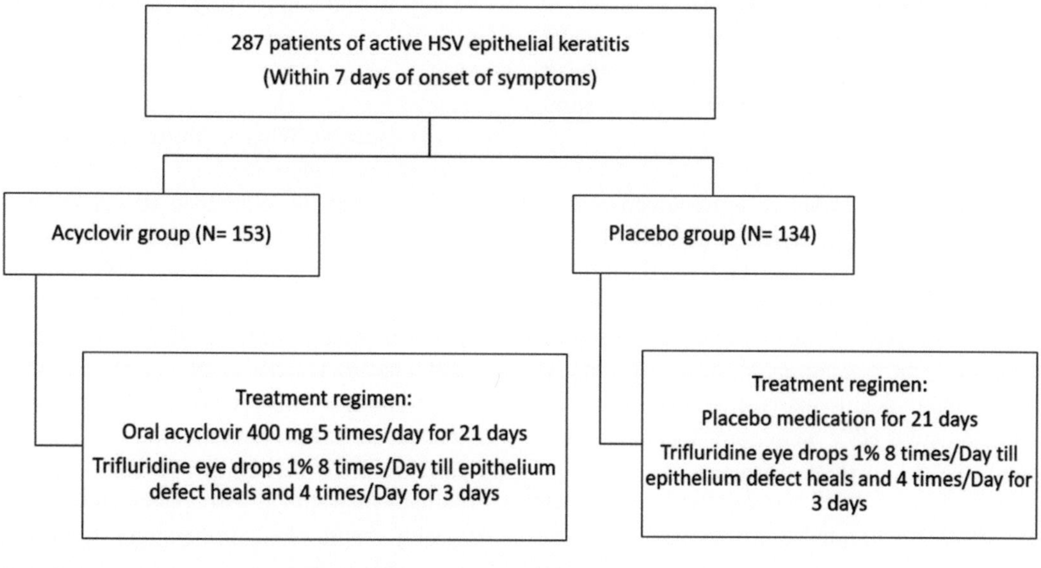

Flowdiagram 4.4 Showing simplified protocol of HEDS -EKT trial

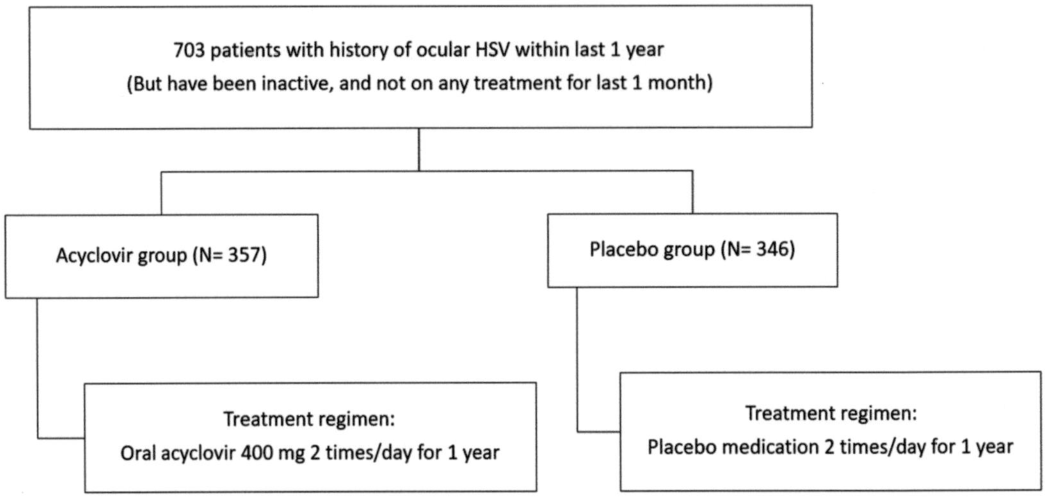

Flowdiagram 4.5 Showing simplified protocol of HEDS -APT trial

Table 4.5 Results of HEDS—APT trial

Study outcomes	Acyclovir group	Placebo group
Ocular HSV recurrence	19%	32%
Recurrence of HSV stromal keratitis	14%	28%
More than 1 HSV recurrence	4%	9%
Non-ocular HSV recurrence	19%	36%

However, the prophylactic action of low dose acyclovir vanished after cessation of treatment. There was no statistical difference in the recurrence of both ocular and non-ocular HSV between the 2 groups over 6 months of post-treatment period. The results are summarised in Table 4.5.

In the placebo group, 18% developed epithelial keratitis, and 18% developed stromal keratitis. Data analysis showed that the history of epithelial keratitis does not increase the recurrence of the same, but history of stromal keratitis increases the recurrence by 10 times. Demographic details like age, gender, ethnicity, and non-ocular HSV were not associated with a significant risk of HSV recurrence.

(d) *Inference:* Prophylactic low-dose acyclovir reduced the recurrence of ocular HSV by 45% but there is no prolonged protective action once the drug is stopped. Previous episodes of stromal keratitis have increased the risk of recurrence of the same by ten-fold [7–9].

4.2.4.3 HEDS-RFS Trial

It was an epidemiological study conducted to evaluate the effect of psychological (stress, emotional factors), environmental (sunlight exposure, seasonal conditions), ocular (trauma, contact lens wear), and biological (fever, menstruation, systemic infection like upper respiratory tract infection) factors on the recurrences of herpetic eye disease.

(a) *Study question:* What are the triggers/predictors of HSV recurrence?
(b) *Protocol:* Patients older than 18 years of age who were recruited into the HEDS-APT trial were included for this study. 308 patients (155 in the acyclovir group and 153 in the placebo group) were enrolled in the study and filled out a questionnaire at the entry level and also every week for 52 weeks to track acute and chronic stressors.
(c) *Results:* HSV recurrence was noted in 67 patients but only 35 participants had a valid weekly report. None of them reported stress before recurrence.

(d) *Inference:* Despite a small sample size, the study suggested no association of HSV recurrence with psychological stress, systemic infection, eye injuries, contact lens wear, menstrual periods, and sun exposure [10].

4.3 Zoster Eye Disease Study (ZEDS)

ZEDS is a multicentric (95 sites), double-masked, placebo-controlled, randomized clinical trial funded by the National Eye Institute to assess the efficacy of oral valacyclovir in Herpes Zoster ophthalmicus (HZO) [11, 12]. The study was conducted between 2017 and 2024. This study aims to evaluate the role of suppressive oral antiviral therapy in immunocompetent non-pregnant patients of herpes zoster ophthalmicus (HZO) with last episode of active HZO within one year of recruitment.

- *Study Question* To determine whether suppressive oral antiviral treatment delays the occurrence of new or worsening stromal keratitis (SK), endothelial keratitis (EK), iritis, or dendriform epithelial keratitis (DEK) during 12 months of treatment (primary end point)
- If treatment benefit persisted at 18 months (secondary end point).
- Whether development of postherpetic neuralgia varies by treatment group, and whether vaccinations against herpes zoster affect study outcomes and coronavirus disease 19 status.

Protocol Immunocompetent patients of herpes zoster ophthalmicus (HZO) with last episode of active HZO within one year of recruitment were included in the study. A total of 527 participants were recruited and randomized into valacyclovir group (n-266) and placebo group (n-261). Patient received treatment for 12 months. The simplified form of study protocol is shown in Flowdiagram 4.6. Follow-up was done at 12 months and 18 months (6 months after treatment discontinuation). First occurrence within 12 months of new or worsening SK, EK, iritis, or DEK was taken as the primary end point.

Results At 12 months, primary end points occurred in 33% cases in placebo and 28% cases in valacyclovir group [13]. Similarly, at 18 months follow-up, 40% cases in placebo group and 32% cases in valacyclovir group had primary end points. However, a reduction of multiple other secondary end points was noted at 12 months and 18 months. The pain score and dosage of neuropathic pain medication was lower in the treatment group [14] (Table 4.6).

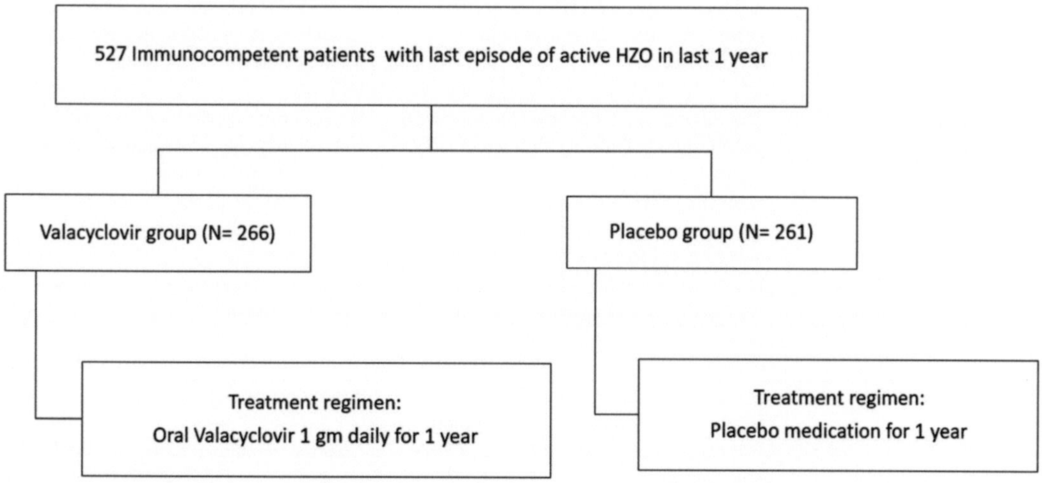

Flowdiagram 4.6 Showing simplified protocol of ZEDS

Inference The suppressive valacyclovir treatment did not show any benefit in the primary outcome. However, the secondary study outcomes showed benefit with treatment at 18 month with decreased frequency of keratitis or iritis and decreased pain score with reduced need for neuropathic pain medication.

Although the primary outcome did not show a benefit of suppressive valacyclovir treatment, secondary study outcomes demonstrated treatment superiority at the 18-month endpoint and a reduced number of multiple episodes of keratitis or iritis at both 12 and 18 months. These results support consideration of 1 year of suppressive valacyclovir treatment for HZO.

Table 4.6 Results of Zoster eye disease study

Study outcome	Valacyclovir group	Placebo group
Primary end point at 12 months	28%	33%
Primary end point at 18 months	32%	40%
Prevalence of postherpetic neuralgia	38%	40%
Total daily dose of neuropathic pain medication		
12 month	271.4 mg/day	363.4 mg/day
18 month	209.0 mg/day	286.2 mg/day
Pain score in participants with <60 yrs age		
12 month	0.3	0.8
18 month	0.2	1.0

4.4 Conclusion

Herpetic Eye Disease Studies (HEDS), a landmark trial and ongoing research like the Zoster Eye Disease Study (ZEDS), have significantly advanced our understanding of viral keratitis. Their results have helped us to refine the management strategies for herpetic eye diseases, focusing on the optimal use of antiviral agents, corticosteroids, and their combinations. The results of ZEDS trial are expected to provide further insights into the efficacy of suppressive antiviral therapy in preventing HZO-related keratitis and post-herpetic neuralgia.

4.5 Summary

The various trials have been summarized in Table 4.7.

Table 4.7 Showing clinical trials in viral keratitis with their outcomes

Type of ocular HSV	Study question	Findings
HSV stromal keratitis	Are *topical steroids* effective in HSV stromal keratitis along with topical trifluridine?	*Yes*, it helps in faster clinical resolution, reduction in disease progression, and fewer treatment failures.
	Should *oral acyclovir* be added to topical steroids and trifluridine regimen in HSV stromal keratitis?	Non-necrotizing type—*no benefit*; Necrotizing type—Inadequate sample size to assess the benefit.
HSV Iridocyclitis	Does *oral acyclovir* aid in better resolution of HSV iritis in patients already using topical steroids and trifluridine?	*May be beneficial* but small sample size to assess the statistical significance.
HSV epithelial keratitis	Does early treatment of HSV epithelial keratitis with *oral acyclovir* prevent progression to stromal keratitis and iridocyclitis?	*No*, does not prevent progression to stromal keratitis.
HSV recurrence	Is *low-dose oral acyclovir* prophylaxis helpful in preventing HSV recurrence?	*Yes*, reduces recurrence by 45%.
	What are the *triggers/predictors* of HSV recurrence?	*None of the factors* were confirmed as triggers.

Key Points

1. Oral acyclovir in active epithelial keratitis does not prevent progression to stromal keratitis or iridocyclitis.
2. Topical corticosteroids in combination with antiviral therapy have shown a beneficial effect in stromal keratitis, leading to faster resolution and fewer treatment failures.
3. In HSV stromal keratitis, adding oral acyclovir to the standard treatment regimen did not show consistent benefit, especially in patients already receiving topical corticosteroids.
4. Stromal keratitis/iritis variant of ocular HSV has a higher risk of recurrence when compared to epithelial keratitis.
5. Low-dose oral acyclovir prophylaxis reduces ocular HSV recurrence by 45%.
6. The role of external and behavioural factors in HSV recurrence remains inconclusive.
7. Low dose valacyclovir prophylaxis in patients of Herpes zoster ophthalmicus does not reduce the recurrence rate or risk of post-herpetic neuralgia.

References

1. Valerio GS, Lin CC. Ocular manifestations of herpes simplex virus. Curr Opin Ophthalmol. 2019;30:525–31.
2. Sibley D, Larkin DFP. Update on herpes simplex keratitis management. Eye. 2020;34:2219–26.
3. Wilhelmus KR, Gee L, Hauck WW, Kurinij N, Dawson CR, Jones DB, et al. Herpetic eye disease study: a controlled trial of topical corticosteroids for herpes simplex stromal keratitis. Ophthalmology. 1994;101:1883–96.
4. Barron BA, Gee L, Hauck WW, Kurinij N, Dawson CR, Jones DB, et al. Herpetic eye disease study. A controlled trial of oral acyclovir for herpes simplex stromal keratitis. Ophthalmology. 1994;101:1871–82.
5. A controlled trial of oral acyclovir for iridocyclitis caused by herpes simplex virus. The Herpetic Eye Disease Study Group. Arch Ophthalmol Chic Ill 1960. 1996;114:1065–72.
6. A controlled trial of oral acyclovir for the prevention of stromal keratitis or iritis in patients with herpes simplex virus epithelial keratitis. The Epithelial Keratitis Trial. The Herpetic Eye Disease Study Group. [published correction appears in Arch Ophthalmol 1997 Sep;115(9):1196]. Arch Ophthalmol. 1997;115(6):703–12.
7. Acyclovir for the prevention of recurrent herpes simplex virus eye disease. Herpetic Eye Disease Study Group. N Engl J Med 1998;339:300–306.
8. Predictors of recurrent herpes simplex virus keratitis. Herpetic Eye Disease Study Group. Cornea 2001;20:123–128.
9. Herpetic Eye Disease Study Group. Oral acyclovir for herpes simplex virus eye disease: effect on prevention of epithelial keratitis and stromal keratitis. Arch Ophthalmol. 2000;118:1030–6.
10. Herpetic Eye Disease Study Group. Psychological stress and other potential triggers for recurrences of herpes simplex virus eye infections. Arch Ophthalmol. 2000;118:1617–25.
11. Cohen EJ, Jeng BH, Troxel AB, Lee M, Shakarov G, Hochman J, et al. Enrollment in the zoster eye disease study. Cornea. 2020;39:1480–4.
12. Cohen EJ, Hochman JS, Troxel AB, Colby KA, Jeng BH, ZEDS Trial Research Group. Zoster Eye Disease Study: rationale and design. Cornea. 2022;41:562–71.
13. Cohen EJ, Troxel AB, Liu M, et al. Low-dose valacyclovir in herpes zoster ophthalmicus: the zoster eye disease randomized clinical trial. JAMA Ophthalmol. 2025;143(4):269–76.
14. Warner DB, Jeng BH, Kim J, et al. Low-dose valacyclovir for postherpetic neuralgia in the zoster eye disease study: a randomized clinical trial. JAMA Ophthalmol. 2025;143(4):277–85.

5 Dry Eye Disease and Viral Keratitis

Lagnajeeta Banerjee, Priyanka, Poorva Shrivastava, Rishika Sharma, and Bhavana Sharma

Abstract

DED is a multifactorial disease caused due to pathological alteration in the homeostasis of ocular surface. Various pathophysiological factors have been implicated in causation of dry eye disease with varying severity. The ocular surface derangements are reflected in tear volume reduction, neurosensory abnormalities, ocular surface inflammation, angiogenesis and damage and high osmotic pressure of the tear film. Viral keratitis has long been implicated as a major causative factor of dry eye disease attributed mainly to neurosensory abnormalities. It causes inflammation of the ocular surface, lacrimal glands and corneal neuropathy, thereby causing dry eye disease of varying severity. Understanding the pathogenesis of post-viral keratitis dry eye disease will aid us in diagnosis and individualised treatment for the patient.

Keywords

Dry eye disease · Ocular surface · Lubricants · Corneal nerves

L. Banerjee · Priyanka · B. Sharma (✉)
AIIMS Bhopal, Bhopal, Madhya Pradesh, India

P. Shrivastava
ASG Eye Hospital, Bhopal, Madhya Pradesh, India

R. Sharma
MGM Medical College and Hospital, Aurangabad, India

5.1 Introduction

Ocular surface is described as the interface between the eye and the external environment. It is a functional unit comprising of the cornea, conjunctiva, eyelids and eyelashes, lacrimal and meibomian glands and the tear film [1]. TFOS DEWS II Definition and Classification Subcommittee defines dry eye as a multifactorial disease of the ocular surface characterised by a loss of homeostasis of the tear film, and accompanied by ocular symptoms, in which tear film instability and hyperosmolarity, ocular surface inflammation and damage and neurosensory abnormalities play etiological roles [2]. As such, ocular homeostasis is a prerequisite to prevent dry eye disorder. It is upheld by the tear film, continuity of the ocular epithelial surface and the rich corneal nerve plexus which maintains feedback regulation of the ocular surface.

Viral infections have long been known to induce ocular surface inflammation especially conjunctival inflammation, keratitis, and tear film instability in addition to morphological and functional changes of the lacrimal glands. The consequent accumulation of inflammatory mediators, stagnant tear film, decreased level of mucins, further damage the junctional complexes and cause resultant destruction of the ocular surface epithelia. The interplay of above factors predisposes the eye to clinical manifestations of DED.

B. Sharma et al. (eds.), *Viral Keratitis*, https://doi.org/10.1007/978-981-95-3148-6_5

This chapter intends to describe pathophysiology, risk factors, causative agents and treatment outcomes of DED induced by viral keratitis.

5.2 Epidemiology and Risk Factors

Epidemiological factors pertaining to dry eye disease particularly the prevalence data and risk factors greatly vary depending on the study population, systemic causes, ocular infections, occupational considerations and the environmental influences. The prevalence rate of DED has been reported to be 9.1% with slight preponderance towards females and older individuals [3]. Risk factors which have been implicated primarily are inflammation, infections, electronic products, diabetes mellitus, laser-assisted in situ keratomileusis (LASIK), and derangements in sex hormones [4–7].

The current incidence of herpes simplex ocular disease is estimated at 1.8 million people globally [8]. Similarly, it has been shown that around 20% cases of VZV infection are complicated by Herpes Zoster Ophthalmicus annually [9].

Systemic infections with viruses, such as HSV, VZV, SARS-CoV-2, HIV, HBV and Epstein-Barr virus (EBV) [10], induce inflammation and consequent functional derangements of the lacrimal glands and ocular surface resulting in DED. There have been reports of increased prevalence of DED in patients with COVID-19 [11].

Viruses may either directly disrupt the corneal epithelial functioning or may indirectly cause dry eye by affecting the lacrimal gland. Additionally, they trigger autoimmune reaction by neoantigen expression and molecular mimicry [12]. Several factors can increase the risk of developing dry eye disease after viral keratitis:

- Severity of Infection: More severe cases of viral keratitis lead to greater damage to the ocular surface and thus, increases the risk of DED.
- Recurrent Infections: Recurrent episodes of viral keratitis, particularly in cases of HSV, are associated with higher rates of DED.
- Age: Older individuals may be more susceptible to both viral keratitis and dry eye disease probably due to age related immunosuppression.
- Immunocompromised States: Conditions or treatments that weaken the immune system can increase the risk and severity of viral keratitis and subsequent dry eye disease.

5.3 Pathophysiology

Viral infections in body tissues activate the innate immune system which recognises viral antigens, such as viral nucleic acids, to activate innate defence pathways, leading to inflammation, apoptosis and impaired cellular regeneration. Viral keratitis can potentially cause derangement of ocular surface homeostasis at several levels. The ocular surface is exposed to the external environment and extremely vulnerable to viral infection which can induce inflammation of the ocular surface, neurosensory abnormalities and reduce tear secretion from the lacrimal gland (LG), consequently triggering ocular morphological and functional changes and resulting in dry eye disease (DED) [12]. The pathophysiology of dry eye following viral keratitis is simplified in the Flowdiagram 5.1.

Flowdiagram 5.1 Showing Pathophysiology of Dry eye in viral keratitis.

Viral infection
↓
Activated innate immunity due to presence of viral nuclei acids
↓
Inflammation and apoptosis of corneal and conjunctival cells
↓
Reduced cell proliferation
↓
Morphological and functional changes on lacrimal gland and ocular surface
↓
Dry eye disease

The factors can be further explained as:

- Direct corneal Damage: Viral keratitis especially those caused by herpes simplex virus and varicella zoster virus directly damage the epithelium and corneal nerves with consequent effect on the trophic functions of cornea and ocular surface.
- Decreased Tear Production: The inflammation caused by viral keratitis can affect the lacrimal glands directly resulting in decreased aqueous production, leading to dry ocular surface with improper lubrication.
- Tear Film Instability: The tear film is a complex tri-layered structure consisting of lipid, aqueous and mucin that protects and lubricates the ocular surface. Viral keratitis can disrupt the composition and stability of the tear film. This disruption may lead to increased tear evaporation, reduced tear resurfacing across the ocular surface and decreased tear film stability.
- Inflammatory Response: The presence of the virus in the cornea triggers an inflammatory response. This inflammatory cascade involves the release of cytokines, chemokines and other inflammatory mediators. These molecules not only contribute to tissue damage but also affect the function of corneal epithelium, goblet cells and lacrimal glands.
- Neurological Damage: Viral infections, particularly the Herpes Simplex Virus, can affect corneal nerve endings. This can disrupt the neural feedback loop that regulates tear production from lacrimal glands and maintenance of the tear film, contributing to DED.
- Persistent Symptoms: Even after the acute phase of viral keratitis resolves, the damage caused to the cornea and tear film can persist. This chronic instability can lead to ongoing dry eye symptoms.

5.4 Clinical Presentation

5.4.1 Symptoms

Patients present with persistent dryness and discomfort in the affected eye(s), foreign body sensation and grittiness. There can be blurring of vision especially during exacerbations or flare-ups. Photophobia and other non-specific symptoms of ocular surface inflammation are also noted.

5.4.2 Clinical Features

Signs of inflammation are usually present on the lids like hyperaemia, with or without squamous metaplasia which indicates the chronicity of the condition. Conjunctival hyperaemia in the form of conjunctival/circumcorneal congestion, conjunctivochalasis and surface erosions may be present. Corneal involvement may be seen in the form of erosions, epithelial defects, superficial punctate keratopathy, vascularisation, pigmentation, healed scars/opacities and isolated islands of subepithelial fibrosis Figs. 5.1 and 5.2.

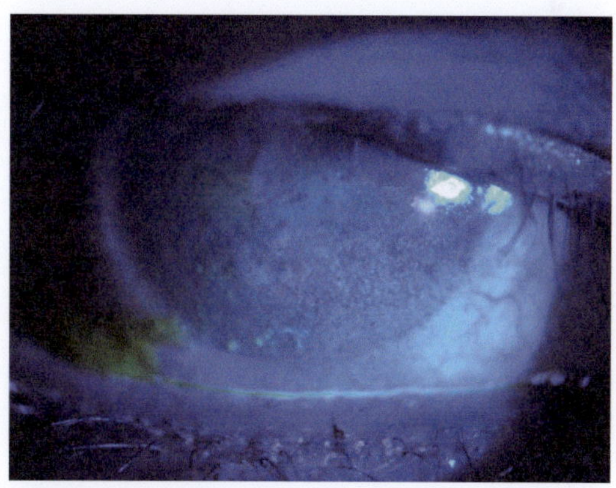

Fig. 5.1 Slit lamp image showing severe dry eye disorder post-HSV keratitis with superficial punctate erosions with decreased tear meniscus

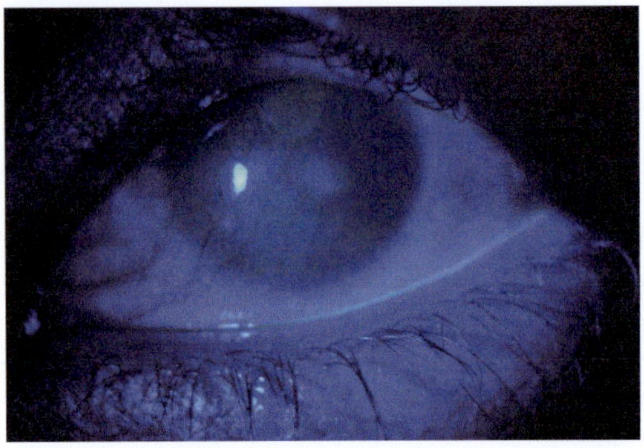

Fig. 5.2 Slit lamp image showing vascularised corneal opacity with bad ocular surface and decreased tear meniscus

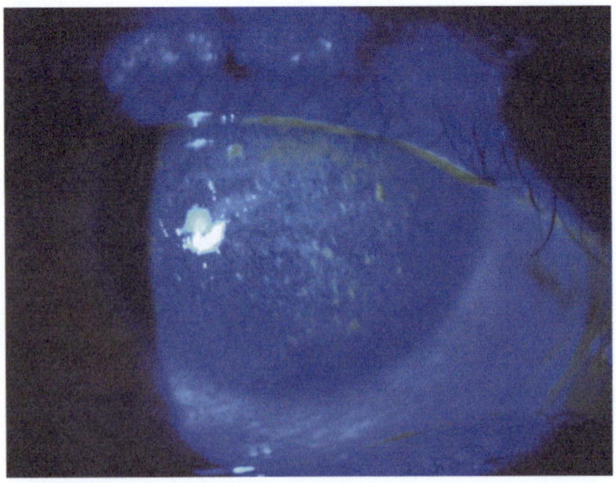

Fig. 5.3 Slit lamp image showing HZO-induced superficial punctate erosions, mucous plaques with bad ocular surface

Severe cases may present with extensive surface erosions and bad ocular surface Fig. 5.3.

It is important to do careful tear film assessment for decreased tear meniscus height and presence of filaments, schirmer's test to measure tear secretion while fluorescein staining of ocular surface is done for tear breakup time Fig. 5.4.

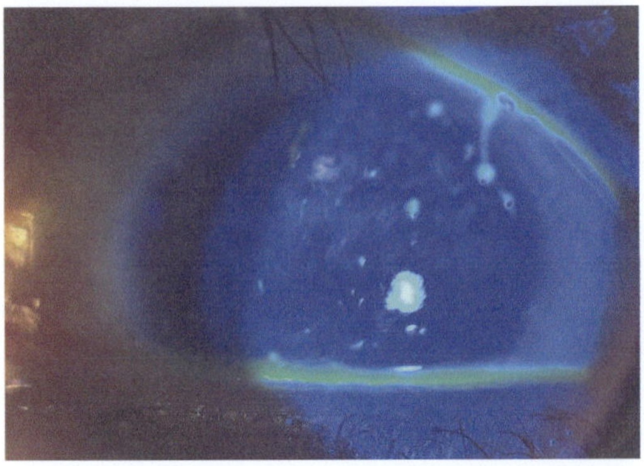

Fig. 5.4 Slit lamp image showing HZO-induced filamentary keratitis and moderate dry eyes

5.5 Viral Agents Implicated in Causation of DED

5.5.1 HSV

HSV can have a varied range of manifestations, including reduction in tear film meniscus and corneal nerve dysfunction in patients of ocular HSV infection [13]. Multiple studies have been conducted in the past decade which show that eyes with neurotrophic corneal ulcer and interstitial herpetic keratitis have ocular surface derangement then normal eyes. Latent stromal herpetic keratitis has also been shown to cause bilateral dry eye disease presumably due to disturbed trigeminal nerve conduction and recurrent episodes of keratitis [13].

5.5.2 VZV

VZV infections have been shown to affect corneal sensory nerves, thereby causing hypoesthesia and neurotrophic keratopathy. This in turn leads to reduced blink rate, increased corneal exposure and delayed epithelial healing [14]. However these patients have minimal symptoms of dry eye due to reduced sensations and as such are at increased risk of developing sterile corneal ulcerations which can easily become superinfected. A recent artificial intelligence based analysis done in 2022 revealed changes in the morphology of meibomian glands post-craniofacial herpes zoster, indicating predisposition to dry eye disease [15].

5.5.3 Adenovirus

Adenoviral keratitis, specifically by serotypes 3, 4, and 7 among others, can contribute to the development of dry eye disease through any of the above mechanisms, most commonly due to loss of conjunctival goblet cells.

Sometimes the presence of subepithelial conjunctival scars in patients with fulminant disease leads to inadequate surface lubrication, corneal irritation and exaggerated dry eye symptoms [16].

5.5.4 Other Viruses

5.5.4.1 SARS-CoV-2

Studies have shown that patients affected by SARS-CoV-2 showed decreased meibomian gland function, reduced tear film thickness and shorter tear film break-up time [12]. SARS-CoV-2 binds to ACE2 receptors present on various tissues including meibomian glands causing decreased size of goblet cells their dysfunction, resultant thinned out lipid layer and squamous epithelial changes [17, 18]. SARS-CoV-2 incites ocular surface inflammation which can further alter the ocular surface microbiome and may lead to persistence of symptoms of dry eye disease [19].

5.5.4.2 HIV

HIV-mediated cellular infiltration and ischaemic damage of the lacrimal and meibomian gland leads to continued inflammation of the ocular surface and dry eye disease with disease progression. HIV patients have been shown to have greater meibomian gland dropout as compared to control population and it negatively correlates with the disease severity of HIV at diagnosis [20].

5.5.4.3 Hepatitis B and C

Hepatitis B virus has been shown to cause cellular inflammation of Meibomian glands. Study conducted on patients with Hepatitis B infection reflected that though the aqueous layer of the tear film was normal, the meibum contained clear fluid which predisposes to non-obstructive meibomian gland dysfunction [21]. This is in contrast to HCV infection which causes aqueous deficient dry eye disease. HCV RNA has been detected in tear of patients affected with systemic HCV infection. HCV causes death of corneal epithelial cells and conjunctival fibroblasts, causing ocular inflammation and DED. HCV also affects the microvasculature of the lacrimal gland due to B-cell lymphocytic infiltration consequently causing tear film instability [21].

5.5.4.4 Ebstein Barr Virus (EBV)

EBV primarily involves oropharyngeal tissues, lacrimal glands and B-lymphocytes. It is a ubiquitous virus which remains latent in the salivary glands. EBV enters corneal epithelial cells and increases levels of proteins like MMP-9 in a cascade mechanism which interferes with corneal epithelial integrity and functioning [12]. EBV also causes B-cell lymphoproliferation in the lacrimal gland leading to severe aqueous deficient DED.

5.5.4.5 Human T-Cell Leukemia Virus Type 1

HTLV-1 is responsible for numerous ocular pathologies most notably sclerouveitis, interstitial keratitis and dry eye disease. HTLV-1 affects CD4 + T cells and causes release of pro-inflammatory cytokines which result in ocular inflammation [22]. HTLV-1 has been shown to cause corneal thinning and consequent corneal opacities which may further exacerbate ocular surface inflammation and deficient tear production [23].

5.6 Treatment

Management of viral infection induced dry eye disease typically involves a multifaceted approach aimed at controlling the viral infection, managing symptoms, reducing inflammation and ocular surface restoration. This includes antiviral medications, anti-inflammatory eye drops, lubricating agents/artificial tears, and in some cases, advanced therapies such as punctal plugs or stimulants for tear production.

Tear supplements serve as the main stay of treatment, being crucial in ocular surface lubrication and restoration (Table 5.1). Various preservative free ocular surface lubricants can be prescribed for long-term use in patients with viral keratitis in addition to other treatments as require [24].

Systemic and topical antiviral agents in appropriate dosage are effective in controlling viral activity especially in herpes simplex keratitis and herpes zoster thereby disease progression and severity.

Table 5.1 Ocular surface lubricants

Categories	Examples	Mode of action
Viscosity enhancing agents	PVP, PVA Dextran 70 HPMC CMC PEG 400 Propylene glycol	Ocular surface lubrication; improve water retention of tear film
Electrolytes	Sodium chloride Potassium chloride	Improve osmotic balance of ocular surface and tear film
Osmoprotectants	Trehalose Sorbitol glycerin	Prevent apoptosis of corneal and conjunctival epithelial cells
Oily agents and surfactants	Mineral oil	Improve lipid layer of tear film
Anti-oxidants	Vitamin E Co-enzyme q10	Reduce oxidative stress and ocular surface inflammation

Topical antiviral agents are epitheliotoxic, can cause damage to goblet cells and hence should be used for short duration, mainly to reduce viral activity and increase the remission period. We recommend minimal dosage of topical antiviral agents like Acyclovir 3% / Ganciclovir 15% for duration not more than 1–2 months if the patient has co-existing DED. Careful evaluation of signs of epithelial toxicity, ocular surface inflammation should be done to discontinue topical antiviral agents accordingly. On the other hand, systemic antiviral agents can be used for prolonged durations of 6 months to a year as per the requirement in dosage of Acyclovir 400 mg 3 times a day or Valacyclovir 1 g twice a day.

Ocular surface inflammation is controlled by agents like non-steroidal anti-inflammatory agents, steroidal agents, immunomodulators, hormonal agents and antibiotics to inhibit inflammatory mediators and provide relief from the symptoms of DED.

Topical steroids namely Loteprednol (0.5%), Fluorometholone (0.1%), Prednisolone acetate (1%) and dexamethasone (0.1%) are used depending on the severity of DED and the viral activity. Steroids are effective at mitigating corneal inflammation, decreasing tear osmolarity and corneal epitheliopathy in addition to prevention of long-term scarring [25].

Cyclosporin A (CsA), used in the concentration of 0.05%, inhibits the activation of T lymphocytes and effectively controls ocular inflammation in moderate to severe DED in addition to being an effective long-term substitute for topical steroids in potential steroid responders. Tacrolimus, a calcineurin inhibitor, is used topically in concentration of 0.03% and aids in reducing ocular inflammation and improving conjunctival cell counts.

Furthermore other anti-inflammatory therapeutic agents like Rebamipide 2% ophthalmic solution four times a day for 12 weeks provide symptomatic relief from dry eye by increasing the number of conjunctival goblet cells on the ocular surface in addition to suppressing the T cell activation and cytokine production [26].

Macrolide group of antibiotics like Tetracyclines can also be used to improve symptoms of dry eye disease as they have both antibacterial and anti-inflammatory properties.

Punctual occlusion is indicated in patients with moderate to severe DED to retain residual tears and improve tear meniscus height, leading to consequent symptomatic improvement and resolution of epitheliopathy. Punctal occlusion can be temporary, for example, plugs, or can be permanent as with the help of electrocautery or argon laser.

5.7 Conclusion

DED caused by viral infection of ocular surface remains an important and potentially serious complication. Various pathophysiological mechanisms have been implicated, mainly neurotrophic influences, meibomian gland and goblet cell involvement and impaired epithelial healing. Timely treatment by way of antiviral agents, ocular lubricants and surface restoration is the mainstay of treatment.

Key Points

- Dry eye disease is one of the most common complications of viral keratitis.
- Viral infections induce ocular surface inflammation especially conjunctival inflammation, keratitis, and tear film instability in addition to morphological and functional changes of the lacrimal glands.
- Multiple treatment modalities are currently available such as tear supplements, steroids, and newer drugs like Rebapimide as adjuncts to antiviral therapy.
- Therapeutic approach to DED is case-specific and combination of various medical and surgical treatment may be needed.

References

1. Knop E, Knop N. Anatomy and immunology of the ocular surface. Chem Immunol Allergy. 2007;92:36–49.
2. Craig JP, Nichols KK, Akpek EK, Caffery B, Dua HS, Joo CK, et al. TFOS DEWS II definition and classification report. Ocul Surf. 2017;15(3):276–83.
3. Vehof J, Snieder H, Jansonius N, Hammond CJ. Prevalence and risk factors of dry eye in 79,866 participants of the population-based lifelines cohort study in The Netherlands. Ocul Surf. 2021;19:83–93.
4. Toda I. Dry eye after LASIK. Invest Ophthalmol Vis Sci. 2018;59(14):DES109–15.
5. Chen Y, Chauhan SK, Lee HS, Saban DR, Dana R. Chronic Dry Eye disease is principally mediated by effector memory Th17 cells. Mucosal Immunol. 2014;7(1):38–45.
6. Schaumberg DA, Dana R, Buring JE, Sullivan DA. Prevalence of dry eye disease among US men: estimates from the physicians' health studies. Arch Ophthalmol. 2009;127(6):763–8.
7. Li S, Tang L, Zhou J, Anchouche S, Li D, Yang Y, et al. Sleep deprivation induces corneal epithelial progenitor cell over-expansion through disruption of redox homeostasis in the tear film. Stem Cell Rep. 2022;17(5):1105–19.
8. McCormick I, James C, Welton NJ, Mayaud P, Turner KME, Gottlieb SL, et al. Incidence of herpes simplex virus keratitis and other ocular disease: global review and estimates. Ophthalmic Epidemiol. 2022;29(4):353–62.
9. Minor M, Payne E. Herpes Zoster Ophthalmicus. In: StatPearls [Internet]. Treasure Island (FL): StatPearls Publishing; 2024 [cited 2024 Aug 16]. Available from: http://www.ncbi.nlm.nih.gov/books/NBK557779/
10. Schiller JT, Lowy DR. An introduction to virus infections and human cancer. Recent Results Cancer Res. 2021;217:1–11.
11. Saldanha IJ, Petris R, Makara M, Channa P, Akpek EK. Impact of the COVID-19 pandemic on eye strain and dry eye symptoms. Ocul Surf. 2021;22:38–46.
12. Wu M, Sun C, Shi Q, Luo Y, Wang Z, Wang J, et al. Dry eye disease caused by viral infection: past, present and future. Virulence. 2024;15(1):2289779.
13. Lobo AM, Agelidis AM, Shukla D. Pathogenesis of herpes simplex keratitis: the host cell response and ocular surface sequelae to infection and inflammation. Ocul Surf. 2019;17(1):40–9.
14. Kalogeropoulos CD, Bassukas ID, Moschos MM, Tabbara KF. Eye and periocular skin involvement in herpes zoster infection. Med Hypothesis Discov Innov Ophthalmol. 2015;4(4):142–56.
15. Yu X, Jia X, Zhang Z, Fu Y, Zhai J, Chen N, et al. Meibomian gland morphological changes in ocular herpes zoster patients based on AI analysis. Front Cell Dev Biol. 2022;10:1094044.
16. Bialasiewicz A. Adenoviral Keratoconjunctivitis. Sultan Qaboos Univ Med J. 2007;7(1):15–23.
17. Partridge LJ, Urwin L, Nicklin MJH, James DC, Green LR, Monk PN. ACE2-independent interaction of SARS-CoV-2 spike protein with human epithelial cells is inhibited by unfractionated heparin. Cells. 2021;10(6):1419.
18. Bozkurt E, Özateş S, Muhafız E, Yılmaz F, Calıskan O. Ocular surface and conjunctival cytology findings in patients with confirmed COVID-19. Eye Contact Lens. 2021;47(4):168–73.

19. Sarkar D, Soni D, Nagpal A, Khurram F, Karkhur S, Verma V, et al. Ocular manifestations of RT-PCR-confirmed COVID-19 cases in a large database cross-sectional study. BMJ Open Ophth. 2021;6(1):e000775. https://doi.org/10.1136/bmjophth-2021-000775.
20. Nguyen BN, Chung AW, Lopez E, Silvers J, Kent HE, Kent SJ, et al. Meibomian gland dropout is associated with immunodeficiency at HIV diagnosis: implications for dry eye disease. Ocul Surf. 2020;18(2):206–13.
21. Li S, Li A, Ruan F, Zhang W, Chen J, Huang C, et al. Evaluation of the clinical characteristics of Dry Eye secondary to different types of liver diseases. Ophthalmol Ther. 2023;12(5):2493–503.
22. Buggage RR, Levy-Clarke GA, Smith JA. New corneal findings in human T-cell lymphotrophic virus type 1 infection. Am J Ophthalmol. 2001;131(3):309–13.
23. Kamoi K. HTLV-1 in ophthalmology. Front Microbiol. 2020;11:388.
24. Labetoulle M, Benitez-del-Castillo JM, Barabino S, Vanrell RH, Daull P, Garrigue JS, et al. Artificial tears: biological role of their ingredients in the management of dry eye disease. Int J Mol Sci. 2022;23(5):2434. https://doi.org/10.3390/ijms23052434.
25. Mohanty A, Behera HS, Barik MR, Kaur A, Sharma S, Das S, et al. Microsporidia-induced stromal keratitis: a new cause of presumed immune stromal (interstitial) keratitis. Br J Ophthalmol. 2023;107(5):607–13.
26. Mohamed HB, Abd El-Hamid BN, Fathalla D, Fouad EA. Current trends in pharmaceutical treatment of dry eye disease: a review. Eur J Pharm Sci. 2022;175:106206.

Section I

Herpes Simplex Keratitis

6 Epidemiology and Pathophysiology

Neet Mehta and Anubha Rathi

Abstract

Herpes simplex keratitis (HSK) is a viral infection affecting the cornea, caused primarily by herpes simplex virus (HSV), most commonly HSV type 1. It is one of the leading causes of corneal blindness worldwide. HSK typically manifests as recurrent, corneal inflammation, which, if untreated, can lead to various ocular complications. Given its potential impact on visual function and quality of life, early diagnosis and treatment are paramount for preventing complications and preserving vision. A comprehensive understanding of HSK's epidemiology, risk factors, clinical manifestations, and management strategies is imperative in this regard. Moreover, public health efforts aimed at raising awareness, promoting early diagnosis, and implementing preventive measures can help reduce the burden of HSK and its associated complications on both individuals and communities.

Keywords

Herpes simplex · keratitis · HSV · corneal ulcer

N. Mehta · A. Rathi (✉)
L V Prasad Eye Institute,
Hyderabad, Telangana, India

6.1 Epidemiology of HSV Keratitis

6.1.1 Epidemiology

6.1.1.1 Incidence and Prevalence

Herpes Simplex Virus (HSV) is widespread globally, with humans serving as its sole natural reservoir. Despite being a major cause of corneal blindness worldwide, herpes simplex keratitis (HSK) remains significantly underreported for several reasons, including a lack of definite diagnostic criteria, subclinical and relatively less painful nature of the disease [1–3], Less microbiological data is available as diagnosis in most cases is based on clinical features. The pooled data of epidemiology studies based in USA and Europe estimate the global burden of HSV Keratitis in 2016 to be 1.7 million cases amounting to an incidence of 24.0 cases per 100,000 person-year, which included 9.2 newly diagnosed cases and 14.8 recurrent keratitis [4]. Most of the data from developing countries have been an extrapolation from the developed country studies which might not provide an accurate depiction [1]. A study by Pramod et al. showed a prevalence of HSK to be 7.8% in southern India [5]. Das et al. conducted a big data analysis of 8308 patients of HSV in a tertiary eye care set up in southern India (May 2012 to August 2019) [3]. This has been the largest electronic medical records-driven data analysis of HSK. Out of the total number of patients seen in cornea depart-

B. Sharma et al. (eds.), *Viral Keratitis*, https://doi.org/10.1007/978-981-95-3148-6_6

ment, 1.95% and 0.34% had HSK at the tertiary and secondary centre eye care facilities respectively. Immune stromal keratitis (59.58%) was the most common, followed by epithelial keratitis (21.08%), endothelitis (13.35%) and kerato-uveitis (2.88%) being the least common. This was unlike other studies which showed a predominance of epithelial involvement which can be attributed to referrals to higher centres [6–8].

6.1.2 Host–Parasite Relationship

HSV responsible for keratitis exists as two types—type 1 (HSV-1) and type 2 (HSV-2). HSV-1 is primarily spread through direct contact with infected secretions (such as saliva, tears, or lesions) and becomes latent in the trigeminal ganglion, leading to manifestations in the oral, ocular, and neurological regions [9]. Conversely, HSV-2 is mainly transmitted through sexual contact, remains latent in the sacral ganglia, and typically causes genital disease [10].

6.1.3 Age

Age indirectly influences the immune status of individuals. Young children with their more robust immune systems are capable of mounting a severe inflammatory reaction against the virus, resulting in a more severe presentation, often with a bilateral involvement and a higher recurrence rate (45–50%) as compared to adults (18%) [11–13].

6.1.4 Gender

Certain studies conducted in India (3,5) have indicated a higher incidence of males being affected compared to females, which is unlike some of the studies where female preponderance was noted [14, 15].

6.1.5 Laterality

HSK usually presents as a unilateral disease. Almost 92.91% cases had unilateral presentation according to one study [3]. Bilateral presentation usually restricted to children or patients with a history of atopy.

6.1.6 Immune Status

The immune status plays an important role in impacting the disease presentation.

6.1.6.1 Depressors of Cell-Mediated Immunity (CMI)

Conditions that depress the CMI can make the host more prone to acquiring HSK [16]. These high-risk groups include organ transplant recipients, diabetics, active measles infection and HIV-infected individuals [17–20].

6.1.6.2 Overactive/Stressed Immune System

Certain conditions can mount an exaggerated or a heightened immune response to a pathogen. These include younger age group [11, 12], history of atopy [21, 22], fever [23], upper respiratory tract infections [24], menstruation [25], and psychological stress [26]. Atopy, especially atopic dermatitis with atopic blepharitis, has been associated significantly with a shorter time to recurrence in cases of HSK [22]. Another study indicates that the recurrence rate increases nearly tenfold when HSK is kinked with atopic conjunctival disease [21].

6.1.6.3 Iatrogenic Factors

Certain induced conditions make the cornea more prone to HSK. These includes use of topical medication like prostaglandin analogues [27], contact lens use [28], LASIK, photorefractive or therapeutic keratectomy (PRK/PTK) [29–31], YAG laser capsulotomy or iridotomy [32], cataract surgery [33], and corneal transplantation [34].

6.1.7 Socio-Economic Strata

Population belonging to lower socio-economical strata and those from rural background have a higher prevalence of HSK [35, 36]. A study by Das et al. [3] showed 52.31% of cases reporting from rural community, with a further higher incidence in agricultural workers amongst all other professions.

6.1.8 History of Previous Attacks

According to HEDS study, the number of recurrences of HSK was strongly associated with the number of past episodes of the same, especially, stromal keratitis. Hence, a past occurrence of HSV stromal keratitis and a high frequency of prior episodes (of any type) elevate the likelihood of future recurrences. Additionally, it is noted that short intervals between past attacks correlated with a shorter interval between future attacks [37, 38].

6.2 Pathophysiology of HSV Keratitis

6.2.1 Viral Entry into the Corneal Cells

HSV-1 virus surface bears various glycoproteins that have an important role in the viral entry into the host corneal cells. These glycoproteins bind to the heparan sulphate (HS) on the host cornea cells, which in turn promotes the viral capsid penetration into the host cytoplasm [39]. Some important host surface glycoprotein receptors include herpes virus entry mediator (HVEM), nectin-1, and PILR-α [40]. Once the virus invades the host cells it can either cause a primary or a recurrent infection.

6.2.2 Primary Infection

Primary infection with HSV can occur at any time in life. This is generally transmitted via airborne droplets than a direct inoculation. Most primary infections are subclinical and may manifest as a prodromal symptom of mild fever, malaise, and upper respiratory tract infection. At times, primary infection can manifest as blepharitis or follicular conjunctivitis, which are usually self-limiting and with no severe consequences. According to Leopold et al. [2], a single primary infection may not allow the parasite to establish itself and repeated subclinical infection are needed for the host to maintain a constant level of antibodies. During this phase, the virus being neurotrophic in nature, travels via the corneal nerves to reach the trigeminal sensory ganglion and enters latency.

6.2.3 Recurrence from Latent Disease

This is the more common type presenting to the clinics with the textbook signs and symptoms of HSK. This occurs due to reactivation of the latent virus from the trigeminal ganglia which then travel retrograde to reach the cornea [41]. It can involve the epithelium (dendritic and geographic ulcer), stroma (immune stromal keratitis), combination of stromal with epithelial component (necrotizing stromal keratitis), endothelium (endothelial keratitis—disciform, diffuse, and linear pattern), and anterior chamber involvement (HSV uveitis). Pathophysiology of HSK can be divided as per its various levels of involvement. Corneal involvement in HSK can be due to either the direct damage by the virus or secondary inflammatory induced corneal damage or a combination of both.

6.2.4 Immune-Mediated Processes

HSV virus on infecting the corneal epithelial cells initiates an initial innate immune response by binding to the toll-like receptors on the cell surface. This stimulates production of various cytokines and chemokines that recruit various inflammatory cells (Neutrophils, dendritic cells, natural killer cells, macrophages, etc.), which gradually infiltrate the stroma for eliminating the virus. Further, once the antigen presenting cells (APC) transmit the information to the helper T cells (Th1 and TH17) via the major histocompatibility complex-II (MHC-II), the adaptive immune response is triggered. It is interesting to note that not all individuals infected with HSV-1 develop symptoms, this can be because the virus needs to effectively evade the barriers of the host immune system which generates the various grades of susceptibility amongst various individual.

6.2.5 Host Factors

6.2.5.1 Toll-Like Receptors (TLR), Cytokines and Chemokines

Binding of the viral antigens to the TLRs on the corneal epithelial cell surface initiates a cellular cascade of innate inflammatory response. Type 1 Interferons (IFN-a and IFN-b) are responsible for early control of viral replication due to their antiviral properties [42, 43]. Type II Interferon (IFN-γ) along with IL-2 is responsible for infiltration of neutrophils and activation of APCs [44]. Various other interleukins have been a major driver in corneal inflammation in HSK. These include IL-1, IL-6, and TNF-a. Out of these IL-6 and IL-17 have additional role in promoting corneal neovascularization through stimulating VEGF production [45–47].

6.2.5.2 Heparanase

This host cell enzyme, helps in viral spread by removing heparan sulphate on the cell surface and promoting release of the viral progeny [48].

6.2.6 Innate and Adaptive Response

6.2.6.1 Neutrophils

These are the predominant response to the viral entry and are seen to infiltrate the cornea in two distinct phases. The first wave is thought to be at 2 to 5 days post infection (dpi). The second wave coincides with the appearance of the clinical symptoms, starting around 8 to 9 dpi, reaching a peak around 21 dpi. This wave contributes to a significant tissue damage observed in HSK [49, 50].

6.2.6.2 Dendritic Cells, Macrophages and Natural Killer Cells

Dendritic cells are potent antigen presenting cells that present non-self-antigens to the T cells in the lymph nodes. Macrophages and natural killer cells form a surveillance system contributing to phagocytosis of the pathogen and elimination of unhealthy cells respectively [51].

6.2.6.3 CD4 + T and CD8+ T Cells

CD4+ T cells are the major contributors of lesions in stromal keratitis. These are responsible for the production of IL-2 and IFN- γ and are responsible for the second wave of neutrophil recruitment [52, 53]. CD8+ (or cytotoxic) T cells generally function in the control of viral infections by sensing and targeting infected cells leading to their destruction [54].

6.2.7 Viral Evasion Mechanisms

The HSV virus has devised various mechanisms to evade the host immune factors [55]. These includes downregulation of the host surface TLRs, RIG-like receptors, cytosolic DNA sensing pathways, disrupting of mechanisms like MHC I antigen presentation [56], autophagy [57], endoplasmic reticulum stress [58], and necroptosis [59].

6.2.8 HSK and Neovascularization

Corneal neovascularization has always been a long-term complication of HSK, leading to vision loss and further increasing risk for graft rejection. This angiogenesis occurs to increase in production or unopposed action of various growth factors especially vascular endothelial growth factor (VEGF) [60]. Apart from this the neutrophilic infiltration in HSK produce matrix metalloproteases - 9 (MMP-9), which promotes new vessel formation by breaking down the extracellular matrix [61].

6.2.9 HSK and Ocular Surface

Multiple studies have pointed out the occurrence of a decrease in the corneal sub-basal plexus [62] leading to poor blink rate, tear film hyperosmolarity, reduction in tearing and tear stability, in both the eyes despite unilateral involvement of HSK in those subjects. These patients thus were at a higher risk of having dry eye disease as compared to normal individuals [63–65].

6.3 Pathogenesis of Various Presentations of HSK

Based on the above immune response and direct virus-associated tissue damage, HSK can involve various layers of the cornea. Broadly they can be divided as the following:

6.3.1 Epithelial Keratitis

The viral infected epithelial cells show cellular swelling and can eventually lyse [66], which on cellular culture have shown to form syncytia that further enables cell to cell viral spread [67]. Initially they present as punctate keratopathy that coalesce to form a dendritic pattern. This pattern is seen as the virus has a tendency to follow the pattern of the underlying sub-basal plexus of corneal nerves [68]. The central epithelium sloughs off staining positive with fluorescein, while the actively multiplying virus are typically seen at the borders or terminal bulbs of the dendritic lesions staining positive with rose Bengal (Dual staining). These lesions may progress further to give a geographic ulcer especially in case of immunocompromised hosts or patients inadvertently using topical steroids. Epithelial involvement in HSK can also present as a marginal keratitis which needs to be differentiated from bacterial causes of marginal keratitis.

6.3.2 Stromal Keratitis

Stromal involvement can be immune stromal or necrotizing stromal keratitis. Immune stromal, as the name suggests, involves predominantly a recurrent stromal inflammation to the retained viral antigen mounting an antigen-antibody-complement cascade. Though it is majorly an immune-mediated inflammatory process, there can be presence of viral particles in the stroma. Sometimes, stromal keratitis is accompanied with epithelial ulceration leading to a more aggressive form of disease. This, often masquerading as a bacterial or fungal infection, is known as necrotizing stromal keratitis.

6.3.3 Endothelitis and Uveitis

This is associated with active viral replication in the anterior chamber. This is characterized with presence of localized corneal oedema, underlying Keratic precipitates (KP), and an increased in intra-ocular pressure (IOP). Based on distribution of KPs, they can be classified as disciform, diffuse, and linear types [69].

6.3.4 Metaherpetic Ulcer

This is a serious long-term complication of HSK, presenting as neurotrophic corneal ulcer. Factors involved in its pathogenesis include loss of corneal sensation because of prior attacks of HSK, chronic inflammation, decreased tear production and topical medication toxicity. These unlike the classical dual staining, show a reverse staining pattern with the base staining with rose Bengal and edges with fluorescein.

6.3.5 Other Manifestations

HSV infection has also been associated with conditions like Acute retinal necrosis (ARN) [70], Iridocorneal endothelial (ICE) syndrome [71], few cases of Episcleritis and scleritis [72], Posner Schlossman syndrome [73], and Fuchs heterochromic iridocyclitis [74].

6.4 Conclusion

Herpes simplex keratitis can manifest in diverse forms and may be accompanied by several associated co-morbidities. Knowledge about epidemiological and pathophysiological factors remains an important determinant for disease management. It is crucial to thoroughly inquire about detailed patient history, enabling tailored planning for subsequent management, follow-ups, and patient counselling.

Key Points

- Herpes simplex keratitis is among the leading causes of corneal blindness.
- The prevalence of herpes simplex keratitis varies with age, gender, and socio-economic status with a predilection to affect the younger and male individuals more.
- Herpes simplex virus-1 primarily causes keratitis through reactivation after a latent phase in the trigeminal ganglion.
- The host's immune status, both adaptive and innate immunity, amongst other factors, determines the severity of the recurrence.

References

1. Farooq AV, Shukla D. Herpes simplex epithelial and stromal keratitis: an epidemiologic update. Surv Ophthalmol. 2012;57(5):448–62.
2. Leopold IH, Sery TW. Epidemiology of herpes simplex keratitis. Investig Ophthalmol. 1963;2:498–503.
3. Das AV, Satyashree G, Joseph J, Bagga B. Herpes simplex virus keratitis: electronic medical records driven big data analytics report from a tertiary eye institute of South India. Int Ophthalmol. 2023;43(12):4669–76.
4. McCormick I, James C, Welton NJ, Mayaud P, Turner KME, Gottlieb SL, et al. Incidence of herpes simplex virus keratitis and other ocular disease: global review and estimates. Ophthalmic Epidemiol. 2022;29(4):353–62.
5. Pramod N. Herpes simplex keratitis in South India Clinico-Virological correlation. Jpn J Ophthalmol. 1999;43(4):303–7.
6. Labetoulle M, Auquier P, Conrad H, Crochard A, Daniloski M, Bouee S, et al. Incidence of herpes simplex virus keratitis in France. Ophthalmology. 2005;112(5):888–895.e1.
7. Liesegang TJ. Epidemiology of ocular herpes simplex: incidence in Rochester, Minn, 1950 through 1982. Arch Ophthalmol. 1989;107(8):1155.
8. Young RC. Incidence, recurrence, and outcomes of herpes simplex virus eye disease in Olmsted County, Minnesota, 1976–2007: the effect of oral antiviral prophylaxis. Arch Ophthalmol. 2010;128(9):1178.
9. Whitley RJ, Roizman B. Herpes simplex virus infections. Lancet. 2001;357(9267):1513–8. https://doi.org/10.1016/S0140-6736(00)04638-9.
10. Gupta R, Warren T, Wald A. Genital herpes. Lancet. 2007;370(9605):2127–37. https://doi.org/10.1016/S0140-6736(07)61908-4.
11. Chong EM, Wilhelmus KR, Matoba AY, et al. Herpes simplex virus keratitis in children. Am J Ophthalmol. 2004;138:474–5.
12. Hsiao CH, Yeung L, Yeh LK, et al. Pediatric herpes simplex virus keratitis. Cornea. 2009;28:249–53.
13. HEDS. Predictors of recurrent herpes simplex virus keratitis. Herpetic Eye Disease Study Group. Cornea. 2001;20:123–8.
14. Miserocchi E, Fogliato G, Bianchi I, Bandello F, Modorati G. Clinical features of ocular herpetic infection in an Italian referral center. Cornea. 2014;33(6):565–70.
15. Smith JS, Robinson NJ. Age-specifc prevalence of infection with herpes simplex virus types 2 and 1: a global review. J Infect Dis. 2002;186(Suppl 1):S3–28.
16. Mandell, ed. Mandell, Douglass, and Bennetts principles and practice of infectious disease. 7th ed. Elsevier; 2009.
17. Papanicolaou GA, Meyers BR, Fuchs WS, et al. Infectious ocular complications in orthotopic liver transplant patients. Clin Infect Dis. 1997;24:1172.
18. Geerlings S, Hoepelman A. Immune Dysfuction in patients with diabetes Mellitis. FEMS Immunol Med Microbiol. 1999;26:259–65.
19. Ukety TO, Maertens K. Ocular ulcerative herpes following measles in Kinshasa, Zaire. Curr Eye Res. 1991:10.
20. Young TL, Robin JB, Holland GN, et al. Herpes simplex keratitis in patients with acquired immune deficiency syndrome. Ophthalmology. 1989;96:1476–9.
21. Safir M, Mimouni M. Atopic disease as a risk factor for recurrent herpetic keratitis. Microorganisms. 2024;12(1):220.
22. Omatsu Y, Shimizu Y, Haruki T, Inoue Y, Miyazaki D. Effect of atopic conditions on development and recurrences of infectious keratitis. Allergol Int. 2024;S1323893024000091
23. Keddie F. Herpes simplex following artificial fever therapy. JAMA. 1941;117:1327–30.
24. Friedman E, Katcher A, Brightman V. Incidence of recurrent herpes labialis and upper respiratory infection: a prospective study of the influence of biologic, social, and psychologic predictors. Oral Surg Oral Med Oral Pathol. 1977;43:873–8.

25. Guinan M, MacCalman J, Kern E, et al. The course of untreated recurrent genital herpes simplex infection in 27 women. N Engl J Med. 1981;304:759–63.
26. Goldmeier D, Johnson A, Jeffries D, et al. Psychological aspects of recurrences of genital herpes. J Psychosom Res. 1986;30:601–8.
27. Deai T, Fukuda M, Hibino T, et al. Herpes simplex virus genome quantification in two patients who developed herpetic epithelial keratitis during treatment with antiglaucoma medications. Cornea. 2004;23:125–8.
28. Mucci JJ, Utz V, Galor A, et al. Recurrence rates of herpes simplex virus keratitis in contact lens and non-contact lens wearers. Eye Contact Lens. 2009;35:185–7.
29. Jain V, Pineda R. Reactivated herpetic keratitis following laser in situ keratomileusis. J Cataract Refract Surg. 2009;35:946–8.
30. Fagerholm P, Ohman L, Orndahl M. Phototherapeutic keratectomy in herpes simplex keratitis. Clinical results in 20 patients. Acta Ophthalmol. 1994;72:457–60.
31. Keskinbora. Long-term results of multizone photorefractive keratectomy for myopia of - 6.0 to −10.0 diopter. J Cataract Refract Surg. 2000;26:1484–91.
32. Hou YC, Chen CC, Wang IJ, et al. Recurrent herpetic keratouveitis following YAG laser peripheral iridotomy. Cornea. 2004;23:641–2.
33. Barequet IS, Wasserzug Y. Herpes simplex keratitis after cataract surgery. Cornea. 2007;26:615–7.
34. Sterk CC, Jager MJ, Swart-vd Berg M. Recurrent herpetic keratitis in penetrating keratoplasty. Doc Ophthalmol. 1995;90:29–33.
35. Das AV, Chaurasia S, Joseph J, Roy A, Das S, Fernandes M. Clinical profle and microbiological trends of therapeutic keratoplasty at a network of tertiary care ophthalmology centers in India. Int Ophthalmol. 2022;42(5):1391–9.
36. Hochberg CH, Schneider JA, Dandona R, Lakshmi V, Kumar GA, Sudha T, et al. Population and dyadic-based seroincidence of herpes simplex virus-2 and syphilis in southern India. Sex Transm Infect. 2015;91(5):375.
37. HEDS. Acyclovir for the prevention of recurrent herpes simplex virus eye disease. Herpetic Eye Disease Study Group. N Engl J Med. 1998;339:300–6.
38. Shuster JJ, Kaufman H, Nesburn A. Statistical analysis of the rate of recurrence of herpesvirus ocular epithelial disease. Am J Ophthalmol. 1981;91:328–31.
39. Shukla D, Spear PG. Herpesviruses and heparan sulfate: an intimate relationship in aid of viral entry. J Clin Invest. 2001;108:503–10.
40. Agelidis AM, Shukla D. Cell entry mechanisms of HSV: what we have learned in recent years. Future Virol. 2015;10:1145–54. https://doi.org/10.2217/fvl.15.85.
41. Lobo AM, Agelidis AM, Shukla D. Pathogenesis of herpes simplex keratitis: the host cell response and ocular surface sequelae to infection and inflammation. Ocul Surf. 2019;17(1):40–9.
42. Hendricks RL, Weber PC, Taylor JL, Koumbis A, Tumpey TM, Glorioso JC. Endogenously produced interferon alpha protects mice from herpes simplex virus type 1 corneal disease. J Gen Virol. 1991;72(Pt 7):1601–10.
43. Macrophages Ellermann-Eriksen S. and cytokines in the early defence against herpes simplex virus. Virol J. 2005;2:59.
44. Tang Q, Chen W, Hendricks RL. Proinflammatory functions of IL-2 in herpes simplex virus corneal infection. J Immunol. 1997;158(3):1275–83.
45. Biswas PS, Banerjee K, Kinchington PR, Rouse BT. Involvement of IL-6 in the paracrine production of VEGF in ocular HSV-1 infection. Exp Eye Res. 2006;82(1):4654.
46. Bryant-Hudson KM, Gurung HR, Zheng M, Carr DJ. Tumor necrosis factor alpha and interleukin-6 facilitate corneal lymphangiogenesis in response to herpes simplex virus 1 infection. J Virol. 2014;88(24):14451–7.
47. Suryawanshi A, Veiga-Parga T, Reddy PB, Rajasagi NK, Rouse BT. IL-17A differentially regulates corneal vascular endothelial growth factor (VEGF)-A and soluble VEGF receptor 1 expression and promotes corneal angiogenesis after herpes simplex virus infection. J Immunol. 2012;188(7):3434–46.
48. Hadigal SR, Agelidis AM, Karasneh GA, et al. Heparanase is a host enzyme required for herpes simplex virus-1 release from cells. Nat Commun. 2015;6:6985.
49. Daheshia M, Kanangat S, Rouse BT. Production of key molecules by ocular neutrophils early after herpetic infection of the cornea. Exp Eye Res. 1998;67(6):619–24. [PubMed: 9990326]
50. Thomas J, Gangappa S, Kanangat S, Rouse BT. On the essential involvement of neutrophils in the immunopathologic disease: herpetic stromal keratitis. J Immunol. 1997;158(3):13831391.
51. Lanier LL. Evolutionary struggles between NK cells and viruses. Nat Rev Immunol. 2008;8(4):259–68.
52. Rowe AM, St Leger AJ, Jeon S, Dhaliwal DK, Knickelbein JE, Hendricks RL. Herpes keratitis. Prog Retin Eye Res. 2013;32:88–101.
53. Hendricks RL. Immunopathogenesis of viral ocular infections. Chem Immunol. 1999;73:120–36.
54. Germain RN. T-cell development and the CD4-CD8 lineage decision. Nat Rev Immunol. 2002;2(5):309–22.
55. Su C, Zhan G, Zheng C. Evasion of host antiviral innate immunity by HSV-1, an update. Virol J. 2016;13:38.
56. Ahn K, Meyer TH, Uebel S, et al. Molecular mechanism and species specificity of TAP inhibition by herpes simplex virus protein ICP47. EMBO J. 1996;15(13):3247–55.
57. Orvedahl A, Alexander D, Tallóczy Z, et al. HSV-1 ICP34.5 confers Neurovirulence by targeting the Beclin 1 autophagy protein. Cell Host Microbe. 2007;1(1):23–35.

58. Li S, Kong L, Yu X. The expanding roles of endoplasmic reticulum stress in virus replication and pathogenesis. Crit Rev Microbiol. 2015;41(2):150–64.
59. Huang Z, Wu SQ, Liang Y, et al. RIP1/RIP3 binding to HSV-1 ICP6 initiates necroptosis to restrict virus propagation in mice. Cell Host Microbe. 2015;17(2):229–42.
60. Zheng M, Deshpande S, Lee S, Ferrara N, Rouse BT. Contribution of vascular endothelial growth factor in the neovascularization process during the pathogenesis of herpetic stromal keratitis. J Virol. 2001;75(20):9828–35.
61. Lee S, Zheng M, Kim B, Rouse BT. Role of matrix metalloproteinase-9 in angiogenesis caused by ocular infection with herpes simplex virus. J Clin Invest. 2002;110(8):1105–11.
62. Hamrah P, Cruzat A, Dastjerdi MH, et al. Corneal sensation and subbasal nerve alterations in patients with herpes simplex keratitis: an in vivo confocal microscopy study. Ophthalmology. 2010;117(10):1930–6.
63. M'Garrech M, Rousseau A, Kaswin G, et al. Impairment of lacrimal secretion in the unaffected fellow eye of patients with recurrent unilateral herpetic keratitis. Ophthalmology. 2013;120(10):1959–67.
64. Jabbarvand M, Hashemian H, Khodaparast M, Rafatnejad A, Beheshtnejad A, Salami A. Do unilateral herpetic stromal keratitis and neurotrophic ulcers cause bilateral dry eye? Cornea. 2015;34(7):768–72.
65. Reynaud C, Rousseau A, Kaswin G, M'Garrech M, Barreau E, Labetoulle M. Persistent impairment of quality of life in patients with herpes simplex keratitis. Ophthalmology. 2017;124(2):160–9.
66. Tabery HM. Early epithelial changes in recurrent herpes simplex virus keratitis: a noncontact photomicrographic study in vivo in the human cornea. Acta Ophthalmol Scand. 1998;76(3):349–52.
67. Thakkar N, Jaishankar D, Agelidis A, et al. Cultured corneas show dendritic spread and restrict herpes simplex virus infection that is not observed with cultured corneal cells. Sci Rep. 2017;7:42559.
68. Remeijer L, Osterhaus A, Verjans G. Human herpes simplex virus keratitis: the pathogenesis revisited. Ocul Immunol Inflamm. 2004;12(4):255–85.
69. Inoue Y. Review of clinical and basic approaches to corneal endotheliitis. Cornea. 2014;33(Suppl 11):S3–8.
70. Hoogewoud F, Rossi D, Stappler T, Guex-Crosier Y. Acute retinal necrosis: a mini review. Front Ophthalmol. 2022;2:916113. https://doi.org/10.3389/fopht.2022.916113.
71. Alvarado JA, Underwood JL, Green WR, Wu S, Murphy CG, Hwang DG, Moore TE, O'Day D. Detection of herpes simplex viral DNA in the iridocorneal endothelial syndrome. Arch Ophthalmol. 1994;112(12):1601–9.
72. Bhat PV, Jakobiec FA, Kurbanyan K, Zhao T, Foster CS. Chronic herpes simplex scleritis: characterization of 9 cases of an underrecognized clinical entity. Am J Ophthalmol. 2009;148(5):779–789.e2.
73. Yamamoto S, Pavan-Langston D, Tada R, Yamamoto R, Kinoshita S, Nishida K, Shimomura Y, Tano Y. Possible role of herpes simplex virus in the origin of Posner-Schlossman syndrome. Am J Ophthalmol. 1995;119(6):796–8. https://doi.org/10.1016/s0002-9394(14)72788-6. PMID: 7785697
74. Barequet IS, Li Q, Wang Y, O'Brien TP, Hooks JJ, Stark WJ. Herpes simplex virus DNA identification from aqueous fluid in Fuchs heterochromic iridocyclitis. Am J Ophthalmol. 2000;129(5):672–3.

Laboratory Diagnosis

7

Arpita Kulshrestha and Chintan Malhotra

Abstract

Herpes simplex virus (HSV) keratitis is a leading cause of vision impairment worldwide; however, early diagnosis and timely treatment has good prognosis. Currently, there are no set diagnostic criteria, and most ophthalmologists depend on characteristic clinical findings and history for diagnosis. The varying and often atypical presentations of HSV keratitis necessitate the use of alternative laboratory diagnostic methods for an accurate diagnosis and exclusion of other infective etiologies. Viral culture, the "gold standard" for HSV diagnosis, has largely been replaced by polymerase chain reaction (PCR). Real-time PCR has high sensitivity and specificity for HSV detection in both corneal scrapings and tear samples. Other more rapid but less sensitive methods include immunofluorescent assay (IFA), ELISA for antibody detection and cytologic examination. Novel, yet less explored, techniques like the multiplex dot hybridization (MDH) assay, ICP0 protein detection in tears, and immunochromatographic assays (ICGA) for both the detection of HSV-DNA (AmpliVue) and glycoprotein D antigens may be used as adjuncts or preliminary diagnostic tools in clinical settings.

A. Kulshrestha · C. Malhotra (✉)
PGI Chandigarh, Chandigarh, India

Keywords

HSV keratitis · Laboratory diagnosis · PCR · Immunofluorescent assay · Viral culture

7.1 Introduction

Herpes simplex virus (HSV) keratitis is a leading cause of vision loss globally, with an incidence of 1.5 million cases every year worldwide [1]. Despite being a globally significant ocular condition, the current diagnosis of HSV keratitis is based largely on clinical findings and history. There are no fixed diagnostic criteria as the clinical presentation of HSV varies vastly.

HSV keratitis may present a diagnostic dilemma to ophthalmologists, as differential diagnoses are often complicated by other infective etiologies, including bacterial or fungal keratitis, or merely a persistent epithelial defect. It could be easily misdiagnosed and treated as *Acanthamoeba* keratitis due to its atypical presentations and ring infiltrates [2]. Although treatment is frequently commenced without laboratory diagnosis, confirmation of HSV should be attempted if an ulcer does not have a classic dendritic appearance, particularly if it is the first episode without a prior confirmed diagnosis. Laboratory diagnosis is also of value in cases with a past history of HSV keratitis with a new epithelial defect which does not have characteristic features. Laboratory investigation is also help-

B. Sharma et al. (eds.), *Viral Keratitis*, https://doi.org/10.1007/978-981-95-3148-6_7

Table 7.1 Laboratory diagnosis of HSV keratitis

I. *Detection of HSV DNA* Polymerase chain reaction (PCR) Immunochromatographic assay- AmpliVue™, ELVIS™ Multiplex dot hybridization (MDH) assay
II. *Detection of HSV antigens* Immunofluorescent assay (IFA) Immunochromatographic assay (ICGA) kit Infected cell protein 0 (ICP0) detection
III. *Antibody detection with ELISA*
IV. *Cytology*
V. *Viral culture*

ful for the exclusion of conditions that require alternative treatment regimens such as varicella-zoster virus, cytomegalovirus, Epstein–Barr virus and human herpesvirus-6 [3].

Viral culture, which was once considered the gold standard for the detection of viruses has now been replaced with newer molecular diagnostic techniques such as real-time polymerase chain reaction (PCR) and enzyme-linked immunosorbent assay (ELISA). Novel, yet less explored, techniques include the multiplex dot hybridization (MDH) assay, ICP0 protein detection in tears, and immunochromatographic assays (ICGA) for both the detection of HSV-DNA (AmpliVue™) and glycoprotein D antigens which are a part of the HSV envelope [4] (Table 7.1).

7.2 Sample Collection

Clinical samples for HSV keratitis can be obtained from tears, corneal epithelial cells, conjunctival cells and aqueous humour tap (Table 7.2). Tear samples can be collected using Schirmer strips, which are placed in lower fornix for five minutes or through a pipette [4]. Corneal epithelial cells can be obtained by corneal scrapings, corneal/conjunctival swabs, or corneal impression membranes [5]. Aqueous tap may be considered in cases of suspected HSV endotheliitis. Fluorescein staining should be avoided prior to immunofluorescent assays. Likewise, Rose Bengal and lissamine green also reduce the sensitivity of PCR and should be avoided prior to sample collection [6].

Table 7.2 Sample collection for HSV keratitis

Tear samples
Corneal scraping
Corneal swab
Conjunctival swab
Corneal impression membranes
Aqueous tap

7.3 Detection of HSV DNA

7.3.1 Polymerase Chain Reaction

Polymerase chain reaction (PCR) is a molecular technique that generates millions of copies of a particular DNA sequence from a few copies of template DNA. PCR identification of HSV DNA has a sensitivity of up to 100% and has become the mainstay in laboratory confirmation of HSV keratitis [7]. It also has the advantage of detecting DNA of other pathogens such as acanthamoeba, VZV, and other viruses, in cases with atypical clinical presentation.

There are various types of PCR assays available, the most common being conventional PCR, quantitative or real-time PCR (qPCR), reverse transcriptase PCR (RT-PCR), and multiplex PCR. Real-time PCR allows for monitoring of the amplified DNA as the amplification progresses by using fluorescent-tagged primers (Fig. 7.1). It has the advantage of being faster than conventional PCR as it excludes the post-amplification process and has improved sensitivity as it enables quantification of viral DNA, even from exceedingly low viral DNA levels [8]. Joseph et al. observed that real-time PCR was superior in detecting HSV-1 (78%) compared to conventional PCR [9].

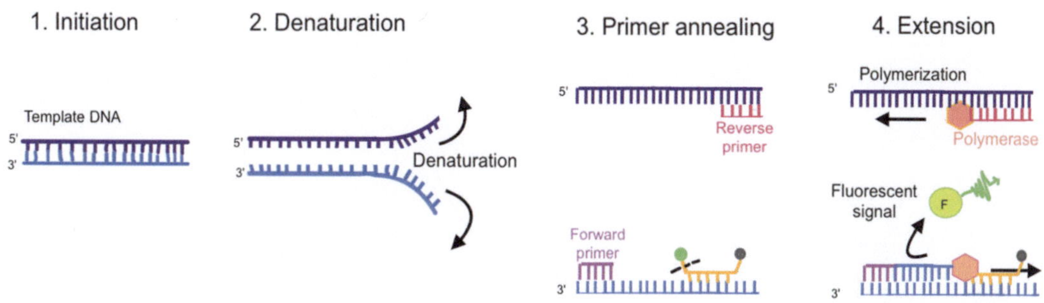

Fig. 7.1 Real time PCR: Allows monitoring of amplified DNA with fluorescent-tagged primers

The site of sample collection plays an important role in determining the diagnostic accuracy. Corneal scrapings have a higher sensitivity compared to tear samples, corneal impression membranes, and conjunctival swabs [5, 10, 11]. HSV DNA detection with tear samples alone may lead to a lower positive detection rate of 20% [4]. In necrotizing stromal keratitis, Ma et al. found a higher detection rate (46.4%) in corneal scrapings compared to tear samples (13.3%) as well as a higher viral load in the former [12]. Similar findings have been reported in another study with an HSV detection rate of 36.7% with corneal scrapings vs. 14% for tear samples [10]. Thus, tear sample collection may be used as a supplementary diagnostic tool, especially in cases where corneal scrapings are not possible. Although a few studies have demonstrated the presence of HSV DNA in the aqueous humour of eyes with HSV endotheliitis, the detection rate was found to be very low (0–12%) [13, 14].

PCR is a more sensitive detection tool when compared to other conventional methods such as immunofluorescent assay (IFA) and cytological examinations. The positive detection rate with PCR is much higher (46–78%) compared to IFA (14–23%) and cell cultures (7–11%) [10, 15]. For cytological examination, it has been reported that typical features of HSV were seen in only 40% of qPCR positive cases [16]. However, one major drawback of conventional PCR is that while it provides evidence for the presence of viral DNA, it does not distinguish between latent and infectious virus. This may explain the low specificity (65–67.9%) of PCR in several studies [7, 17]. This can be overcome by quantifying DNA levels using real-time PCR as levels are significantly higher in patients with clinical viral keratitis.

7.3.2 Immunochromatographic Assays

AmpliVue™ is a commercially available immunochromatographic assay that is Food and Drug Administration (FDA) cleared for the detection of HSV (1 and 2) from symptomatic patients with cutaneous or mucocutaneous lesions from oral, genital, and facial sources [18].

The assay utilizes helicase-dependent amplification (HDA) of gene sequences specific to HSV-1 and HSV-2 and a self-contained disposable amplification detection device that allows for visual evaluation of the results without any analytical instrumentation. The presence of HSV DNA is detected as a coloured line on a lateral flow strip (Fig. 7.2). AmpliVue™ is moderately sensitive (84%) and highly specific (100%) for HSV detection in corneal and conjunctival samples [18]. It has the advantage of providing test results within one hour.

ELVIS™ (Enzyme-linked virus inducible system) is another commercially available assay based on histological staining of induced beta-galactosidase production within infected cells. AmpliVue™ has however been documented to have a much higher sensitivity than ELVIS™ for HSV detection (64.7% vs. 0) [19].

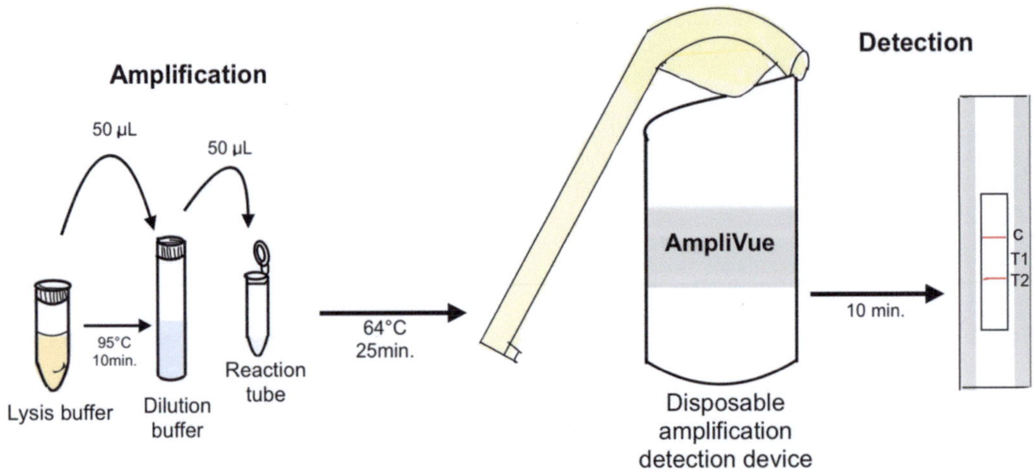

Fig. 7.2 Diagrammatic representation of AmpliVueTM assay: HSV DNA is extracted, amplified and detected as coloured lines on lateral flow strip

7.3.3 Multiplex Dot Hybridization (MDH) Assay

This assay uses a series of oligonucleotide probes that are specific for different genes found in different microorganisms. These probes are fixed on a nylon membrane and made to react with PCR-amplified DNA samples. The hybridization reaction results in the formation of coloured spots that can be read by the naked eye. For HSV-1 and HSV-2, the specific probes are designed from conserved sequences of long unique region 30 (UL30 gene).

Kuo et al. found high sensitivity (93.3%) and specificity (100%) for HSV-specific MDH assay when compared with real-time PCR as the standard test [20]. This assay has the advantage of simultaneous detection of multiple pathogens in the sample. It may serve as a rapid test for HSV detection as it generates results within one day and does not require any specialized technician.

7.4 Antigen Detection

7.4.1 Immunofluorescent Assay

Indirect immunofluorescent assay (IFA) is performed by introducing antibodies to infected cell samples that can recognize and bind to HSV antigens specifically. Fluorophore-tagged secondary antibodies are subsequently introduced to the sample, that bind to the primary antibodies and examination is done under a fluorescent microscope (Fig. 7.3).

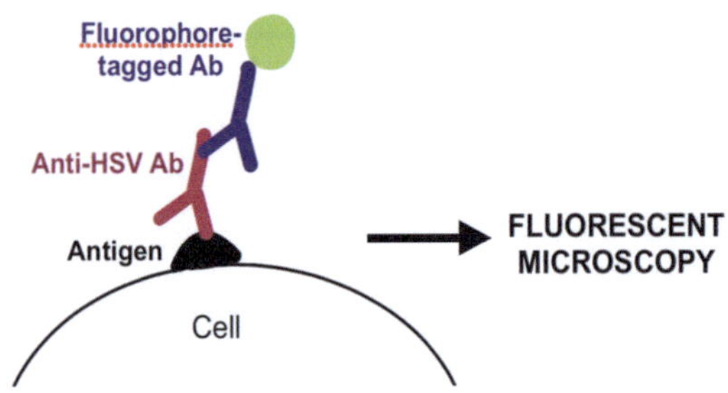

Fig. 7.3 Indirect immunofluorescence: Fluorophore-tagged antibodies bind to HSV-specific antibodies and examined under a fluorescent microscope

Both corneal scrapings and tear samples can be analyzed with IFA, with higher positivity rates than the former [10]. However, fluorescent staining of the tear film should be avoided prior to sample collection, as this can interfere with the fluorescein-conjugated antibodies.

One of the limitations of IFA is its susceptibility to cross-reactivity with other microorganisms, thereby increasing its risk of rendering false positives. When compared to PCR, the sensitivity (85.7%) and specificity of IFA is lower (85.3%).

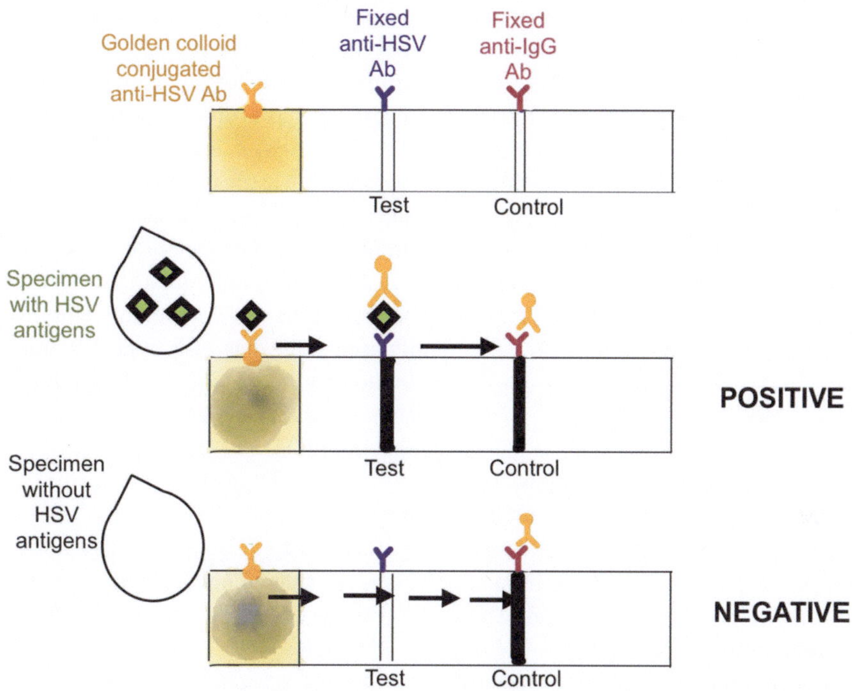

Fig. 7.4 ICGA kit: Golden colloid conjugated Ab against glycoprotein D antigen are detected by colorimetric reaction on lateral flow strip

However, IFA detects 33.3% more positive cases than viral culture [9, 21]. Although IFA is a rapid test for the detection of the herpes virus, a combination of PCR and IFA would result in a more reliable and accurate result [10].

7.4.2 Immunochromatographic Assay (ICGA) Kit

ICGA kit utilizes monoclonal antibodies against the glycoprotein D antigen that is present in the HSV envelope and is essential for infectivity. The colorimetric reaction is seen as an observable line in the lateral flow strip (Fig. 7.4).

This kit can be performed as an "in-the-office" diagnostic test within 15 minutes and does not require specialized equipment and expertise. It has moderate sensitivity and high specificity for HSV detection in corneal scrapings with a 46.7% positive concordance between final clinical diagnosis and ICGA and a 100% negative concordance rate [22].

7.4.3 Infected Cell Protein 0 (ICP0) Detection

Infected cell protein 0 (ICP0) is an acute phase protein of HSV-1 that is expressed in the early phase of the disease. It regulates the ubiquitin-proteasome pathway to degrade target proteins and plays an important role in viral reactivation from latency.

Morshige N et al. have observed ICP0 in 4 out of 7 tear films of patients with HSV keratitis with a 57.1% positive detection rate [23]. A lower detection rate may be related to the time of detection in the course of the disease [23].

7.5 Antibody Detection- ELISA

Serum detection of IgG and IgM antibodies is typically of limited use in the diagnosis of HSV infection, given the widespread ubiquity of HSV and that HSV keratitis is not a primary infection but a reactivation of latent infection [6].

ELISA can be used for quantitative analysis of HSV-1 specific secretory immunoglobulin A (sIgA) antibody detection in tear samples. Huang et al. found that the tear sIgA–positive rate was 36.59% in stromal keratitis and that the positivity of sIgA was a potential factor for predicting the risk of herpes keratitis recurrence [24]. A combination of real-time PCR for HSV DNA with ELISA for sIgA may be performed in conjunction for higher sensitivity for HSV detection [25, 26].

7.6 Cytology

A Tzanck smear with Giemsa stain shows characteristic multinucleated giant cells and intranuclear eosinophilic HSV inclusions. However, sensitivity is much lower than PCR and immunofluorescent assay (IFA) [27]. Cytological examination of corneal smears could only identify typical HSV features in 40% of qPCR positive cases [16].

7.7 Viral Culture

The gold standard for HSV diagnosis is virus culture. In addition to diagnosis, it allows viricidal drug sensitivity testing, strain identification, and epidemiological tracing. Virus isolation is done in a confluent monolayer of Hep-2 cells/Vero cells that are then examined for the development of a cytopathic effect. After obtaining a sample it is required to be kept at 4 °C until plated on the cell monolayer, and isolation can take up to 10 days. Although virus isolation on culture has 100% specificity, it has very low sensitivity (7–11%) [10]. With very low virus isolation rates, culture is not performed routinely, other than in reference laboratories and research settings [28].

7.8 Conclusion

A common cause of global vision loss, herpes simplex virus affects about 1.5 million people annually. Due to the myriad of presentations, and the possibility for various differentials, diagnosis may often be challenging, especially in atypical disease morphology. A myriad of diagnostic modalities has evolved over the decades to facilitate diagnosis viz. real-time PCR, immunochromatographic assays, multiplex dot hybridization, and immunofluorescent assays. These tests, albeit preferred over the older viral culture, have respective advantages and limitations. PCR continues to be among the most commonly employed modality used in the diagnosis of HSV even though it is limited by its inability to distinguish latent and active infections despite high sensitivity and specificity.

Key Points

- Laboratory diagnosis of HSV keratitis should be considered in cases with atypical presentations and to exclude other infective etiologies.
- Corneal scrapings have a higher sensitivity compared to tear samples, corneal impression membranes, and conjunctival swabs.
- Real-time PCR is a more sensitive detection tool when compared to other conventional methods such as immunofluorescent assay (IFA), cytological examination, and culture.
- A combination of real-time PCR with IFA or ELISA can improve the sensitivity of HSV detection.
- Rapid methods such as the MDH assay, ICGA kits, and ICP-0 detection can act as adjuncts or preliminary "in-the-office" diagnostic tools.

References

1. Farooq AV, Shukla D. Herpes simplex epithelial and stromal keratitis: an epidemiologic update. Surv Ophthalmol. 2012;57(5):448–62.
2. Poon SHL, Wong WHL, Lo ACY, Yuan H, Chen CF, Jhanji V, et al. A systematic review on advances in diagnostics for herpes simplex keratitis. Surv Ophthalmol. 2021;66(3):514–30.
3. Venugopal A, Christy J, Raut V, Preethi P, Patwardhan V, Veeramma V, et al. Viral keratitis, surgical intervention in viral keratitis, challenges in diagnosis and treatment of viral keratitis, HSV, HZV. Semin Ophthalmol. 2024;39:340–52.

4. Lee SY, Kim MJ, Kim MK, Wee WR. Comparative analysis of polymerase chain reaction assay for herpes simplex virus 1 detection in tear. Korean J Ophthalmol KJO. 2013;27(5):316–21.
5. Brunner M, Somerville T, Corless CE, Myneni J, Rajhbeharrysingh T, Tiew S, et al. Use of a corneal impression membrane and PCR for the detection of herpes simplex virus type-1. J Med Microbiol. 2019;68(9):1324–9.
6. Sibley D, Larkin DFP. Update on herpes simplex keratitis management. Eye. 2020;34(12):2219–26.
7. Subhan S, Jose RJ, Duggirala A, Hari R, Krishna P, Reddy S, et al. Diagnosis of herpes simplex virus-1 keratitis: comparison of Giemsa stain, immunofluorescence assay and polymerase chain reaction. Curr Eye Res. 2004;29(2–3):209–13.
8. Mackay IM. Real-time PCR in virology. Nucleic Acids Res. 2002;30(6):1292–305.
9. Joseph Ruben J, Madhuri Guda SJ, Sontam B, Bagga B, Konduri R, Sharma S. Evaluation of multiplex real-time polymerase chain reaction for the detection of HSV-1 & 2 and VZV in the diagnosis of viral keratitis. Invest Ophthalmol Vis Sci. 2017;58(8):3604.
10. Satpathy G, Mishra AK, Tandon R, Sharma MK, Sharma A, Nayak N, et al. Evaluation of tear samples for Herpes Simplex Virus 1 (HSV) detection in suspected cases of viral keratitis using PCR assay and conventional laboratory diagnostic tools. Br J Ophthalmol. 2011;95(3):415–8.
11. McGilligan VE, Moore JE, Tallouzi M, Atkinson SD, O'Neill H, Feeney S, et al. A comparison of the clinical and molecular diagnosis of herpes simplex keratitis. Open J Ophthalmol. 2014;04(03):65–74.
12. Ma JX, Wang LN, Zhou RX, Yu Y, Du TX. Real-time polymerase chain reaction for the diagnosis of necrotizing herpes stromal keratitis. Int J Ophthalmol. 2016;9(5):682–6.
13. Abu Dail Y, Daas L, Flockerzi E, Munteanu C, Kahlert J, Smola S, et al. PCR testing for herpesviruses in aqueous humor samples from patients with and without clinical corneal endothelial graft rejection. J Med Virol. 2024;96(3):e29538.
14. Kakimaru-Hasegawa A, Kuo CH, Komatsu N, Komatsu K, Miyazaki D, Inoue Y. Clinical application of real-time polymerase chain reaction for diagnosis of herpetic diseases of the anterior segment of the eye. Jpn J Ophthalmol. 2008;52(1):24–31.
15. Guda SM, Sontam B, Bagga B, Ranjith K, Sharma S, Joseph J. Evaluation of multiplex real-time polymerase chain reaction for the detection of herpes simplex virus-1 and 2 and varicella-zoster virus in corneal cells from normal subjects and patients with keratitis in India. Indian J Ophthalmol. 2019;67(7):1040.
16. Erdem E, Harbiyeli İİ, Öztürk G, Oruz O, Açıkalın A, Yağmur M, et al. Atypical herpes simplex keratitis: frequency, clinical presentations and treatment results. Int Ophthalmol. 2020;40(3):659–65.
17. Kaye SB. Human herpesviruses in the cornea. Br J Ophthalmol. 2000;84(6):563–71.
18. Kowalski RP, Karenchak LM, Dhaliwal DK, Mammen A. AmpliVue is a practical and timely test for the detection of HSV from keratitis specimens. Eye Contact Lens. 2018;44(Suppl 1):S244–8.
19. Granato PA, Alkins BR, Yen-Lieberman B, Greene WH, Connolly J, Buchan BW, et al. Comparative evaluation of AmpliVue HSV 1+2 assay with ELVIS culture for detecting herpes simplex virus 1 (HSV-1) and HSV-2 in clinical specimens. J Clin Microbiol. 2015;53(12):3922–5.
20. Kuo MT, Fang PC, Yu HJ, Chao TL, Chien CC, Chen SH, et al. A multiplex dot hybridization assay for detection and differentiation of Acanthamoeba and herpes keratitis. Invest Ophthalmol Vis Sci. 2016;57(4):2158–63.
21. Satpathy G, Behera HS, Sharma A, Mishra AK, Mishra D, Sharma N, et al. A 20-year experience of ocular herpes virus detection using immunofluorescence and polymerase chain reaction. Clin Exp Optom. 2018;101(5):648–51.
22. Inoue Y, Shimomura Y, Fukuda M, Miyazaki D, Ohashi Y, Sasaki H, et al. Multicentre clinical study of the herpes simplex virus immunochromatographic assay kit for the diagnosis of herpetic epithelial keratitis. Br J Ophthalmol. 2013;97(9):1108–12.
23. Morishige N, Yamada N, Morita Y, Nakamura Y, Nishida T, Sonoda KH. Detection of ICP0 protein in tear fluid of individuals with active herpetic epithelial keratitis. Jpn J Ophthalmol. 2011;55(6):591–4.
24. Huang F, Wang Z, Zhang C. Tear HSV-specific secretory IgA as a potential indicator for recurrent stromal herpes simplex keratitis: a preliminary study. Cornea. 2013;32(7):987–91.
25. Shoji J, Sakimoto T, Inada N, Kamei Y, Matsubara M, Takamura E, et al. A diagnostic method for herpes simplex keratitis by simultaneous measurement of viral DNA and virus-specific secretory IgA in tears: an evaluation. Jpn J Ophthalmol. 2016;60(4):294–301.
26. Qiu J, Huang F, Wang Z, Xu J, Zhang C. The evaluation of diagnostic efficiency for stromal herpes simplex keratitis by the combination of tear HSV-sIgA and HSV-DNA. Graefes Arch Clin Exp Ophthalmol Albrecht Von Graefes Arch Klin Exp Ophthalmol. 2017;255(7):1409–15.
27. Farhatullah S, Kaza S, Athmanathan S, Garg P, Reddy SB, Sharma S. Diagnosis of herpes simplex virus-1 keratitis using Giemsa stain, immunofluorescence assay, and polymerase chain reaction assay on corneal scrapings. Br J Ophthalmol. 2004;88(1):142–4.
28. Athmanathan S, Reddy SB, Nutheti R, Rao GN. Comparison of an immortalized human corneal epithelial cell line with Vero cells in the isolation of Herpes simplex virus-1 for the laboratory diagnosis of Herpes simplex keratitis. BMC Ophthalmol. 2002;2:3.

Congenital Herpes

8

Brindha Periasamy, Bhavana Sharma, Pooja Bang, and Priyanka

Abstract

Congenital herpes is a serious condition resulting from maternal HSV transmission to the foetus or newborn. The infection can lead to a spectrum of systemic and ocular manifestations, ranging from isolated mucocutaneous lesions to more severe outcomes like keratitis, chorioretinitis, or optic atrophy. Early diagnosis and prompt antiviral treatment are crucial to prevent potentially blinding complications. This chapter discusses the pathophysiology, clinical presentation, diagnosis, and management of congenital herpes, emphasizing the need for comprehensive care in affected neonates.

Keywords

Congenital infection · Ocular manifestations Neonatal HSV · Ophthalmia neonatorum

8.1 Introduction

Congenital herpes is a group of anomalies that an infant may acquire as a result of maternal HSV infection, which gets transmitted to the foetus or newborn. The estimated annual incidence of congenital herpes ranges between 1.6 and 8.4 per 100,000 live births [1]. The risk of maternal transmission to the child is considerably high with HSV-1, which can lead to significant neonatal morbidity [2, 3]. Neonates may present with several systemic and ocular manifestations of varying severity. Ocular manifestations in neonatal HSV can include isolated mucocutaneous lesions, blepharoconjunctivitis or keratitis, chorioretinitis, or optic atrophy. The mode of infection can be categorized as:

8.1.1 Primary Herpes Virus

Primary herpes virus infections occur mainly in utero and can cause microcephaly, microphthalmos, colobomas, and optic nerve involvement in addition to other ocular affections. Herpes simplex eye disease is a spectrum of ocular morbidities seen in infants with congenital syphilis. It can result in keratitis, corneal ulceration, cataracts, secondary glaucoma, anterior uveitis, vitritis, chorioretinitis, salt and pepper fundus, and optic atrophy. In acute phase, blepharoconjunctivitis is the most frequent manifestation in neonates, which is commonly associated with epithelial keratitis [4] (Figs. 8.1, 8.2, and 8.3). Given the non-specificity of clinical signs in neonatal patients, it is often challenging to diagnose and treat such patients. Corneal involvement is generally unilateral in most cases, which is an impor-

B. Periasamy · B. Sharma (✉) · Priyanka
AIIMS Bhopal, Bhopal, Madhya Pradesh, India

P. Bang
AIIMS Nagpur, Nagpur, Maharashtra, India

B. Sharma et al. (eds.), *Viral Keratitis*, https://doi.org/10.1007/978-981-95-3148-6_8

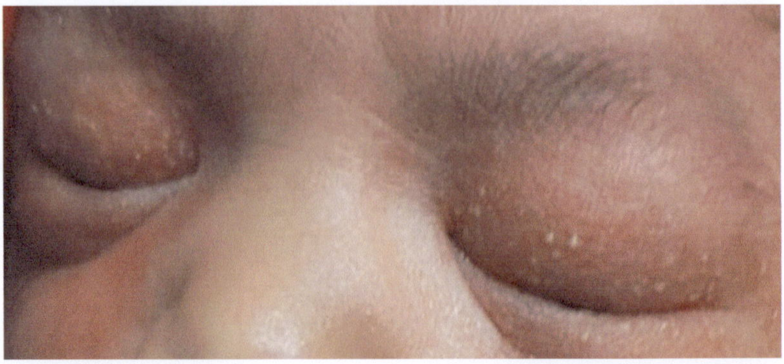

Fig. 8.1 Primary HSV infection showing vesicles and severe lid edema

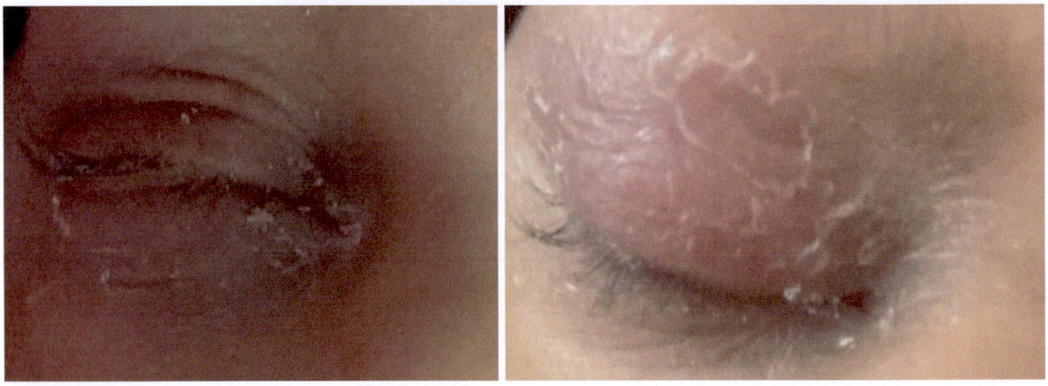

Figs. 8.2 and 8.3 Seven days post treatment showing epidermal excoriation and resolved vesicles

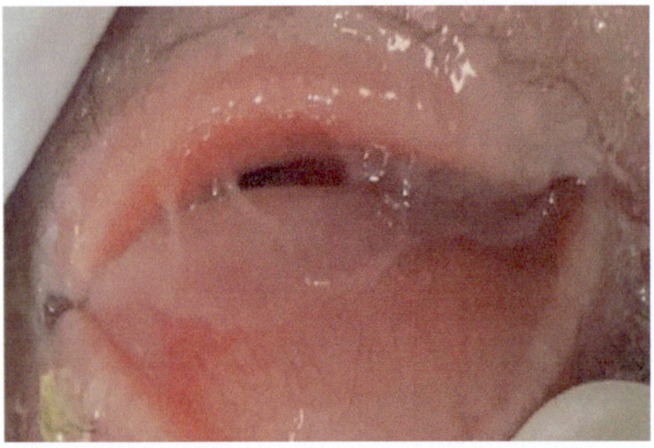

Fig. 8.4 HSV blepharitis with secondary bacterial infection and severe mucopurulent discharge

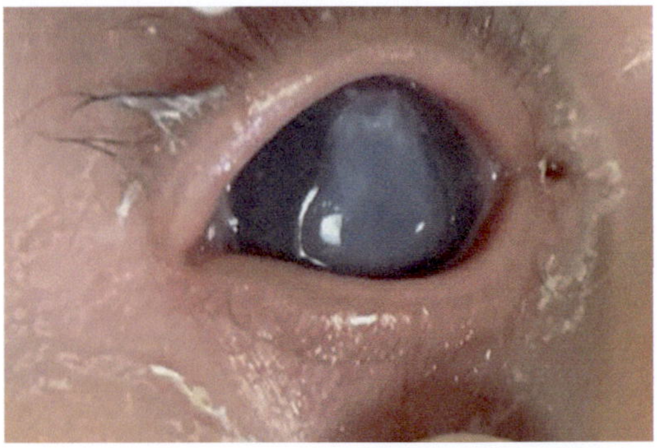

Fig. 8.5 One-week post treatment showing resolving blepharitis and healing of corneal ulcer with formation of maculo leucomatous opacity

tant diagnostic differentiator along with presence of epithelial defect and no improvement with instated topical antibiotics (Figs. 8.4 and 8.5).

8.1.2 Cross Infection with Herpes Virus

Cross infection typically occurs at the time of delivery with a potential to cause Ophthalmia neonatorum in addition to carrying a serious risk of systemic infection for the newborn. This risk may be high during the initial infection of the mother (33–50%), but is considered to be low in reinfection because of the protective effect of maternal antibodies.

Pathophysiology

Neonates are at higher risk of infection due to predisposing factors like decreased tear production, lack of IgA in tears, deficient immune function, absence of lymphoid tissue in conjunctiva, and decreased lysozyme activity. Risk factors include premature rupture of membranes, prolonged delivery, prematurity, poor prenatal care, poor hygiene conditions, history of midwife interference, and infected mothers.

8.1.2.1 Herpes Simplex Ophthalmia Neonatorum

Herpes simplex ophthalmia neonatorum refers to blepharoconjunctivitis, with or without keratitis, in newborn infants caused by active HSV infection acquired through an infected birth canal. The global prevalence of ophthalmia neonatorum is estimated to be around 10 per 100,000 live births [5]. However, genital HSV infection in mothers often goes misdiagnosed or underdiagnosed due to mild clinical symptoms and subsequent underreporting. This underdiagnosis can lead to HSV-induced ophthalmia neonatorum being misdiagnosed as well, resulting in prolonged illness and potentially vision-threatening complications [6].

Asymptomatic neonates born to women with active genital lesions at the time of delivery should be carefully evaluated and tested for HSV infection [7].

The onset of herpes simplex ophthalmia neonatorum typically occurs within the first 28 days of life. The disease is characterized by severe conjunctival inflammation, intense congestion, follicular reaction, chemosis, and associated discharge. Neonatal HSV eye infections can have potentially blinding sequelae, requiring a high index of suspicion in such cases [8]. Thus, ocular involvement in children born to mothers with genital herpes should be evaluated carefully and promptly treated for viral ophthalmia neonatorum.

8.1.2.2 HSV Congenital Infection

Congenital HSV infections of the eye may occur in association with systemic herpes infection or local skin lesions. The onset of signs and symptoms typically occurs between the first and fourth weeks of life [5]. The most common presenting sign is typical vesicular lesions on an erythematous base. The hallmark of the disease is keratoconjunctivitis of varying severity. Ocular infection can be unilateral or bilateral, with variable signs and symptoms including vesicles on the lid margins, eyelid edema or preseptal cellulitis, conjunctival chemosis, and congestion, with or without conjunctival membranes. In severe cases, involvement of cornea in the form of haze, edema, infiltration, and ulcer may be seen. Recurrences have been reported in up to 90% of patients [9].

8.2 Diagnosis

Neonatal ocular HSV is diagnosed primarily by clinical features seen in children born to infected mothers. However, the virus isolated from the culture of the tissue specimens from skin, conjunctiva, and other involved body fluids remains the gold standard for specific diagnosis. After the virus is inoculated into the cell culture system and grows, it may then be further identified as HSV-1 or HSV-2. In addition, polymerase chain reaction & ELISA of conjunctival swabs allows for the rapid diagnosis of HSV in the clinical setting, with a reported sensitivity of 80%. Tzank smear can be done to identify multinucleated giant cells in any lesion that may be suspicious of HSV. Other laboratory tests which can be done to evaluate systemic functions and may be suggestive of HSV infection, include leukopenia, thrombocytopenia, elevated liver enzymes, hypoglycaemia, and elevated protein in the CSF.

8.3 Management

Differential diagnoses for congenital HSV infection include ophthalmia neonatorum caused by gonococcal or chlamydial infections. Gonococcal ophthalmia neonatorum is characterized by intense inflammation, membranous conjunctivitis, and profuse purulent discharge, which distinguishes it from the milder presentation of chlamydial infection. The discharge in gonococcal infection is initially copious, becoming purulent, and is often associated with significant lid edema.

Given that neonates have immature immune systems, they should be treated intensively in the same vein as immunocompromised patients. Any delay in initiating treatment may lead to the progression of the disease to a disseminated form. Ocular involvement in neonatal HSV can be effectively treated with both systemic and local antiviral agents.

Treatment should be started at earliest with systemic Acyclovir, in recommended dose of 20 mg/kg three times daily for 14 days. Treatment is to be extended for 1–2 weeks more in cases with CNS involvement. Patients may present with recurrences which should be carefully monitored. There are recommendations of suppressive therapy with a lower dose of Acyclovir (300 mg/m^2/dose TDS) for 6 months to prevent recurrences. In cases with prolonged treatments, liver and kidney function tests in addition to hemogram should be advised every month.

Prognosis varies based on the extent of the disease. Congenital HSV-infected infants should be evaluated by a paediatrician and ophthalmologists to assess the extent and severity of involvement. MRI of the brain should be performed to evaluate the CNS involvement if any. Infants should be treated with intravenous (IV) acyclovir 20 mg/kg/dose every 8 hours for a total of 21 days. At the completion of treatment, blood PCR should be done to ensure the virus has been eliminated. If the results are positive, the infant should be treated for another seven days or until a negative result is obtained. After IV treatment, suppressive therapy should be given with oral acyclovir 300 mg/m^2 per dose three times per day for six months [10].

8.4 Conclusion

Preventive measures directed towards maternal care by way of disease awareness, systemic evaluation, and aseptic measures in addition to early diagnosis and timely initiation of antiviral therapy are important measures for timely treatment and complications mitigation. The infant should be followed up not only by the paediatrician but also by the ophthalmologist for evaluation of the recurrence of symptoms, complications, or sequelae. Caesarean delivery for women known to have active genital lesions present at term has been shown to decrease transmission. Oral acyclovir or valacyclovir during the last few weeks of pregnancy to women with a history of genital HSV may prevent recurrences at the time of delivery.

Key Points

- Congenital herpes can present with severe ocular manifestations and requires early diagnosis and treatment.
- Systemic acyclovir is the primary treatment for neonatal HSV infection, with suppressive therapy recommended to prevent recurrences.
- Preventive measures, including caesarean delivery for active genital lesions, can significantly reduce the risk of neonatal transmission.

References

1. Sánchez Pujol MJ, Docampo Simon A, Sanguino L, Blanes M, Betlloch I. Herpes simplex virus infection in neonates born to asymptomatic mothers: a case series. Cureus. 2022;14:e32393.
2. Rząd M, Nitsch-Osuch A, Tyszko P, Goryński P, Bogdan M, Lewtak K. Congenital herpes simplex virus infection among hospitalized infants in Poland. Ann Agric Environ Med. 2021;28(4):612–6. https://doi.org/10.26444/aaem/142999.
3. Kidszun A, Bruns A, Schreiner D, et al. Characteristics of neonatal herpes simplex virus infections in Germany: results of a 2-year prospective nationwide surveillance study. Arch Dis Child Fetal Neonatal Ed. 2022;107(2):188–92.
4. Jesus J, Almeida I, Matias M, Chibante J, Costa Ferreira C. Neonatal Type-2 unilateral herpes simplex Blepharokeratoconjunctivitis after cesarean delivery. Acta Sci Ophthalmol. 2021;1(1):6–9.
5. Pinninti SG, Kimberlin DW. Neonatal herpes simplex virus infections. Paediatr Clin North Am. 2013;60(2):351–65.
6. Scott HJ, Kimberlin DW. Neonatal herpes simplex virus infection: epidemiology and treatment. Clin Perinato. 2015;42(1):47–59.

7. Kimberlin DW, Baley J, Committee on infectious diseases, committee on fetus and newborn: guidance on management of asymptomatic neonates born to women with active genital herpes lesions. Pediatrics 2013;131(2).
8. Matos RJC, Peres JMS, Cortesão D. Management of neonatal herpes simplex infection: a rare case of blepharoconjunctivitis and concurrent epithelial and stromal keratitis. Ocul Immunol Inflamm. 2016;26(4):625–7.
9. Boyd RL, Ward R, Kasman LM. Herpes simplex Neonatorum. In: StatPearls. Treasure Island, FL: StatPearls Publishing; 2023.
10. Kimberlin DW, Whitley RJ, Wan W, et al. Oral acyclovir suppression and neurodevelopment after neonatal herpes. N Engl J Med. 2011;365(14):1284–92.

9 Primary Ocular Infections

Rakhi Kusumesh, Prabhakar Singh, Vijay Sharma, and Bhavana Sharma

Abstract

HSV-1 infection remains the primary cause of herpetic eye diseases across all age groups and acquired during childhood and adolescence and is markedly more widespread than HSV-2 infection. Most primary infections are subclinical. HSV infection in children poses a significant diagnostic challenge due to difficulties in examination and a high risk of amblyopia from corneal scarring. Primary infection generally occurs through the oropharyngeal mucosa on exposure to secretions of an individual shedding HSV. Most of the cases are diagnosed clinically based on the clinical features, antecedent history, and high degree of suspicion. Considering the significant morbidity caused by HSV, particularly in children, prompt diagnosis, close monitoring, and appropriate antiviral therapy are essential to reduce the impact of this ocular herpes simplex infections and to improve the outcomes.

R. Kusumesh (✉)
Indira Gandhi Institute of Medical Science, Patna, India

P. Singh
AIIMS Kalyani, Kalyani, West Bengal, India

V. Sharma
AFMC, Pune, Maharashtra, India

B. Sharma
AIIMS Bhopal, Bhopal, Madhya Pradesh, India

Keywords

HSV · Primary · Congenital
Blepharoconjunctivitis

9.1 Introduction

Herpetic infections in the eye exhibit characteristics similar to herpetic diseases elsewhere in the body. A primary distinction between primary and recurrent disease is the presence or absence of immune responses at the onset. Primary infections occur in hosts susceptible to herpes simplex virus (HSV) who lack existing HSV antibodies [1, 2]. Typically, primary herpes manifests early in life, between 6 months to 5 years, following the decline of maternally acquired antibodies. HSV type 1 is predominantly responsible for initial infections in children and remains the primary cause of herpetic eye diseases across all age groups. The incubation period for HSV ranges from 3 to 12 days. While HSV-1 is the more common cause, HSV-2 also plays a role in neonatal infections, occasionally leading to ocular herpes through exposure during birth [3, 4]. In recent times, primary HSV infections are increasingly observed later in life, typically during adolescence or early adulthood. This shift is attributed to improved hygiene and social conditions, while there is an increased likelihood of acquiring HSV-2 through sexual contact. HSV-2 is suspected to cause more severe diseases compared to HSV-1.

B. Sharma et al. (eds.), *Viral Keratitis*, https://doi.org/10.1007/978-981-95-3148-6_9

Most primary infections are subclinical but may include systemic symptoms such as fever, pharyngitis, rhinitis, malaise, and lymphadenopathy. It is estimated that 98% of primary ocular HSV infections remain undiagnosed because they are either subclinical or present only as mild conjunctivitis. Less than 2% of those infected develop noticeable ocular disease. The condition typically affects one eye but can appear bilaterally in 5.8% to 26% of cases [1, 2, 5, 6]. Systemic antiviral treatment is crucial during a primary HSV episode to prevent the spread of the virus within the eye and to nearby ganglionic tissue.

HSV infection in children poses a significant diagnostic challenge due to difficulties in examination, and a high risk of amblyopia from corneal scarring [7]. Therefore, children tend to have poorer visual outcomes when affected, necessitating more frequent monitoring. This necessitates early recognition and treatment by ophthalmologists, including intensive medical treatment, regular refraction tests, and occlusion therapy to ensure favourable visual outcomes [8].

9.2 Epidemiology

Humans are the only known natural reservoir of HSV, and seroprevalence studies indicate that HSV-1 and HSV-2 infections are common worldwide, in both developed and developing countries [9]. Research on HSV ocular infections in children has been somewhat limited due to the small numbers of patients in individual studies. However, data suggest that by the age of 5, around 20–40% of children in the United States show serological evidence of HSV-1 infection. Despite significant improvements in perinatal care, HSV ocular infections continue to be associated with considerable morbidity. The estimated annual incidence of these infections varies, ranging from 1.6 to 8.4 per 100,000 live births [10, 11].

Seroprevalence rates for both HSV-1 and HSV-2 range from 50% to 90% in the general population, affecting both adults and children. Notably, seroconversion rates vary significantly across socioeconomic groups. Children under 5 from lower socioeconomic backgrounds experience seroconversion rates approximately 30% higher than those from middle socioeconomic standings [12].

9.3 Mode of Transmission

Primary infection generally occurs through the oropharyngeal mucosa on exposure to secretions of an individual shedding HSV. HSV-1 causes orofacial and eye infections by contact from an infected individual, while HSV-2 causes genital disease transmitted sexually [13].

Neonatal/Congenital HSV While both HSV types contribute to neonatal infections, HSV-1 is more commonly transmitted from mother to child. Transmission routes for these infections are not always clear, but it is estimated that about 85% of infected infants acquire the virus during childbirth (intrapartum), 10% are infected after birth (postnatally), and 5% acquire the virus while in the uterus (in utero) [14, 15].

9.4 Pathophysiology

The initial infection of ocular tissues with HSV typically occurs during first exposure to the virus. After the initial infection, the body responds by producing circulating antibodies and sensitized lymphocytes. In healthy individuals, general immune defences including macrophages, natural killer cells, and interferon work together to limit this primary infection. However, immunocompromised individuals, including newborns, are at a higher risk of widespread viral infection due to their weaker immune systems. This can lead to more severe symptoms, delayed healing, and a heightened risk of herpes infections [16, 17].

Typically, the primary infection within the eyes is either subclinical—showing no noticeable symptoms—or presents symptoms that are not distinctly recognized as herpes. The extent to which HSV spreads within the eye may vary depending on how it interacts with neurons or myelin, which affects the severity at the initial site of entry and the potential for the disease to affect other dermatomes [18]. The mucocutaneous junction near the epidermis is often the first site of infection. Following this, the virus travels as an unenveloped particle up the axon to the trigeminal ganglion. Typically, ocular herpes simplex represents a recurrence of a latent virus, not a new infection. True primary ocular disease, characterized by a primary infection confirmed by seroconversion, is relatively rare.

9.5 Risk Factors

The risk factors and triggers for the occurrence or recurrence of herpes simplex virus (HSV) infections in children continue to be subjects of ongoing research and discussion. Key risk factors include:

- *Altered immune System*: Children with compromised immune systems are more susceptible to both primary infections and recurrences of HSV [19].
- *Atopic individuals*: Those with atopic conditions may have depressed Th1-cell functions, making them more vulnerable to HSV infections [20].
- *Trauma*: Physical injury to the eye or surrounding areas can facilitate the entry and activation of HSV.
- *Primary maternal infections near term*: Neonatal herpes can occur if the mother has a primary HSV infection close to delivery, as there isn't sufficient time for the mother to develop an effective immune response and pass protective antibodies to the newborn [21].

9.6 Clinical Features and Management of Primary Ocular Herpes

From the previous section, it is evident that the spread of disease is by direct contact, commonly from infected saliva or genital secretions. The first acquisition of HSV results in the proliferation of virus in mucosa or skin which subsequently spread to dorsal root ganglia through neurons. Approximately two-thirds of all primary HSV infections are asymptomatic or unidentified, so the first presentation of the disease to an ophthalmologist may or may not be the primary disease. Primary infection in neonates' manifests as ophthalmia neonatorum and in children as blepharoconjunctivitis (Fig. 9.1).

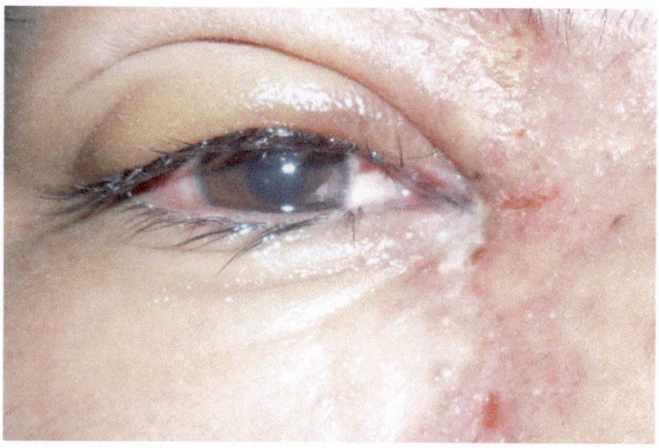

Fig. 9.1 Primary HSV infection showing characteristic cutaneous vesicular eruption and edema over the lids with surface excoriation and reactionary conjunctivitis

A study on primary ocular herpes suggests its varied presentations in the form of moderate to severe conjunctivitis (84%), moderate to severe blepharitis (38%), dendritic ulcers (15%), and disciform keratitis (2%); with bilateral involvement in 20% cases. HSV-2 virus from an infected birth canal can manifest as neonatal conjunctivitis.

9.6.1 Congenital HSV Infection

In utero (congenital) HSV transmission has been found to occur with both primary and recurrent maternal HSV infections. It is characterized by a triad of clinical manifestations present at birth: 1. Cutaneous findings (active lesions, scarring, aplasia cutis, hyperpigmentation or hypopigmentation) 2. Neurologic findings (microcephaly, intracranial calcifications, hydranencephaly) 3. Ocular findings (chorioretinitis, microphthalmia, optic atrophy).

9.6.2 Neonatal Conjunctivitis

Neonatal conjunctivitis and ophthalmia neonatorum often manifest between 3–15 days of delivery. Keratitis, keratouveitis, vitritis, retinitis, and optic neuritis may follow conjunctivitis [13].

9.6.3 Keratitis

In the acute phase, conjunctivitis is the most frequent ophthalmologic symptom in neonates and is often associated with herpetic epithelial keratitis. Symptoms of HSV keratitis in children include tearing, burning, decreased vision, swollen eyelids, and photophobia. Corneal epithelial disease starts as a painful punctate epithelial keratopathy that progresses to dendritic epithelial ulcers or geographic ulcers. Up to 76% of children with HSV keratitis develop damage to the corneal nerves leading to decreased corneal sensation and neurotrophic keratitis, contributing to corneal scarring [2, 12]. Primary keratitis normally heals up completely and it is the recurrence of the infection that leaves a corneal scar [22].

9.6.4 Blepharoconjunctivitis

Vesicular lesions involve the lid margin and periocular skin and subsequently develop into ulcerative lesions. The lesions persist for 7–10 days and are a potential source of viral shedding. Conjunctival involvement manifests as redness, follicular conjunctivitis, and ulcerative lesions. This is associated with preauricular lymphadenopathy. Diagnosis is largely clinical and a high degree of suspicion is the key to diagnosis. However, clinical diagnosis may be challenging as HSV blepharitis is uncommon and may be confused for the more ubiquitous meibomian gland dysfunction and follicular conjunctivitis can occur without lid lesions and mimic other causes of chronic conjunctivitis [13].

9.7 Differential Diagnosis

Accurate diagnosis of ocular HSV in children can be challenging due to its symptoms overlapping with other eye conditions. Key differential diagnosis include:

9.7.1 Peripheral Keratitis and Corneal Neovascularization

These conditions involve inflammation and blood vessel growth in the cornea, which can also be seen in HSV infections.

9.7.2 Staphylococcal Blepharokeratoconjunctivitis

This is often misdiagnosed as HSV keratitis in children. It is characterized by infiltrates in the peripheral cornea, typically where the eyelid margins cross the limbus at the 2, 4, 8, and 10 o'clock positions. These infiltrates are usually parallel to the limbus and separated by a clear zone of cornea.

9.7.3 Phlyctenular Keratoconjunctivitis

This condition presents as small, grey, well-defined nodules of lymphoid tissue surrounded by vascular injection, occurring at the conjunctiva, limbus, or cornea.

9.7.4 Neonatal Conjunctivitis

Considering the potential clinical overlap with other etiologies of conjunctival disease, such as gonococcal disease, it is essential to consider HSV infection in cases of neonatal conjunctivitis, especially in patients with an epithelial defect and not improving with empirical treatment.

9.8 Investigations

Laboratory diagnosis is helpful in atypical cases. Most of the cases are diagnosed clinically based on the clinical features, antecedent history, and high degree of suspicion.

9.8.1 Specimen Collection

Specimens from vesicular lesions preferably within the first 3 days (preferably 24 hours) of appearance are specimens of choice. Deroofed vesicles are swabbed with a dacron or rayon swab with a long plastic shaft to collect epithelial cells from the base of the lesion. The swab is then transported to the laboratory in a viral transport media at 4 degrees Celsius [23]. Test sensitivity is better for primary lesions than recurrent lesions [24].

9.8.2 Viral Isolation

Tube culture isolation is considered the gold standard. Cell monolayer adsorption can be done. HSV grows well on cell lines, including Vero, Hep2 cells, rabbit kidneys, and many genetically engineered cell lines. Subsequently, HSV isolate typing can be performed.

9.8.3 Antigen Detection

Viral antigen detection can be an alternative to culture for places with peripheral and smaller laboratories and also in cases with high chances of viral inactivation. Viral antigen detection sensitivity is the same or more than the culture [25].

9.8.4 Tzanck Smear

In case of urgency with no alternative test available, the cytopathic effect of the virus is looked for. Enlarged multinucleated cells with intranuclear inclusions (Wright-Giemsa stain) can be seen.

9.9 Management

Medical management is based on the type of ocular HSV infection and the age of the child. Topical medications currently available in the United States and Europe include trifluridine and ganciclovir, and current oral antivirals include acyclovir, valacyclovir, and famciclovir. In addition to the above medications, acyclovir 3% ophthalmic ointment is available and approved for topical use in Europe [26]. Studies have proven that acyclovir is considered safe in children for neonatal herpes and is well-tolerated. The recommended dosing of acyclovir in children is 12–20 mg/kg/day. Kidney and liver function should be checked biannually for children using oral antivirals [8, 27]. The concentration of commercially available acyclovir suspension is 200 mg/5 ml. Liu S et al. prescribed the suspension in 100-mg increments in order to make dosing more convenient for parents [8]. This is especially important when long-term prophylaxis is recommended, because compliance can be difficult if complicated treatments are recommended.

Treatment of Neonatal Conjunctivitis According to the guidelines from the American Academy of Pediatrics, neonatal ocular herpes (Skin, eye, and mucosa-SEM) should be treated with Intravenous Acyclovir 60 mg/kg/day in three divided doses for 14 days [5]. In suspected CNS involvement the treatment is extended to 21 days [28]. The absolute neutrophil count (ANC) should be followed twice weekly while on parenteral acyclovir therapy. On completion of the course of parenteral acyclovir, suppressive oral acyclovir (300 mg/m^2/dose by mouth three times a day) should be administered for 6 months.

Oral acyclovir should be started on pregnant mothers with infective lesions from 36 weeks of gestation and an elective cesarian section is indicated [13].

Treatment of Blepharoconjunctivitis and/or Keratitis It usually resolves in 2 weeks. Acyclovir eye ointment for keratitis and lid vesicular lesions can be used.

9.10 Differences in Herpetic Keratitis Between Children and Adults

Herpetic keratitis manifests differently in children compared to adults, with several distinct characteristics:

- *Bilateral Involvement*: Children are more likely to experience bilateral herpetic keratitis, either concomitantly or sequentially, with rates ranging from 10% to 21%.
- *Blepharoconjunctivitis Prevalence*: This is a more common manifestation in children than in adults.
- *Severity of Corneal Involvement*: In children, severe inflammation and stromal keratitis are more likely, whereas adults more commonly exhibit dendritic keratitis.
- *Inflammatory Response*: Children may exhibit a robust inflammatory response during HSV stromal keratitis, which can compromise vision and increase the risk of developing amblyopia.
- *Recurrences*: Children are particularly susceptible to recurrent episodes of ocular herpes.
- *Misdiagnosis*: Misdiagnosis is common in pediatric HSV, leading to challenges in appropriate management.

9.11 Conclusion

Primary ocular herpes simplex infection presents significant clinical challenges due to its varied clinical presentations. Understanding the epidemiology, transmission, and pathophysiology of the infection is crucial for effective management and prevention of its long-term effects. Considering the significant morbidity caused by HSV, particularly in children, prompt diagnosis, close monitoring, and appropriate antiviral therapy are essential to reduce the impact of HSV ocular involvement and for better outcomes.

Key Points

1. Primary herpes manifests early in life, between 6 months to 5 years, following the decline of maternally acquired antibodies.
2. 98% of primary ocular HSV infections remain undiagnosed because they are either subclinical or present only as mild conjunctivitis.
3. Most of the cases are diagnosed clinically based on the clinical features, antecedent history, and high degree of suspicion.
4. Accurate diagnosis of ocular HSV in children can be challenging due to its symptoms overlapping with other eye conditions.

References

1. Poirer RH. Herpetic ocular infections of childhood. Arch Ophthalmol. 1980;98:704–6.
2. Hsiao CH, Yeung L, Yeh LK, et al. Pediatric herpes simplex virus keratitis. Cornea. 2009;28(3):249–53.
3. Nahmias AJ, Visintine AM, Caldwell DR, et al. Eye infections with herpes simplex viruses in neonates. Surv Ophthalmol. 1976;21:100–5.
4. Azazi ME, Gunilla M, Marianne F. Late ophthalmologic manifestations of neonatal herpes simplex virus infection. Am J Ophthalmol. 1990;109:1–7.
5. Chong EM, Wilhelmus KR, Matoba AY, et al. Herpes simplex virus keratitis in children. Am J Ophthalmol. 2004;138:474–5.
6. Beigi B, Algawi K, Foley-Nolan A, et al. Herpes simplex keratitis in children. Br J Ophthalmol. 1994;78:458–60.
7. Schwartz GS, Holland EJ. Oral acyclovir for the management of herpes simplex virus keratitis in children. Ophthalmology. 2000;107:278–82.
8. Liu S, Pavan-Langston D, Colby KA. Pediatric herpes simplex of the anterior segment: characteristics, treatment, and outcomes. Ophthalmology. 2012;119:2003–8.
9. Smith JS, Robinson NJ. Age-specific prevalence of infection with herpes simplex virus types 2 and 1: a global review. J Infect Dis. 2002;186(Suppl 1):S3–28.
10. Kylat RI, Addams J, Sobonya RE. Fatal disseminated herpes simplex in a very premature neonate. Autopsy Case Rep. 2018;8(4):e2018050.
11. Sánchez Pujol MJ, Docampo Simon A, Sanguino L, Blanes M, Betlloch I. Herpes simplex virus infection

in neonates born to asymptomatic mothers: a case series. Cureus. 2022;14:e32393.
12. Serna-Ojeda JC, Ramirez-Miranda A, Navas A, et al. Herpes simplex virus disease of the anterior segment in children. Cornea. 2015;34:S68–71.
13. Kanukollu VM, Patel BC. Herpes Simplex Ophthalmicus. [Updated 2023 Apr 17]. In: StatPearls [Internet]. Treasure Island (FL): StatPearls Publishing; 2025 Jan-. Available from: https://www.ncbi.nlm.nih.gov/books/NBK559194/
14. James SH, Kimberlin DW. Neonatal herpes simplex virus infection: epidemiology and treatment. Clin Perinatol. 2015;42(1):47–viii. https://doi.org/10.1016/j.clp.2014.10.005.
15. Kidszun A, Bruns A, Schreiner D, Tippmann S, Winter J, Pokora RM, et al. Characteristics of neonatal herpes simplex virus infections in Germany: results of a 2-year prospective nationwide surveillance study. Arch Dis Child Fetal Neonatal Ed. 2021;107:188–92.
16. Bloomfield SE, Lopez C. Herpes infections in the immunosuppressed host. Ophthalmology. 1980;87(12):1226–35.
17. Binder PS. A review of the treatment of ocular herpes simplex infections in the neonate and immunocompromised host. Cornea. 1984;3(3):178–82.
18. Hill TJ. Ocular pathogenicity of herpes simplex virus. Curr Eye Res. 1987;6:1–7.
19. Wilhelmus KR, Falcon MG, Jones BR. Bilateral herpetic keratitis. Br J Ophthalmol. 1981;65:385–7.
20. Wollenberg A, Wetzel S, Burgdorf WH, Haas J. Viral infections in atopic dermatitis: pathogenic aspects and clinical management. J Allergy Clin Immunol. 2003;112:667–74.
21. Rząd M, Nitsch-Osuch A, Tyszko P, Goryński P, Bogdan M, Lewtak K. Congenital herpes simplex virus infection among hospitalized infants in Poland. Ann Agric Environ Med. 2021;28(4):612–6.
22. Jesus J, Almeida I, Matias M, Chibante J, Costa Ferreira C. Neonatal Type-2 unilateral herpes simplex Blepharokeratoconjunctivitis after caesarean delivery. Acta Sci Ophthalmol. 2021;1(1):6–9.
23. Singh A, Preiksaitis J, Ferenczy A, Romanowski B. The laboratory diagnosis of herpes simplex virus infections. Can J Infect Dis Med Microbiol. 2005;16(2):92–8.
24. Lafferty WE, Krofft S, Remington M, Giddings R, Winter C, Cent A, et al. Diagnosis of herpes simplex virus by direct immunofluorescence and viral isolation from samples of external genital lesions in a high-prevalence population. J Clin Microbiol. 1987;25(2):323–6.
25. Baker DA, Gonik B, Milch PO, Berkowitz A, Lipson S, Verma U. Clinical evaluation of a new herpes simplex virus ELISA: a rapid diagnostic test for herpes simplex virus. Obstet Gynecol. 1989;73(3 Pt 1):322–5.
26. White ML, Chodash J. Herpes simplex viral keratitis: A treatment guideline: compendium of evidence-based eye care. 2014. p. 1–76.
27. Revere K, Davidson SL. Update on management of herpetic keratitis in children. Curr Opin Ophthalmol. 2013;24(4):343–7.
28. Kimberlin DW, Baley J, Committee on Infectious Diseases, Committee on Fetus and Newborn. Guidance on management of asymptomatic neonates born to women with active genital herpes lesions. Pediatrics. 2013;131(2):383–6.

Epithelial Keratitis

10

Sohini Mandal, Sridevi Nair, Brindha Periasamy, and Jeewan Singh Titiyal

Abstract

HSV keratitis can involve all corneal layers including the epithelium which is characterized by epithelial manifestations like dendritic ulcer and geographic ulcer. Most dendritic ulcers heal spontaneously, but treatment with antivirals is essential to prevent complications and reduce viral replication. Early intervention is crucial to minimize inflammation, shorten disease duration, and preserve vision. This chapter provides a detailed overview of HSV epithelial keratitis, including its epidemiology, pathophysiology, clinical manifestations, investigations, and treatment.

Keywords

Epithelial keratitis · HSV keratitis · Dendritic ulcer · Geographic ulcer

10.1 Introduction

HSV infections of the eye are the leading cause of infectious corneal blindness in developed countries [1]. HSV-1 is primarily the cause of infections around the mouth, face, and eyes; while HSV-2 is majorly transmitted sexually and causes genital diseases [2]. HSV-2 could also infect the eyes by contact or spread from lesions present in the genital area. While most infections are unilateral, around 1.3%–12% of affected individuals have bilateral ocular infections. Bilateral infections are seen mostly in immunocompromised patients [3]. HSV recurrence within the cornea causes herpes simplex keratitis. Both primary and recurrent HSV infections can have epithelial keratitis. Epithelial manifestations of herpes simplex keratitis include herpetic dendrites and geographical ulcers. The diagnosis of HSV epithelial keratitis relies on clinical examination, with confirmatory tests such as PCR and viral cultures. Most of the HSV epithelial lesions heal spontaneously, but treatment with antivirals is essential to prevent vision-threatening complications.

10.2 Epidemiology

HSV infection has a seroprevalence of 60%–90% [4]. Every year, about a million people worldwide get HSV epithelial keratitis [5]. According to several scientific studies, epithelial keratitis is the most common type of HSV ocular involvement [6, 7]. Also, dendritic keratitis showed the most frequent recurrences of about 56.3% [8].

S. Mandal · S. Nair · J. S. Titiyal (✉)
R P Centre, AIIMS Delhi, New Delhi, India

B. Periasamy
AIIMS Bhopal, Bhopal, Madhya Pradesh, India

B. Sharma et al. (eds.), *Viral Keratitis*, https://doi.org/10.1007/978-981-95-3148-6_10

10.3 Pathogenesis

Primary infection results after HSV spread via direct contact with the mucous membrane of the host. HSV is transported by primary retrograde infection to the trigeminal ganglion via the first branch of the trigeminal nerve; here, it remains asymptomatic until the reactivation of the virus leads to recurrent infections. Reactivation can be triggered later in life by various stressors, including fever, trauma, immunosuppression, hormonal changes, radiation, or UV exposure. Harrison et al hypothesized that stress stimulates viral gene expression and productive infection during reactivation from the latency stage [9]. Yan et al also postulated that stress can reactivate a dormant HSV infection [10]. Viral replication in the epithelial layer leads to cell lysis and subsequent shedding of cells, contributing to the formation of dendritic ulcers. Histopathologically, dendritic ulcers are characterized by swollen epithelial cells exhibiting ballooning degeneration, with ground-glass nuclei and chromatin marginalization.

10.4 Clinical Features

Both primary and recurrent HSV infection can have epithelial involvement with latter being more common and have classic features. Symptoms include redness, thin watery discharge, irritation, pain, blurring of vision, and photophobia. Ocular pain is more prominent in epithelial keratitis making it the most painful form of HSV keratitis. Primary HSV usually presents as blepharoconjunctivitis which may be associated with corneal microcysts and diffuse punctate keratopathy. Recurrent HSV can have four forms of corneal epithelial disease in which dendritic ulcer and geographic ulcer are the most common forms. (Fig. 10.1a, b).

10.4.1 Corneal Vesicles

This is the earliest manifestation of epithelial keratitis presenting as small vesicles in the epithelium which are raised and clear. They correspond to the skin or mucous membrane vesicular eruptions seen elsewhere in the body. These fluid filled vesicles contain active replicating viruses. With progressive healing owing to antiviral medications, the vesicles tend to disappear leaving a nebular haze at the site of involvement known as ghost images. (Fig. 10.1c) However in immunocompromised cases, the infection gets arrested at the vesicle stage and viruses continue to multiply with subsequent complications.

10.4.2 Dendritic Ulcer

In 24 h, the corneal raised vesicles rapidly coalesce to form dendritic lesions that often mimic the cornea's sub-basal nerve plexus arrangement (Fig. 10.2a, b). The dendritic ulcer is the hallmark of HSV epithelial keratitis. Classic features include linear ulcer with dichotomous branching, terminal bulbs and, swollen borders with intraepithelial cell infiltration. Lesions are better visualized by staining with fluorescein and Rose Bengal dye. Fluorescein dye stains the base of the ulcer whereas rose Bengal dye stains its edges (Fig. 10.2a, b). Recurrence of HSV infection after corneal transplantation is seen only after regeneration of corneal nerves which is usually after 12 months. Hence any epithelial ulcer in graft before 12 months should not be confused with HSV recurrence. Before this time, recurrence if any would be seen in graft host junction or in host cornea.

Figure 10.2c, d show post PK viral epithelial recurrence at the graft host junction and in graft tissue, respectively, with surrounding corneal oedema.

Dendritic ulcer is a true ulcer breaching the epithelial basement membrane. On examination, there will be reduced corneal sensations and they might be associated with eyelid vesicular lesions as well. They can also present as recurrence in a corneal graft performed for a stromal scar. Mild subepithelial haze and scarring may develop after the healing of the lesion.

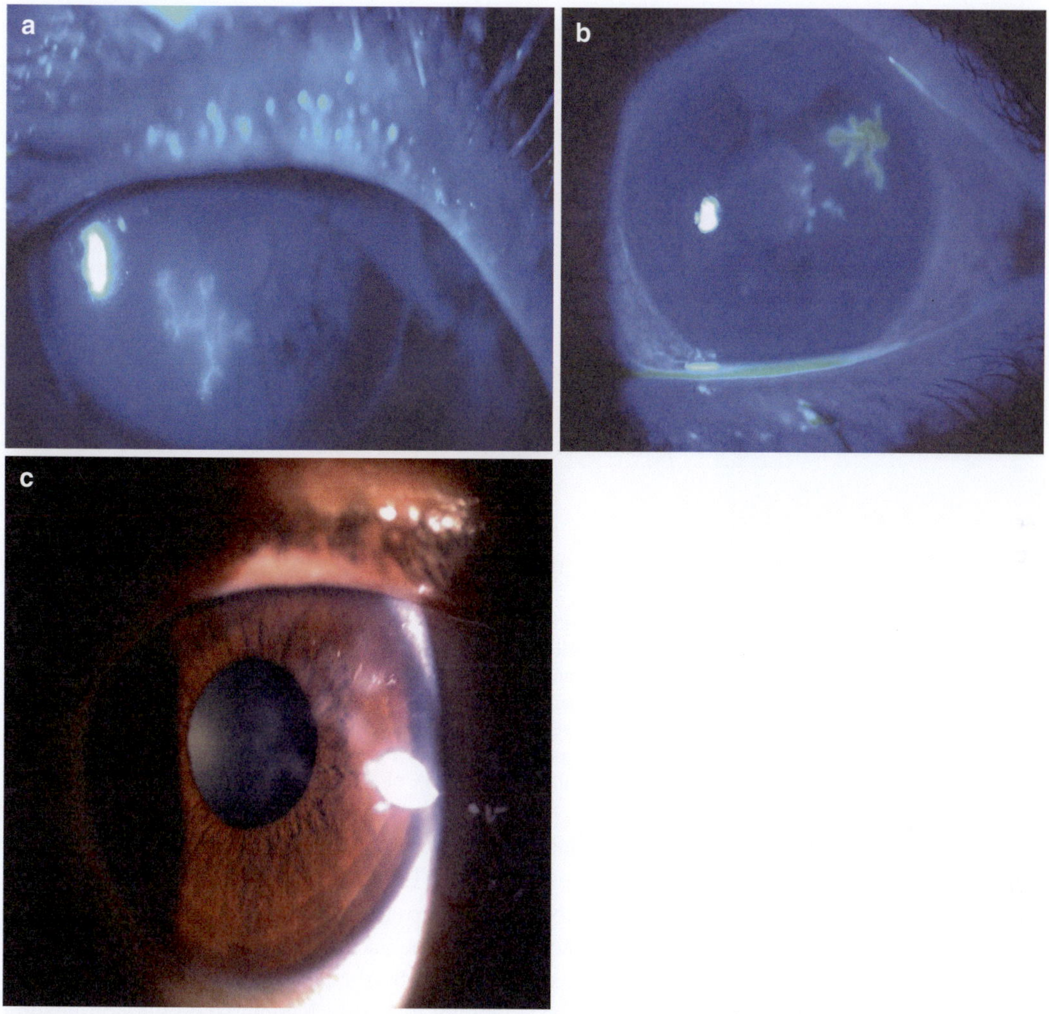

Fig. 10.1 (**a**, **b**) Slit lamp image showing Herpes simplex epithelial keratitis with typical dendritic pattern and few clumps of viral laden vesicles in the centre stained with fluorescein. (**c**) Healed HSV dendritic ulcer showing ghost image

10.4.3 Geographic Ulcer

The virus predominantly replicates at the edges and tips of these dendritic lesions, linear ulcer enlarges leading to the development of larger geographic ulcer with scalloped margins. Immunocompromised patients, atopy, and inadvertent usage of topical corticosteroids in a case of dendrite might result in a geographic/amoeboid ulcer (Fig. 10.2e, f).

10.4.4 Marginal Keratitis

It is an uncommon manifestation of HSV keratitis presenting with marginal dendritic ulcer with underlying anterior stromal infiltrate and adjacent limbal injection. It is important to differentiate this entity from staphylococcal marginal keratitis because improper treatment with topical antibiotics or topical steroids without antiviral cover might lead to central ulcer progression with

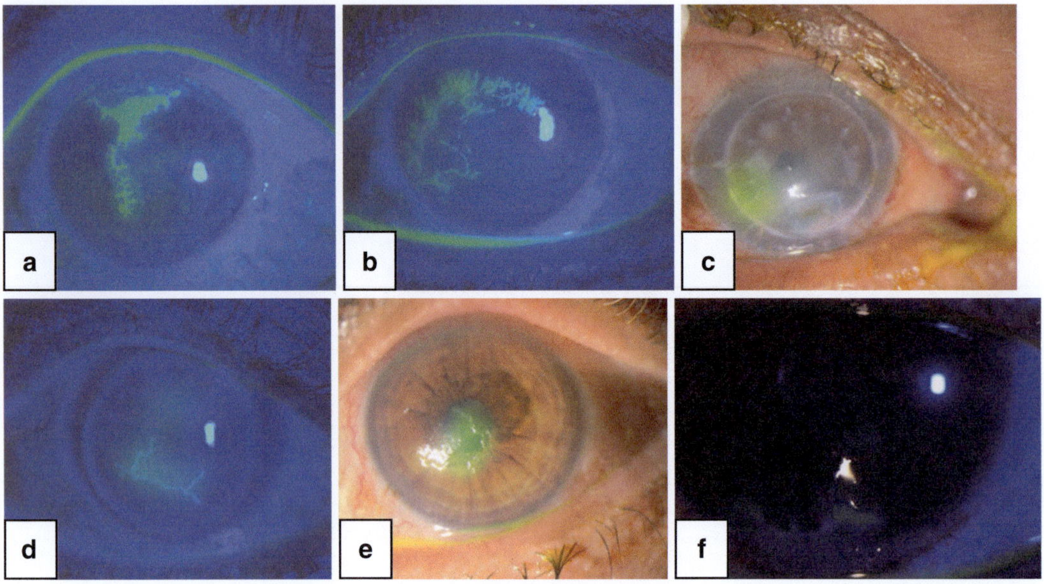

Fig. 10.2 (**a**, **b**) Slit lamp image demonstrates dendritic viral epithelial keratitis with characteristic terminal bulbs better visualized by staining with fluorescein dye and observed in cobalt blue filter. Note the conversion of dendrite to geographic ulcer in the superior half of the cornea in picture 1A; (**c**) Slit lamp image demonstrates viral epithelial recurrence at the graft host junction of a post PK graft with surrounding corneal oedema; (**d**) Slit lamp image demonstrates recurrence of dendritic viral epithelial keratitis in case of post PK graft (**e**) Slit lamp image demonstrates small geographic ulcer in the central cornea due to inadvertent use of topical steroids; (**f**) Slit lamp image showing Herpes simplex dendritic ulcer progressing to stage of geographical ulcer

subepithelial infiltration. Unlike bacterial marginal keratitis, HSV presents as localized infiltrates of varying size and shape which can be multiple and involve both peripheral or any other site. HSV variant is associated with intense vascularization and absence of clear zone between lesion and limbus. HSV Marginal keratitis should be differentiated from the common staphylococcal marginal keratitis. Table 10.1 helps to identify each entity clinically.

10.4.5 Neurotrophic Keratopathy

HSV epithelial keratitis increases the risk of developing neurotrophic keratopathy due to impaired corneal innervation along with reduced tear secretion. This results in failure of re-epithelization augmented by topical medication toxicity. Early signs of this entity include corneal surface irregularity with loss of lustre and punctate epithelial erosions. This often occurs in the interpalpebral area. Classical neurotrophic keratopathy lesion is characterized by a non-healing oval-shaped epithelial defect with smooth borders and heaped up margins (Fig. 10.3a–d). Persistent epithelial defect might progress to develop stromal ulceration called as *neurotrophic ulcer* and this stroma undergoes opacification causing a grey opaque colour, which may or may not be associated with secondary bacterial or fungal infection. Refractory cases may be associated with stromal melting and perforation. Classification and management of neurotrophic keratopathy are explained in detail in Chap. 13.

Table 10.1 Diagnostic differentiators between bacterial and viral marginal keratitis

Features	HSV Marginal keratitis	Staphylococcal marginal keratitis
Location	Any	2,4,8,10 o'clock
Epithelial integrity	Epithelial defect seen	Intact epithelium
Neovascularization	Present	Absent
Progression	Central	Circumferential
Lucid zone	Not present, presence of vascular tuft which reaches up to the lesion.	Present, vascular tuft is not seen.
Eyelid	May have vesicles	Associated with blepharitis

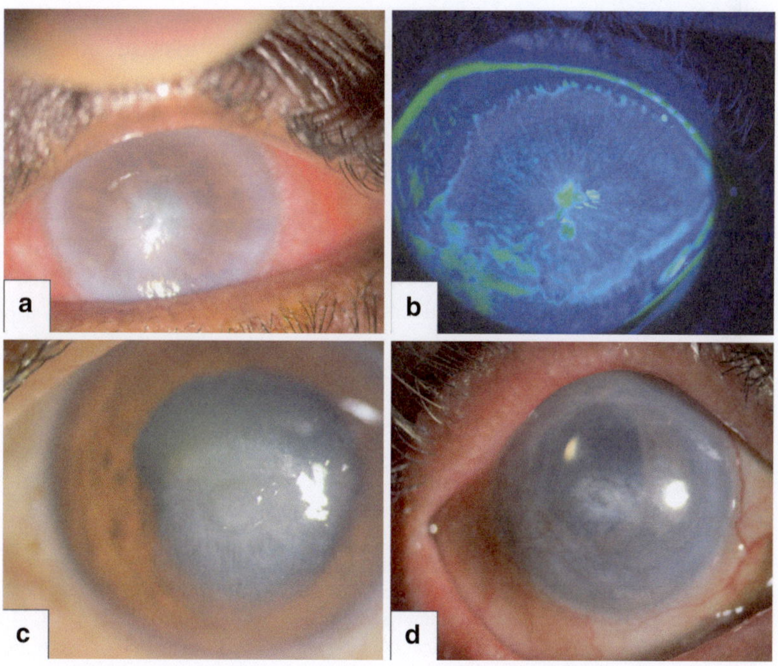

Fig. 10.3 (**a, b**) Slit lamp image shows neurotrophic ulcer with heaped up and rolled margins of the hypertrophic epithelium in the interpalpebral area; the base of the ulcer is taking up fluorescein stain; (**c**) Slit lamp image shows neurotrophic ulcer with early stages of stromal involvement and surrounding corneal oedema; (**d**) Slit lamp image shows neurotrophic ulcer without any stromal involvement

10.5 Investigations

HSV epithelial keratitis is a clinical diagnosis that is based on a thorough slit lamp examination in most of the cases. But, in more ambiguous and intricate cases (and in all cases of neonatal herpetic infections) the definite diagnosis requires microbiological confirmation. Conjunctival swab, corneal scraping, and tear samples can be taken for cytology, PCR assay (Polymerase Chain Reaction), immunofluorescence assay, HSV DNA titres, and viral culture. A Tzanck smear can reveal multinucleated giant cells and intranuclear eosinophilic inclusion bodies

(Cowdry type A). Though tear sample analysis is less invasive, it is significantly less sensitive than corneal scraping due to the dilute nature of tears and the intermittent shedding of the virus [11]. PCR is more likely to identify patients who present with typical lesions or patients who are not on antiviral medications. Rose Bengal and lissamine green dye inhibit the detection of HSV DNA by PCR assay [12]. Sensitivity and specificity for PCR is noted to be higher at 55.8% and 100%, respectively, in tear samples [13, 14]. The sensitivity of PCR declines later during infection. Hence, a negative test does not necessarily mean absence of the virus. Viral culture is considered the gold standard for identifying HSV. When compared to viral culture, clinical diagnosis is only 55%–65% accurate. Unfortunately, culturing HSV is time-consuming. Immunofluorescence tests are rarely used as their sensitivity is much lower than the other methods.

10.6 Differential Diagnosis

Conditions that should be considered while evaluating herpes simplex dendritic ulcers are shown in Table 10.2.

Table 10.2 Diagnostic differentiators for dendritic/pseudodendritic presentations

Herpes zoster keratitis	Punctate keratitis (superficial scattered fluorescein-stained swollen lesions) Pseudodendrites (smaller lesions, non-erosive mucous plaques with minimal staining and absence of terminal bulbs) Skin rash along a dermatome
Other causes of pseudodendrites	Healing corneal abrasion Recurrent corneal erosion Acanthamoeba keratitis Epithelial effects or impressions of soft contact lens use Toxic keratopathy secondary to topical medications Preservative-induced keratopathy

10.7 Epithelial Keratitis Sequelae

(a) Epithelial cell swelling occurs within the first day of infection, leading to the breakdown of the outer corneal layers and subsequent cell death. Type I interferon production by the infected cells helps contain the virus, making the surrounding tissue less susceptible to infection and viral replication. Additionally, HSV-specific antibodies present in the tears and corneal stroma play a crucial role in limiting the spread of the infection within the epithelial layer. These protective mechanisms result in complete resolution of the lesions in some cases.
(b) In cases of immunodeficiency or improper use of corticosteroids, the immune response may be insufficient, allowing the virus to penetrate deeper into the cornea. This can disrupt the corneal layers and result in stromal inflammation which could be necrotizing or immune-mediated.
(c) *HSV Dendritic epitheliopathy* is an abnormal epithelium following the healing of the dendritic ulcer. This can be aggravated by the toxicity of the topical antiviral medications. The healing epithelium has a dendritic shape but shows negative staining on fluorescein dye.
(d) The healing phase of the HSV epithelial keratitis involves corneal scarring which could be severe and vision-threatening. The spectrum of scarring can range from faint subepithelial opacities called "Ghost figures" or "footprints" of HSV to dense stromal scarring. This can be associated with corneal thinning and vision deterioration. The immune response, number of recurrences, and duration of the lesions correlate with the degree of corneal scarring.

10.8 Management

HSV keratitis infections are often self-limiting; however, healing is delayed without antiviral use, and inappropriate treatment can worsen inflammation leading to recurrence and subsequent deterioration in vision. Therefore, it is recommended to initiate treatment at the earliest, to reduce viral replication, subepithelial scarring, and risk of immune-mediated corneal lesions, shorten the disease course, and maintain latency.

Topical antiviral and preservative-free lubricants are the mainstay of treatment. Currently available first-line HSV keratitis antivirals are acyclovir, ganciclovir, trifluridine, vidarabine, penciclovir, and valacyclovir [15, 16]. The treatment regimen is explained in Table 10.3 and an algorithmic approach to a case of epithelial infectious viral keratitis has been illustrated in Flow diagram 10.1.

Table 10.3 HSV epithelial keratitis management

Type of HSV epithelial keratitis	Treatment regimen
Dendritic ulcer/ geographic ulcer	1. Topical antivirals for 14 days Acyclovir 3% eye ointment 5 times/day Or Ganciclovir gel 0.15% 5 times/day Or Trifluridine 1% eye drops Every 2 hourly Or Vidarabine 3% eye ointment 5 times/day 2. Preservative-free lubricants 3. Broad-spectrum topical antibiotics (fluoroquinolones—Ofloxacin0.3%, Moxifloxacin 0.5%)
Marginal ulcer	Same as above and add topical corticosteroids Loteprednol 0.5% or Fluorometholone 0.1% eye drop in 4–6 times dosing as per clinical requirement
Subepithelial scarring	Topical soft corticosteroids in 4–6 times dosing for 2–4 weeks
HSV dendritic epitheliopathy	Stop topical antivirals and use only preservative-free lubricants
Neurotrophic ulcer	1. Preservative-free lubricants 2. Punctal occlusion 3. Autologous serum drops or platelet-rich plasma drops 4. Ulcer debridement and bandage contact lens 5. Oral doxycycline 6. Tarsorrhaphy 7. Amniotic membrane transplantation and tissue adhesives

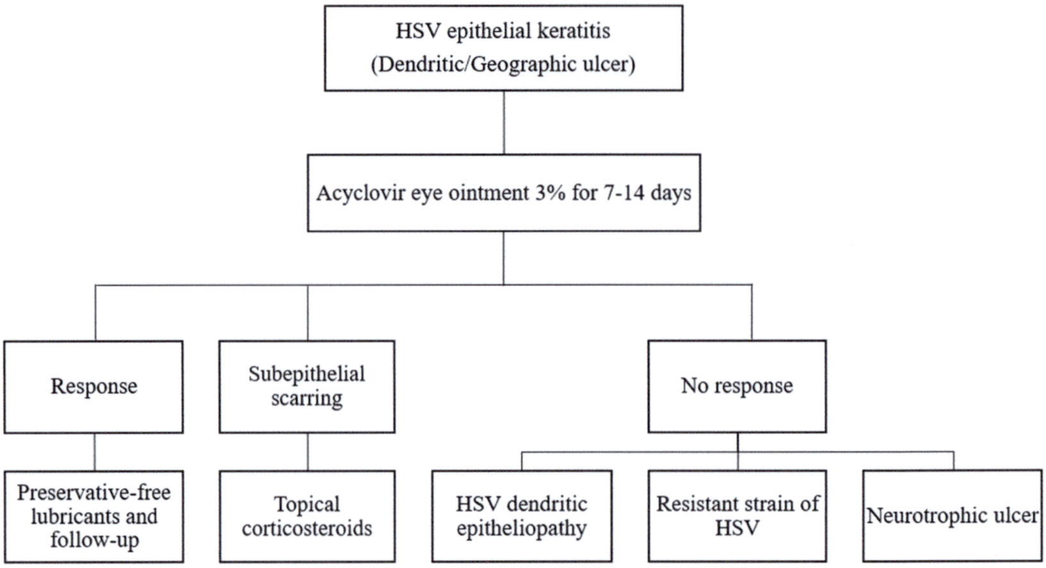

Flow diagram 10.1 Algorithmic approach to a case of epithelial infectious viral keratitis.

10.9 Prognosis

The prognosis of HSV keratitis is generally favourable with therapy. Majority of dendritic ulcers heal spontaneously without treatment. Mild to moderate disease recovers with just 2 weeks of topical therapy reinforced with debridement if needed (Fig. 10.4). Delayed response to treatment or severe recurrent disease may require lowering the HSV load by debriding the ulcer using a sterile cotton-tipped applicator. Mild subepithelial haze and scarring may develop after healing.

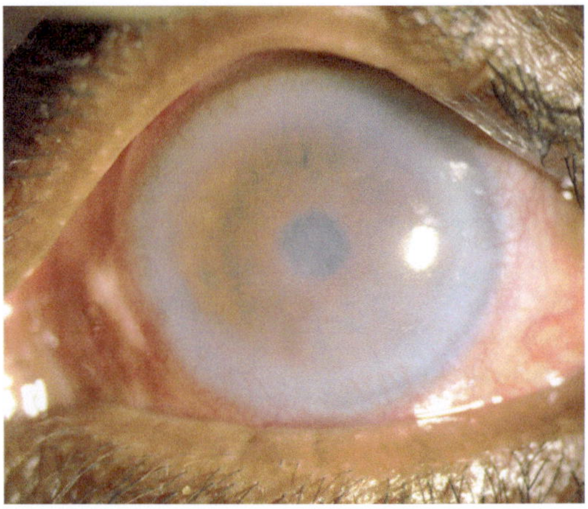

Fig. 10.4 A case of neurotrophic ulcer shown in Fig. 10.3 (**a**, **b**) post treatment with epithelial debridement, preservative free lubricants, and bandage contact lens

10.10 Conclusion

HSV epithelial keratitis is primarily a clinical diagnosis based on the slit-lamp findings. It is essential to differentiate it from HSV mimickers. HSV PCR and viral cultures may help to confirm the diagnosis in ambiguous presentation and paediatric cases. Accurate and prompt diagnosis is necessary to initiate appropriate treatment and prevent vision-threatening complications and recurrences.

Key Points

1. Both primary and recurrent HSV infections can have epithelial involvement.
2. Dendritic and geographic ulcers are the classical and most common forms of HSV epithelial keratitis.
3. The diagnosis of HSV epithelial keratitis is based on clinical examination.
4. Topical antivirals are used to reduce viral replication and prevent complications like scarring and vision loss, although mild cases may heal spontaneously.

References

1. Darougar S, Wishart MS, Viswalingam ND. Epidemiological and clinical features of primary herpes simplex virus ocular infection. Br J Ophthalmol. 1985 Jan;69(1):2–6.
2. Gupta D, Daigavane S. A clinical case of viral Keratitis. Cureus. 2022;14(10):e30311.
3. Tsatsos M, MacGregor C, Athanasiadis I, Moschos MM, Hossain P, Anderson D. Herpes simplex virus keratitis: an update of the pathogenesis and current treatment with oral and topical antiviral agents. Clin Experiment Ophthalmol. 2016 Dec;44(9):824–37.
4. Yadavalli T, Koganti R, Shukla D. Infection-induced porcine ex vivo corneal wound model to study the efficacy of herpes simplex Virus-1 entry and replication inhibitors. Methods Mol Biol. 2021;2193:183–96.
5. Farooq AV, Shukla D. Herpes simplex epithelial and stromal keratitis: an epidemiologic update. Surv Ophthalmol. 2012 Sep;57(5):448–62.
6. Group HEDS. Predictors of recurrent herpes simplex virus keratitis. Cornea. 2001 Mar;20(2):123.
7. Young RC, Hodge DO, Liesegang TJ, Baratz KH. Incidence, recurrence, and outcomes of herpes simplex virus eye disease in Olmsted County, Minnesota, 1976–2007: the effect of oral antiviral prophylaxis. Arch Ophthalmol. 2010 Sep;128(9):1178–83.
8. Labetoulle M, Auquier P, Conrad H, Crochard A, Daniloski M, Bouée S, et al. Incidence of herpes simplex virus keratitis in France. Ophthalmology. 2005 May;112(5):888–95.
9. Harrison KS, Zhu L, Thunuguntla P, Jones C. Antagonizing the glucocorticoid receptor impairs explant-induced reactivation in mice latently infected with herpes simplex virus 1. J Virol. 2019;93(13):e00418–9.
10. Yan C, Luo Z, Li W, Li X, Dallmann R, Kurihara H, et al. Disturbed yin-Yang balance: stress increases the susceptibility to primary and recurrent infections of herpes simplex virus type 1. Acta Pharm Sin B. 2020 Mar;10(3):383–98.
11. Satpathy G, Mishra AK, Tandon R, Sharma MK, Sharma A, Nayak N, et al. Evaluation of tear samples for herpes simplex virus 1 (HSV) detection in suspected cases of viral keratitis using PCR assay and conventional laboratory diagnostic tools. Br J Ophthalmol. 2011 Mar;95(3):415–8.
12. Seitzman GD, Cevallos V, Margolis TP. Rose bengal and lissamine green inhibit detection of herpes simplex virus by PCR. Am J Ophthalmol. 2006 Apr;141(4):756–8.
13. Shoji J, Sakimoto T, Inada N, Kamei Y, Matsubara M, Takamura E, et al. A diagnostic method for herpes simplex keratitis by simultaneous measurement of viral DNA and virus-specific secretory IgA in tears: an evaluation. Jpn J Ophthalmol. 2016 Jul;60(4):294–301.
14. Kowalski RP, Gordon YJ, Romanowski EG, Araullo-Cruz T, Kinchington PR. A comparison of enzyme immunoassay and polymerase chain reaction with the clinical examination for diagnosing ocular herpetic disease. Ophthalmology. 1993 Apr;100(4):530–3.
15. Wilhelmus KR. Antiviral treatment and other therapeutic interventions for herpes simplex virus epithelial keratitis. Cochrane Database Syst Rev. 2015;1(1):CD002898.
16. Vadlapudi AD, Vadlapatla RK, Mitra AK. Update on emerging antivirals for the management of herpes simplex virus infections: a patenting perspective. Recent Pat Antiinfect Drug Discov. 2013 Apr;8(1):55–67.

11 Stromal Keratitis

Saloni Gupta and Radhika Tandon

Abstract

HSV Stromal keratitis is a significant cause of corneal blindness worldwide and is a result of inflammatory response to HSV reactivation within the corneal stroma. If left untreated, it can lead to progressive corneal scarring and neovascularization. This chapter provides review of its etiology, epidemiology, pathophysiology, clinical presentation, and management. The chapter also highlights the role of antiviral therapy in controlling viral replication and the critical importance of anti-inflammatory treatment, particularly corticosteroids, in managing stromal inflammation. Prophylactic strategies, including long-term antiviral suppression, are discussed to prevent recurrences in individuals with a history of recurrent HSV keratitis. This comprehensive overview aims to help in effective management of HSV stromal keratitis, improve patient prognosis, and minimize the risk of vision-threatening complications.

Keywords

Stromal keratitis · Interstitial keratitis · Stromal inflammation

S. Gupta · R. Tandon (✉)
R P Centre, AIIMS Delhi, New Delhi, India

11.1 Introduction

HSV Stromal Keratitis (HSK) is a type of corneal inflammation caused by the Herpes Simplex Virus (HSV), most commonly HSV-1, though HSV-2 can also be implicated [1, 2].

The corneal stroma may be affected through primary or secondary mechanisms as summarized in Table 11.1.

Primary stromal disease from HSV involves the stroma in the form of necrotizing stromal keratitis from direct viral invasion, whereas immune stromal keratitis is the result of an immune reaction within the stroma. Secondary involvement may occur as a sequela to infectious epithelial keratitis, neurotrophic keratitis, or endothelitis.

Necrotizing stromal keratitis is seen as a response to certain stressors, including exposure to ultraviolet light, psychological stress, and hormonal fluctuation. HSV may reactivate from latency to produce infectious virions with recurrent disease at the initial sight of infection.

Non-necrotizing stromal keratitis is an immune-mediated condition in which the primary cause is the inflammatory response to viral antigens that were previously latent in the trigeminal ganglion rather than direct replication of the virus in the stroma. The virus typically causes a primary infection and can later reactivate, especially during times of stress, trauma,

B. Sharma et al. (eds.), *Viral Keratitis*, https://doi.org/10.1007/978-981-95-3148-6_11

Table 11.1 Types and mechanism involve in HSV stromal keratitis

HSV stromal keratitis	Findings
Primary mechanism	
1. Direct viral invasion of stroma	*Necrotizing stromal keratitis* – Epithelial defect with dense stromal infiltration and necrosis.
2. Ag-Ab compliment-mediated immune reaction	*Non-necrotizing/ immune stromal keratitis*—Stromal infiltrate with immune ring Neovascularization, scarring and thinning
Secondary mechanism	
1. *Infectious epithelial keratitis*—Live virus in epithelium incites an immune stromal response.	Dendritic, geographic, or marginal ulcer with stromal scarring.
2. *Neurotrophic keratopathy*—Impaired corneal innervation, damaged basement membrane, epithelial drug toxicity resulting in stromal inflammation	Epitheliopathy with persistent epithelial defect Stromal ulceration and scarring
3. *Endothelitis*—Endothelial immune response leading to secondary stromal involvement	Secondary stromal oedema and scarring Keratic precipitates on endothelium

UV exposure, or immune suppression, leading to keratitis [3].

This condition can result in significant visual impairment if not managed appropriately, due to potential corneal scarring, vascularization, and, in severe cases, corneal perforation [4]. Moreover, recurrent episodes of stromal keratitis can lead to chronic damage and further complications.

11.2 Epidemiology

Stromal keratitis accounts for 20–40% of all cases of HSV-induced keratitis. It is a recurrent condition that can lead to significant morbidity and has a recurrence rate of about 29.5% [5]. It typically develops in adulthood, usually between 20 and 40 years of age. The risk of developing HSV stromal keratitis increases in immunocompromised individuals, exposure to trauma, stress, malnourishment, fever, or intense UV light exposure.

11.3 Etiology

Herpes simplex keratitis can have varied manifestations with herpetic stromal keratitis being a common presentation. HSV Stromal keratitis can result due to a primary infection or most frequently due to reactivation that leads to an immune-mediated inflammatory response [6, 7].

After the initial infection, the virus remains latent in the trigeminal ganglion via the first branch of the trigeminal nerve. In case of reactivation the virus travels back to the cornea along the axon, causing recurrent stromal keratitis. The immune system's response to the virus in the corneal stroma causes inflammation [8] (Flow diagram 11.1).

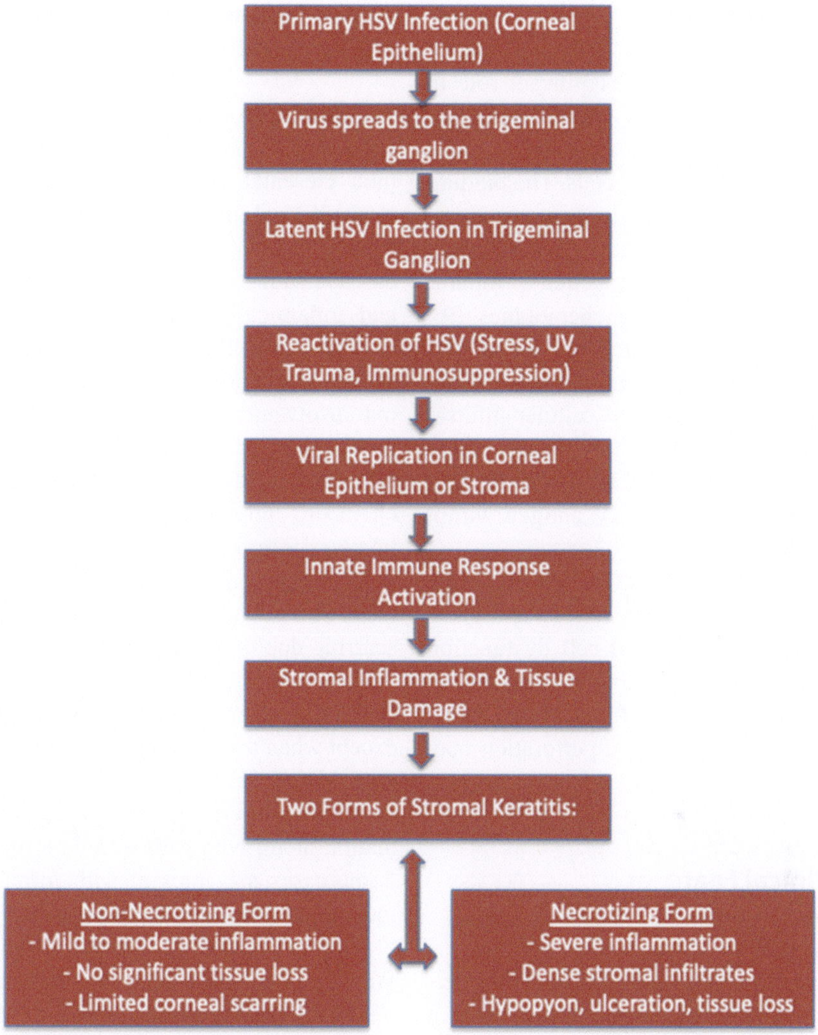

Flow diagram 11.1 showing life cycle and pathogenesis of HSV

11.4 Pathogenesis

The immune system plays a significant role in the pathogenesis of Herpes stromal keratitis. HSV-1 in an infected cornea initiates virus replication in the corneal epithelial cells. The binding of virus to the cell surface induces a cascade of innate immune responses and signal pathway responses, stimulating the production of inflammatory cells, cytokines, and chemokines [9]. They gradually infiltrate into the stroma and results in the characteristic inflammatory reaction and tissue damage due to cellular infiltration, keratocyte apoptosis. CD4 T cells have been implicated which are HSV-specific and driven by the presence of HSV antigen within the stroma [10].

Moreover, Inflammatory cytokines including tumour necrosis factor-alpha (TNF-α) and interleukins also cause endothelial cell dysfunction and keratocyte activation leading to corneal scarring and vascularization [11]. In severe and recurrent cases corneal thinning and perforation may also occur.

11.5 Clinical Features

Stromal keratitis is characterized by intense inflammation of the corneal stroma including cellular infiltration and neovascularization. It is a result of a combination of the viral replication, toxins, virus induced inflammation as well as the host's immunological response [7]. Patients usually present with redness, photophobia, tearing, eye pain, and blurred or decreased vision [4].

Based on different clinical manifestations, HSK is divided into two clinical types: non- necrotizing stromal keratitis and necrotizing stromal keratitis. Other clinical manifestations may be limbal vasculitis, endothelitis with trabeculitis, and immune ring of Wesseley.

11.5.1 Non-necrotizing Stromal Keratitis

The disease process is often referred as immune stromal keratitis of HSV which is a more common presentation. The inflammation is due to retained viral antigen within the stroma, which triggers an antigen-antibody-complement (AAC) cascade with consequent intrastromal infiltration and inflammation Fig. 11.1a–d. The immune system reacts to viral particles in the corneal stroma, causing focal, multifocal, or diffuse stromal involvement, which may manifest as a disciform lesion or ring Fig. 11.2. It may also be associated with stromal oedema and anterior chamber inflammation. Oedema commonly involves inferior region of the corneal stroma, with or without the presence of keratic precipitates. Stromal neovascularization can later cause scarring due to leakage from the blood vessels. However, in this form there is no necrosis and the overlying epithelium is almost always intact except when there is concomitant infectious epithelial keratitis [4, 9].

Varying severity of anterior chamber inflammation along with cells and flare may be seen. Some cases may present with formation of an incomplete or complete immune ring as a result of ring shaped AAC precipitate similar to a Wessely ring, mainly in the mid stroma Fig. 11.2.

HSV stromal keratitis may have a recurring course due to AAC immune complexes manifesting as punctate stromal opacities accompanied by surrounding haze and cellular infiltrate of the stroma. These lesions heal by formation of stromal opacities. Severe inflammation can lead to dense infiltration with subsequent scarring, vascularization and ensuing visual loss. Corneal vascularization remains a hall mark sequalae of stromal keratitis owing to intense inflammatory process. It may present with single or multiple quadrants involvement, and is a

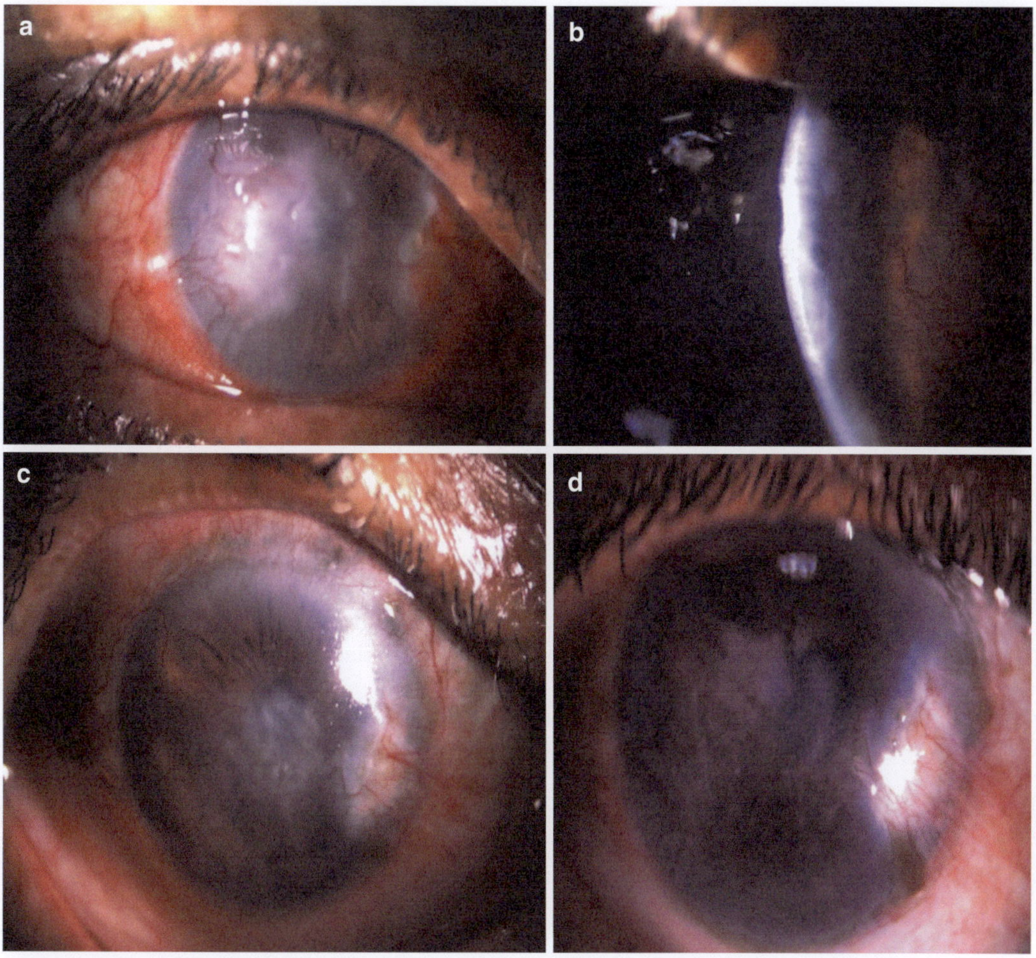

Fig. 11.1 Slit lamp image showing HSV Non necrotizing stromal keratitis. (**a**) Dense stromal infiltrates and neovascularization (**b**) Slit beam showing dense stromal infiltration. (**c, d**) Residual scarring, neovascularization and lipid deposition

significant risk factor for graft rejection. However, treatment of inflammation can result in complete resolution of the blood vessels leaving behind ghost vessels, within the stroma. It is important to note that ghost vessels do not cause any decrease in vision or increased risk penetrating keratoplasty rejection. The clinical course of stromal keratitis is chronic and recurrent which can present with exacerbations of varying severity. Long-term topical corticosteroids may be required to suppress the inflammatory reaction and mitigate relapses.

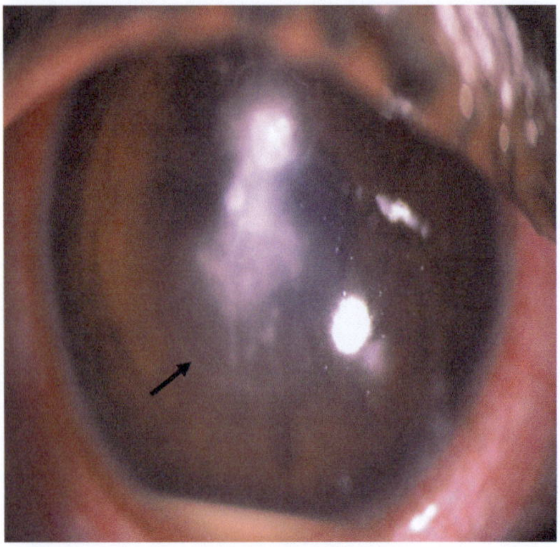

Fig. 11.2 Image showing Wessley's immune ring in non necrotizing stromal keratitis stromal with 2 mm hypopyon

11.5.2 Necrotizing Stromal Keratitis

The necrotizing form of stromal keratitis results from fulminant viral replication in stromal keratocytes and resultant severe host inflammatory response. The clinical findings are necrosis, ulceration, and dense yellow white infiltration of the stroma with an overlying epithelial defect. The combination of replicating virus and severe host inflammatory response leads to destructive stromal involvement. Figure 11.3 Figure As the lesion progresses, it can result in corneal thinning, ulceration, perforation and melt [9, 11]. Neovascularization of the corneal stroma usually extends from the peripheral cornea to the infiltrating site of the central stroma. Chronicity and recurrence of stromal disease can cause complications like corneal scarring, neovascularization, or corneal thinning Fig. 11.4a–f. The disease features are similar to infectious keratitis secondary to microbial invasion. Therefore, bacterial and fungal pathogens must be ruled out while treating necrotizing stromal keratitis.

Lipid keratopathy is an important sequalae of HSV stromal keratitis due to vascularization and can cause scarring and diminution of vision.

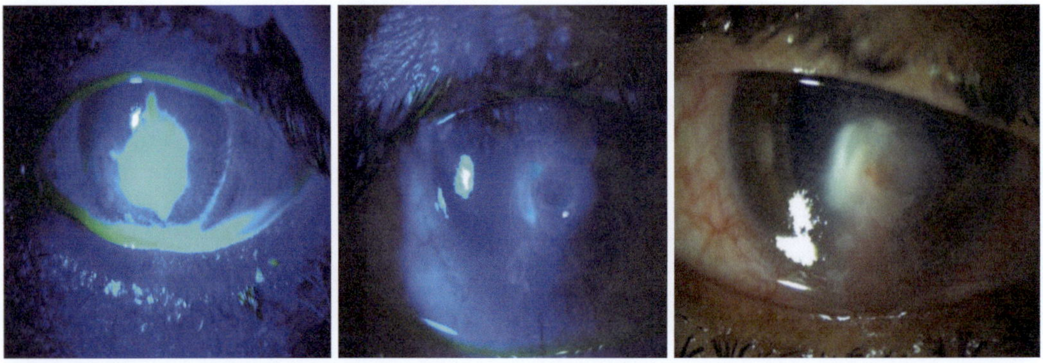

Fig. 11.3 Slit lamp image showing HSV necrotizing stromal keratitis with dense stromal infiltrates central stromal lysis and deep vascularization

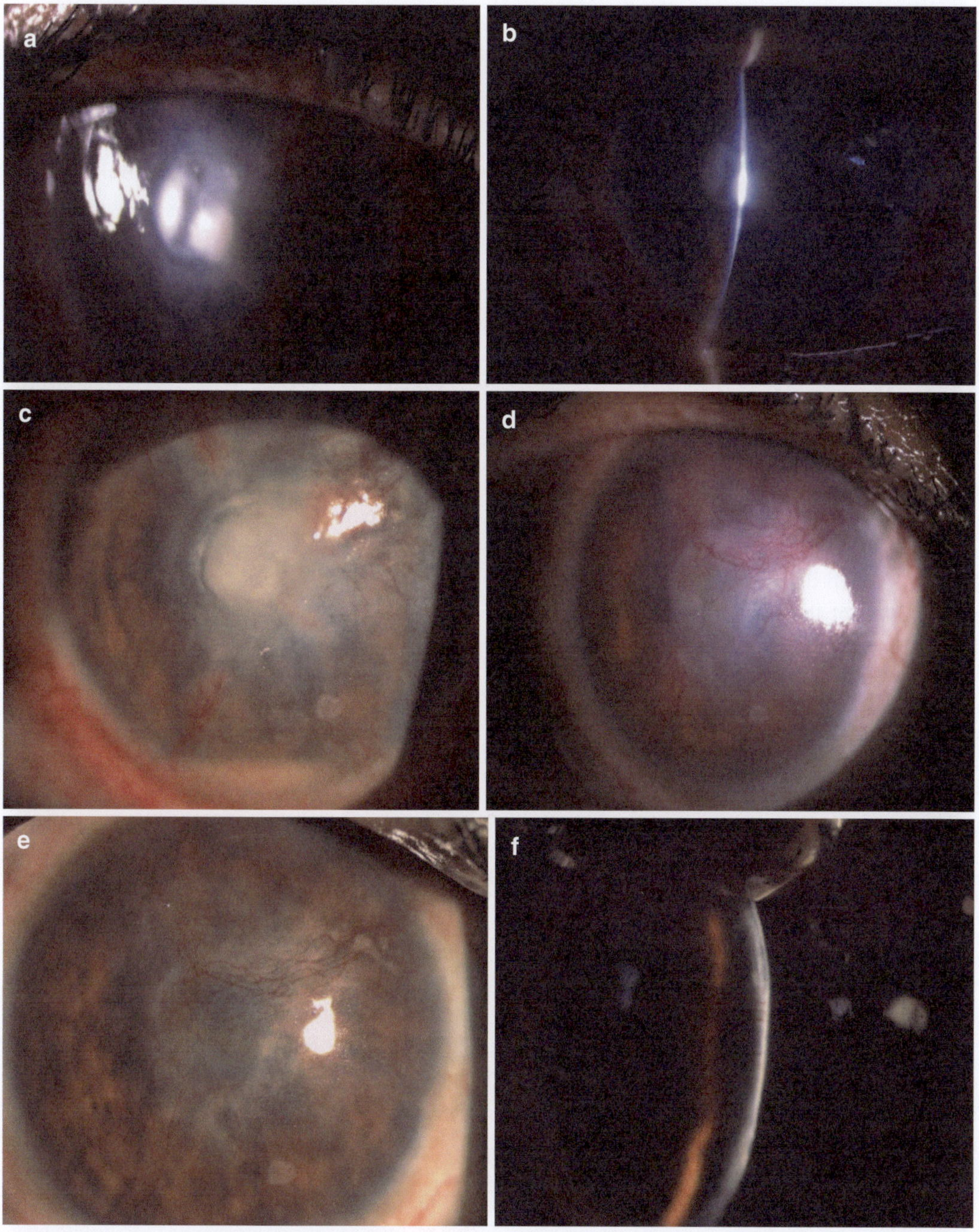

Fig. 11.4 HSV necrotizing stromal keratitis (**a**) Image showing corneal stromal lysis with thinning and ulceration (**b**) Slit beam showing dense stromal infiltrates (**c**) Post treatment image showing arrest of stromal necrosis, healing margins with vascularization and resolving streak hypopyon (**d–f**) Formation of vascularized NMCO after treatment and stromal thinning

11.6 Differential Diagnosis

- Infectious interstitial keratitis caused by.
  - Viruses (Varicella zoster virus, Epstein-Barr virus).
  - Bacteria (Syphilis, Lyme).
  - Acanthamoeba keratitis.
- Immune-mediated etiologies.
  - Sarcoidosis.
  - Cogan Syndrome.

11.7 Diagnosis

The diagnosis of HSV stromal keratitis is predominantly clinical, based on history of recurrent ocular disease and characteristic herpetic lesions as described above. Confirmatory diagnostic tests like PCR analysis, enzyme-linked assays, and viral culture of the tear film may reveal HSV-1 DNA, protein, or live virus, respectively [12].

11.8 Management

The treatment of HSV stromal keratitis is aimed at inhibiting viral replication with oral or topical antiviral medications and reducing inflammatory damage with topical corticosteroids [13].

11.8.1 Non-necrotizing

The main stay of treatment is topical steroids to control inflammation. It is important to keep steroid potency and duration to the minimum required for effective control of inflammation. Topical prednisolone 1% or dexamethasone 0.1% with antiviral cover, four –six times daily is the preferred regimen. It is further tapered over 2–4 weeks with decrease in frequency of administration. Cycloplegics to provide symptomatic relief and vasodilatation is required in addition. For mild disease, a weaker steroid such as fluorometholone 0.1% or loteprednol 0.2% can be given for 2–4 weeks.

The treatment approach differs in the presence of epithelial defect. Steroid intensity should be low and with cover of topical antiviral agents like Acyclovir 3% or Gancyclovir 0.15% eye ointment five times daily, or titrated according to the signs of activity of both. Oral antiviral treatment may be required in recurrences and in immunosuppressed state.

Oral steroids are indicated in severe stromal inflammation as an adjunct, to reduce potential IOP elevation with topical steroids and prevent viral replication in infectious viral keratitis.

Topical cyclosporin 0.05% may be useful, particularly in the presence of epithelial ulceration and to facilitate tapering of topical steroids such as in steroid-related IOP elevation.

Fine needle diathermy and ND YAG laser are recommended for corneal neovascularization and improving vision.

11.8.2 Necrotizing

The management approach for necrotizing HSK is more aggressive due to the potential for rapid progression and complications as compared to non-necrotizing HSK. Mainstay of treatment is systemic and topical antiviral to prevent viral replication. Oral acyclovir in dose of 2 gm per day is the recommended therapeutic regimen and can be administered as 400 mg — 5 times daily followed by 1 gm per day as maintenance dose for another 2–4 weeks. Additionally, Valacyclovir 500 mg — 3 times daily or Famciclovir 250 or 500 mg — 3 times daily for 1–2 weeks can be given. Topical antivirals like Acyclovir 3% or Gancyclovir 0.15% eye ointment five times daily, for 2–4 weeks till complete epithelial regeneration is indicated in addition to cycloplegic for comfort from ciliary spasm. Ocular surface lubricants to facilitate healing and reduce ocular discomfort, topical antibiotics to prevent secondary infection and IOP lowering agents are important adjuncts. Topical steroids are indicated for prevention of scarring, however, after distinct signs of healing and epithelial regeneration with antiviral cover.

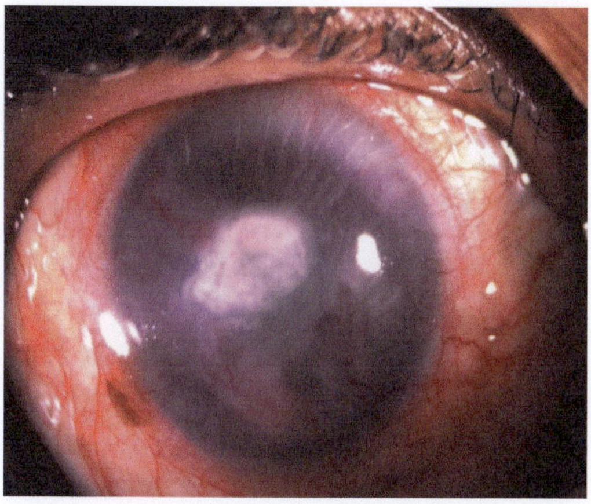

Fig. 11.5 HSV Necrotizing stromal keratitis with central perforation sealed by cyanoacrylate glue and overlay bandage contact lens surrounded by intense deep vascularization

11.8.3 Surgical Therapy

Necrotizing herpetic keratitis with small perforations can be managed by cyanoacrylate gluing and bandage contact lens in addition to amniotic membrane transplantation Fig. 11.5. Conjunctival flap may be useful in patients with ulcers not responding to instated therapy with risk of perforation. In cases where stromal scarring has caused severe visual impairment, corneal transplantation in the form of either full-thickness penetrating keratoplasty or deep anterior lamellar keratoplasty is done for restoring corneal clarity and visual rehabilitation. Deep anterior lamellar keratoplasty is indicated in patients with healthy endothelium and penetrating keratoplasty in full thickness scars that cannot be treated with other modalities. Corneal transplantation should be done after a minimum period of quiescence and inactivity of 6 months and in some cases up to 1 year. This is achieved by the use of perioperative oral acyclovir and topical antivirals for a period of 6–12 months [14].

Treatment summary is mentioned in Table 11.2.

Table 11.2 HSV Stromal keratitis treatment options

Treatment	Dosage
Oral antiviral therapy	Acyclovir 400 mg 5 times/day for 7–14 days *Alternatives:* Valacyclovir 500 mg 3 times/day Famciclovir 250 mg 3 times/day *Maintenance therapy* Acyclovir 400 mg twice daily for recurrent HSK or high-risk patient *to prevent recurrence*
Topical antiviral therapy *Consider if epithelial involvement is present*	Trifluridine or ganciclovir eye drops
Anti-inflammatory therapy *Topical corticosteroids under antiviral cover*	*Necrotizing stromal keratitis:* Prednisolone acetate 1%: Start at 1 drop 4–6 times/day and taper gradually. *Non-necrotizing stromal keratitis:* Prednisolone acetate 1%: Start at 1 drop every 1–2 h, taper gradually over weeks.
Surgical management *In cases of significant scarring causing visual impairment*	Corneal transplantation may be considered.

11.9 Prophylaxis for HSV Keratitis

The primary goal of prophylaxis for Herpes Simplex Virus (HSV) stromal keratitis is to reduce the risk of recurrence and minimize the potential for vision-threatening complications. For high-risk patients such as those with frequent recurrences, previous corneal allografts, or compromised immune systems, long-term or indefinite oral acyclovir prophylaxis is recommended. Oral antiviral prophylaxis should also be considered before scheduled ocular surgery, including photorefractive procedures, in patients with a known history of HSV keratitis, and should continue until corticosteroid therapy is tapered [14,

15]. Prophylactic oral medications are advised for patients with a history of HSK undergoing penetrating keratoplasty. Nutritional deficiencies, long-term use of immunosuppressants, and even SARS-CoV-2 vaccination have been associated with HSK reactivation [13, 15, 16]. Treatment and prophylaxis should be personalized, considering individual patient history and risk factors.

11.10 Conclusion

HSK often results from reactivation of latent HSV affecting the stroma and leads to visual impairment if left untreated. Early diagnosis and appropriate treatment are crucial to prevent long-term complications like corneal scarring, neovascularization, or even blindness. Given the risk of recurrence and complications, a comprehensive approach that includes both medical and preventive strategies is vital in reducing the impact of the disease.

Key Points

1. HSV stromal keratitis is a recurrent, potentially sight-threatening condition that arises due to the immune response to reactivated HSV in the corneal stroma.
2. Factors such as stress, trauma, ultraviolet (UV) exposure, or immune suppression can trigger HSV reactivation.
3. Antiviral agents are the mainstay of treatment in necrotizing HSK while steroids in non-necrotizing variety.
4. Long-term antiviral prophylaxis is required in preventing recurrences, especially in patients with severe stromal involvement and frequent episodes.

References

1. Chaloulis SK, Mousteris G, Tsaousis KT. Incidence and risk factors of bilateral herpetic keratitis: 2022 update. Trop Med Infect Dis. 2022;7(6):92.
2. McCormick I, James C, Welton NJ, Mayaud P, Turner KME, Gottlieb SL, Foster A, Looker KJ. Incidence of herpes simplex virus keratitis and other ocular disease: global review and estimates. Ophthalmic Epidemiol. 2022 Aug;29(4):353–62.
3. Morey JN, Boggero IA, Scott AB, Segerstrom SC. Current directions in stress and human immune function. Curr Opin Psychol. 2015;5:13–7.
4. Lobo AM, Agelidis AM, Shukla D. Pathogenesis of herpes simplex keratitis: the host cell response and ocular surface sequelae to infection and inflammation. Ocul Surf. 2019;17:40–9. https://doi.org/10.1016/j.jtos.2018.10.002.
5. Labetoulle M, Auquier P, Conrad H, Crochard A, Daniloski M, Bouée S, El Hasnaoui A, Colin J. Incidence of herpes simplex virus keratitis in France. Ophthalmology. 2005 May;112(5):888–95.
6. Zhu S, Viejo-Borbolla A. Pathogenesis and virulence of herpes simplex virus. Virulence. 2021 Dec;12(1):2670–702.
7. Sibley D, Larkin DFP. Update on herpes simplex keratitis management. Eye (Lond). 2020 Dec;34(12):2219–26. https://doi.org/10.1038/s41433-020-01153-x.
8. Whitley R, Baines J. Clinical management of herpes simplex virus infections: past, present, and future. F1000Res. 2018;7:F1000.
9. Rowe AM, St Leger AJ, Jeon S, Dhaliwal DK, Knickelbein JE, Hendricks RL. Herpes keratitis. Prog Retin Eye Res. 2013;32:88–101. https://doi.org/10.1016/j.preteyeres.2012.08.002.
10. Verjans GM, Remeijer L, van Binnendijk RS, Cornelissen JG, Völker-Dieben HJ, Baarsma SG, Osterhaus AD. Identification and characterization of herpes simplex virus-specific CD4+ T cells in corneas of herpetic stromal keratitis patients. J Infect Dis. 1998 Feb;177(2):484–8.
11. Gierlikowska B, Stachura A, Gierlikowski W, Demkow U. The impact of cytokines on neutrophils' phagocytosis and NET formation during sepsis-a review. Int J Mol Sci. 2022;23(9):5076.
12. Kowalski RP, Gordon YJ, Romanowski EG, Araullo-Cruz T, Kinchington PR. A comparison of enzyme immunoassay and polymerase chain reaction with the clinical examination for diagnosing ocular herpetic disease. Ophthalmology. 1993 Apr;100(4):530–3.
13. Biswas PS, Rouse BT. Early events in HSV keratitis—setting the stage for a blinding disease. Microbes Infect. 2005;7:799–810. https://doi.org/10.1016/j.micinf.2005.03.003.
14. Gurnani B, Czyz CN, Mahabadi N, Havens SJ. StatPearls [Internet]. Treasure Island (FL): StatPearls Publishing; 2023. Corneal Graft Rejection
15. de Rojas Silva MV, Díez-Feijóo E, Javaloy J, Sánchez-Salorio M. Prophylactic perioperative antiviral therapy for LASIK in patients with inactive herpetic keratitis. J Refract Surg. 2006;22:404–6. https://doi.org/10.3928/1081-597X-20060401-19.
16. Young TL, Robin JB, Holland GN, et al. Herpes simplex keratitis in patients with acquired immune deficiency syndrome. Ophthalmology. 1989;96:1476–9.

Disciform Keratitis

12

Purvasha Narang, Bhavana Sharma, Snehal Nimje, and Aviral Vasudeo

Abstract

Disciform keratitis remains an important vision-threatening entity seen in viral keratitis. This chapter provides a detailed overview of disciform keratitis, including its epidemiology, aetiology, pathophysiology, clinical manifestations, diagnosis, investigations, treatment, and recent advances. Although Herpes Simplex Virus (HSV) is the most common cause of disciform keratitis, other infective agents like varicella-zoster virus (VZV), Adenovirus, Cytomegalo Virus (CMV), and monkey-pox virus are also reported. Patients are typically impacted in their early decades of life; therefore, the condition has a significant influence on quality of life and vision among young, productive adults.

Keywords

Disciform keratitis · Endotheliitis · Viral keratitis · Endothelial keratitis

12.1 Introduction

Disciform keratitis, also sometimes referred to as herpes simplex endothelial keratitis, is characterized by virus-induced endothelial dysfunction leading to a distinctive disc-shaped area of stromal edema and keratic precipitates due to anterior chamber inflammation [1]. HSV disciform keratitis represents a delayed-type hypersensitivity response to HSV-induced membrane surface expression alteration or damage to the underlying endothelium. Thus the opacity in HSV endotheliitis is due to stromal edema without stromal inflammation or neovascularization.

Since it usually presents as round to oval disc-shaped configuration, it is also known as disciform keratitis. Corneal endothelial cell involvement is assumed to be the primary cause, and despite the severe corneal symptoms, there is comparatively little anterior chamber inflammation linked to it. Interestingly, the diagnosis of HSV stromal or endothelial keratitis is made solely on the basis of typical clinical signs in the absence of histopathologic results from a keratoplasty or biopsy. This condition may also lead to significant corneal inflammation and scarring, if not treated adequately.

The original version of the chapter has been revised. A correction to this chapter can be found at https://doi.org/10.1007/978-981-95-3148-6_29

P. Narang · S. Nimje
AIIMS Nagpur, Nagpur, Maharashtra, India

B. Sharma (✉) · A. Vasudeo
AIIMS Bhopal, Bhopal, Madhya Pradesh, India

B. Sharma et al. (eds.), *Viral Keratitis*, https://doi.org/10.1007/978-981-95-3148-6_12

12.2 Etiology

Herpes simplex virus (HSV) is responsible for a variety of ocular symptoms, including endotheliitis, stromal keratitis, and epithelial keratitis. In primary ocular HSV, only 2% of the patients show disciform keratitis. Apart from herpes simplex virus, literature depicts evidence of disciform keratitis due to infection with varicella zoster, adenovirus, CMV, Variola, and Vaccinia virus (used for mass smallpox inoculation) [2–5]. In primary ocular HSV, only 2% of the patients show disciform keratitis [6]. Endotheliitis is one of the HZO-related corneal manifestations in addition to Monkey Pox virus which may also rarely induce disciform keratitis and scarring, compared to other ocular viral infections [7]. There is also evidence of relapsed disciform herpetic keratitis following mRNA COVID-19 vaccination [8].

12.3 Pathogenesis

The immune reaction involving the endothelium leads to secondary stromal edema that may result in scarring. There might be a possible role of live virus. The suggested mechanism is as follows:

12.3.1 Viral Entry and Replication

HSV, a double-stranded DNA virus from the Herpesviridae family, enters ocular endothelial cells by a complex mechanism of viral glycoproteins and receptors. When HSV binds to host cell receptors such as herpesvirus entry mediator (HVEM) and nectin-1, it enters the cell via endocytosis or membrane fusion. Once within the cell, viral capsids move to the nucleus, where viral DNA is duplicated and transcribed, producing viral offspring. The discharge of infectious virions from infected endothelium cells helps to propagate viral infection and maintain inflammation in contiguous manner.

12.3.2 Host Immunological Response

Pathogenesis in viral keratitis is heavily influenced by the host immunological response, which includes both innate and adaptive immune mechanisms causing tissue destruction and inflammation. When viral antigens are recognized, innate immune cells such as macrophages, dendritic cells, and natural killer cells get activated, resulting in the production of proinflammatory cytokines and chemokines. The subsequent recruitment of neutrophils and monocytes enhances the inflammatory response, causing tissue infiltration and injury. Furthermore, HSV-specific CD4+ and CD8+ T lymphocytes help to remove the virus but may also increase tissue harm by releasing cytotoxic mediators.

12.3.3 Corneal Edema

Corneal edema due to endothelial dysfunction is due to poor barrier function, altered cell shape, and diminished pump function. Viral infection of corneal endothelial cells breaks intercellular connections, resulting in increased permeability and fluid buildup inside the corneal stroma. Furthermore, viral-induced death of endothelial cells and loss of cell-to-cell contact disturb the integrity of the endothelium monolayer, impairing its ability to maintain corneal moisture and clarity. Downregulation of endothelial pump activity worsens corneal edema and vision impairment. Hence, the suggested simple classification system based on the location of principle site of HSV infection or involvement should be applied for all cases of HSV keratitis [9].

12.4 Genetics

Seropositive individuals with a history of recurrent HSK are likely to have the CCIL28B genotype. This genotype may be related to incomplete control of the infection and more frequent periodical viral shedding along the first nerve branch of the trigeminal ganglion, which clinically manifests as recurrent herpes keratitis. The clinical manifestation of recurrent HSV-1 infection seems to be influenced by polymorphism of the IL28B genotype. No specific genetic association has been found for disciform keratitis [10].

12.5 Clinical Features

HSV can manifest as various forms of keratitis and the distinctive nature of each of these manifestations can be distinguished upon careful slit-lamp biomicroscopic examination where individual layers of the cornea can be assessed. Often, there will not be a documented history of HSV disease, and the episode of disciform endotheliitis may occur months to years after the episode of infectious epithelial keratitis.

Disciform keratitis has unique clinical characteristics that set it apart from other types of viral keratitis. Patients frequently complain of photophobia, pain, light-halo, ocular discomfort, and blurred vision, all of which may get worse over time.

Impaired visual acuity, circumcilliary congestion, mild to moderate anterior chamber inflammation, and unilateral circumscribed disc-shaped corneal edema ("ground glass" appearance with a definite demarcation between involved and uninvolved cornea) are common clinical presentations of disciform keratitis (Fig. 12.1a–b). The presence of keratic precipitates (KP), which appear as fine, granular or coin-shaped deposits visible on slit-lamp examination, on the corneal endothelium is a defining characteristic of disciform endotheliitis (Fig. 12.2). These KP patterns may have a distinctive "peppered" appearance and are frequently restricted to being behind the disc-shaped distribution in central or paracentral cornea focal pattern. With acute corneal inflammation, KPs may be difficult to see, but with resolution of the edema they become more prominent (Fig. 12.3). Corneal decompensation which is marked by corneal edema may manifest as development of epithelial bullae (Fig. 12.4).

Examination with fluorescein instillation indicates no fluorescein uptake, but the dye can highlight epithelial edema and endothelial dysfunction in all forms.

Anterior Chamber Inflammation with anterior chamber cells and flare is common in patients with HSV endotheliitis emphasizing its immunological nature. In severe cases, an increase of inflammatory cells in the anterior chamber can cause hypopyon. The presence of severe anterior chamber inflammation may necessitate stronger anti-inflammatory treatment. Furthermore, there is frequently elevated intraocular pressure, which

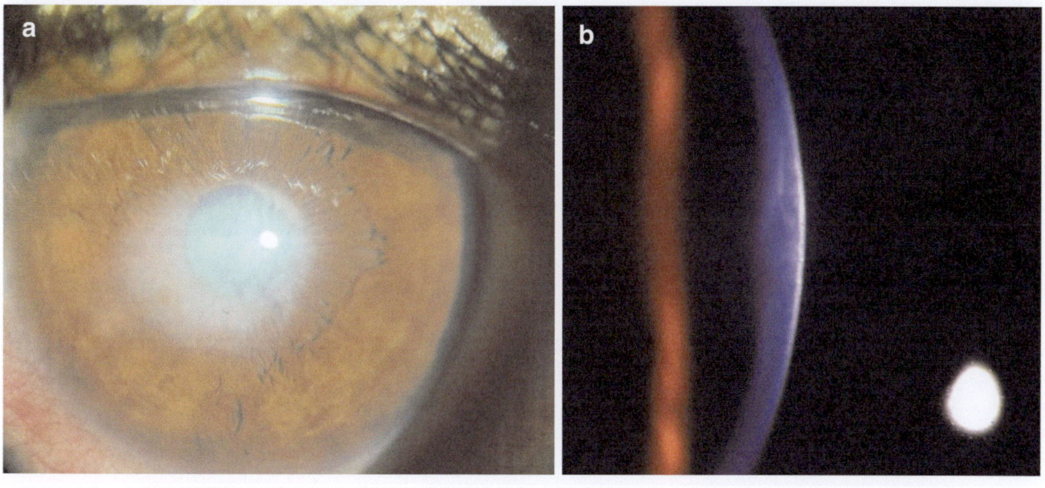

Fig. 12.1 (**a**) Perilimbal injection, central disc-shaped stromal, and endothelial edema along with few DM folds covering pupillary area on diffuse illumination. (**b**) Slit beam showing focal stromal edema in disciform keratitis

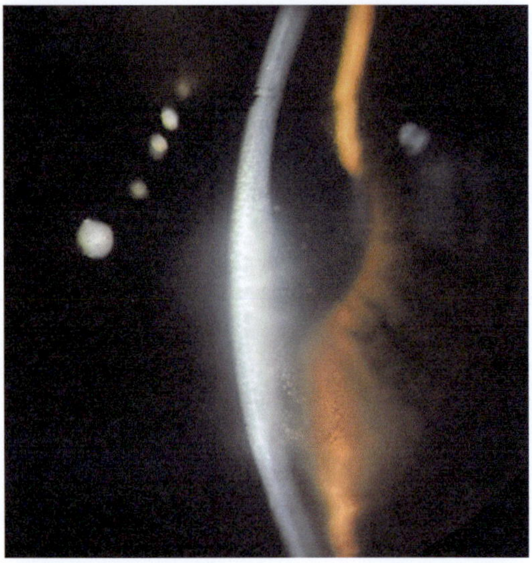

Fig. 12.2 Slit-lamp image with slit section of cornea showing active endotheliitis involving visual axis with surrounding endothelial haze and multiple fresh keratic precipitates along with overlying epithelial and stromal edema

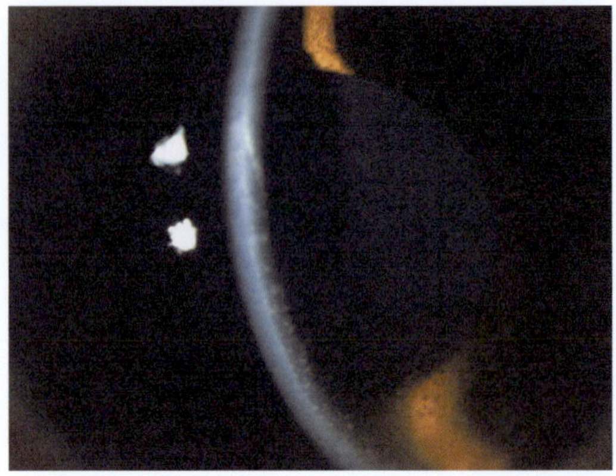

Fig. 12.3 After resolution of central stromal edema, localized keratic precipitates become more evident

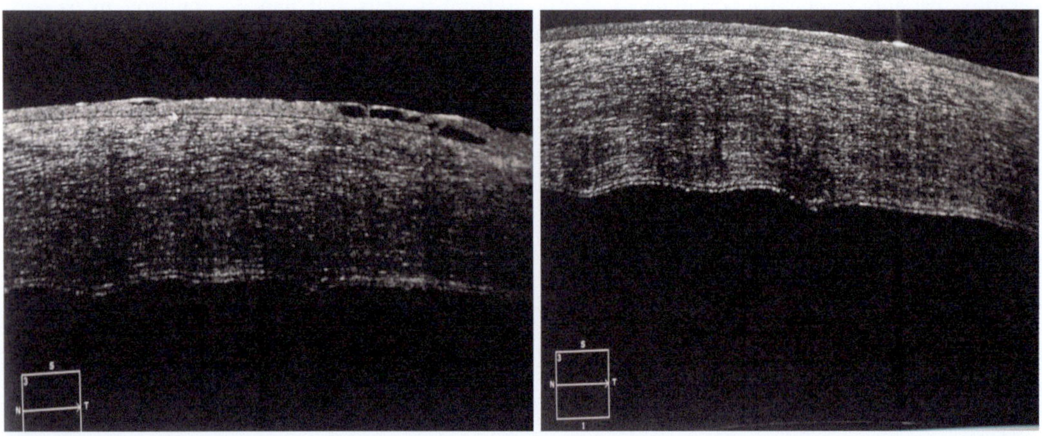

Fig. 12.4 ASOCT image showing stromal edema with epithelium bullae and descemet's folds in diffuse endotheliitis

can be due to a primary trabeculitis or aqueous outflow obstruction by inflammatory cells.

In cases of Herpes Zoster Ophthalmicus (HZO) 10% patients may show disciform keratitis after 3–4 months of disease onset resulting from a direct viral invasion of the endothelium with an immune reaction. Immune rings can also be associated with such disciform keratitis.

12.6 Types and Patterns

Disciform endotheliitis is the most common presentation of endotheliitis, and as mentioned above it is seen as a round or disc-shaped area of stromal edema in central or paracentral cornea. The disease course for endotheliitis generally involves healing after specific treatment, with the pattern of endotheliitis not affecting the healing process. Common sequelae across all types include recurrences of stromal keratitis, endothelial cell loss, and dysfunction. The patterns of viral endotheliitis are disciform, diffuse, and linear (Table 12.1) [6].

12.6.1 The Disciform Keratitis

It derives this name from the edema which is in a strikingly focal, disc-shaped pattern with absence of infiltrates or neovessels and a clear demarcation between involved and uninvolved cornea. Presence of KP is always a rule; however, they may sometimes be not appreciable behind the stromal edema. However with the clearing of edema they are well appreciated. Iritis, aqueous calls/flare, and elevated intraocular pressure (ocular hypertension) may also be seen which can be attributed either to inflammatory cells blocking aqueous outflow or primary trabeculitis Figs. 12.5 and 12.6. The epithelium may have microcystic edema overlying the areas of stromal edema. In more severe cases, epithelial bullae may form. Disciform endotheliitis typically results in minimal endothelial loss,

12.6.2 Diffuse Endotheliitis

It is characterized by widespread stromal edema, underlying KPs over the whole cornea, iritis, aqueous cells/flare with or without raised IOP. Diffuse and intense stromal edema may lead to epithelial edema, microcysts, or bullaes. In severe cases dense cellular infiltration in AC may result into hypopyo. As compared to disciform, diffuse endotheliitis is particularly sensitive to topical steroids with complete resolution of edema and moderate endothelial loss. However inadequate treatment may complicate to loss of vision due to bullous keratopathy, scarring, and neovascularization.

Table 12.1 Types of endotheliitis with diagnostic differentiators

	Disciform	Diffuse	Linear
Epithelium	Microcystic edema in untreated advanced stage	Microcystic edema in untreated advanced stage	Microcystic edema in untreated advanced stage
Stroma	Disc-shaped edema	Stromal edema involving the entire cornea	Stromal edema peripheral to the line of KP
Keratitic precipitates	KP underlying. The stromal edema	Scattered KP over the entire endothelium	Line of KP progressing from the limbus
Clinical course	Usually responsive to topical corticosteroids	Usually responsive to topical and systemic corticosteroids	Require aggressive treatment with topical and systemic antivirals and corticosteroids. Poorer prognosis as compared to other two types

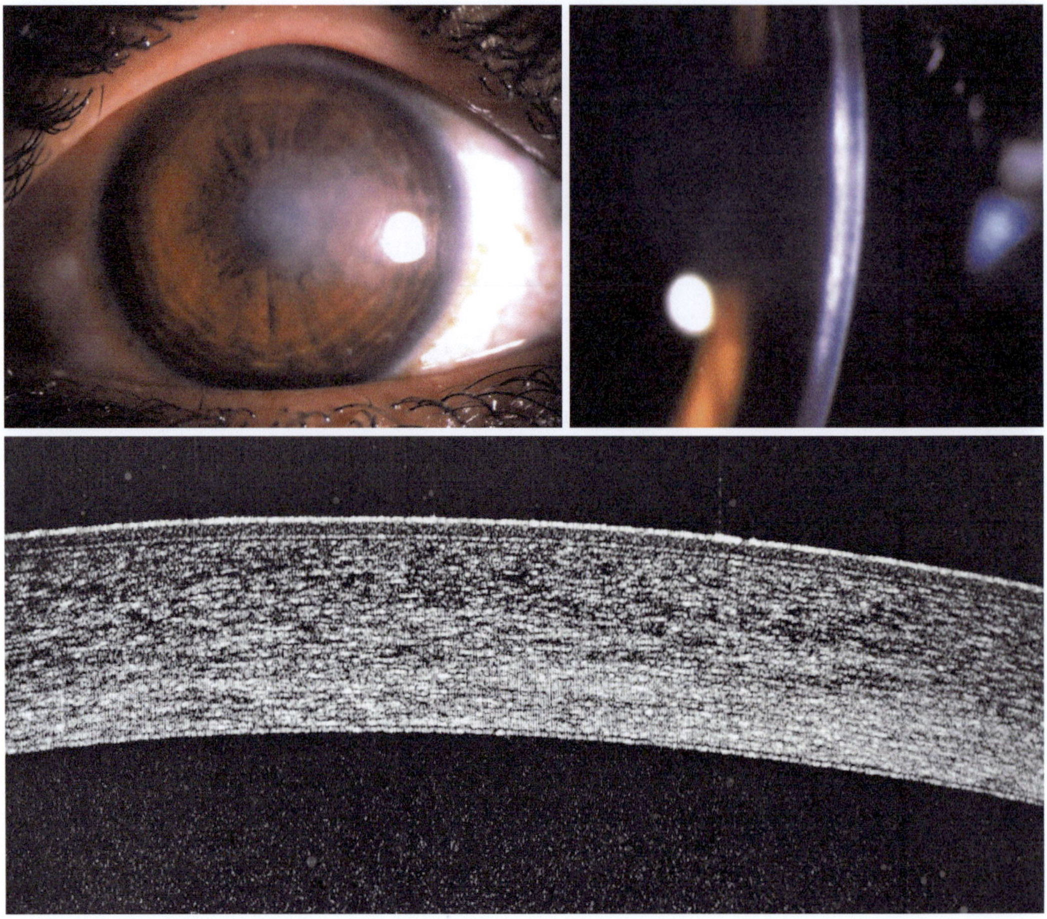

Fig. 12.5 Slit-lamp and AS-OCT Image showing disciform endotheliitis with central stromal edema and posterior haze

12.6.3 Linear Endotheliitis

Presents as stromal edema extending from the limbus with linear KPs along the leading edge and a Khodadoust line. The line of KP can be sectoral or circumferential, moves centrally with clear demarcation between the edematous and non-edematous cornea, and KP located at the leading edge of the edema. As compared to disciform and diffuse endotheliitis, linear endotheliitis is more difficult to treat and often leads to more significant endothelial loss and corneal decompensation, chronic stromal edema, fibrosis, and pre-descemetic neovascularization.

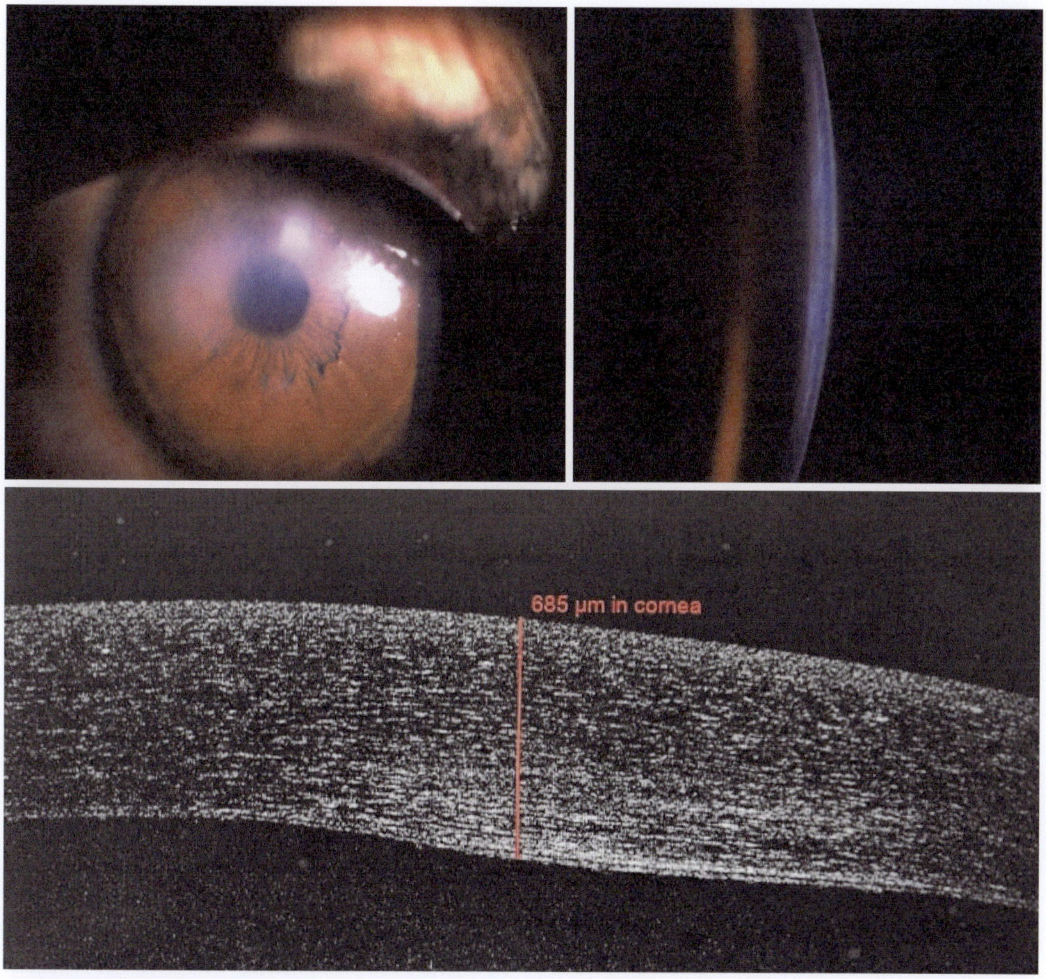

Fig. 12.6 Slit-lamp and AS-OCT Image showing disciform endotheliitis, central disc-shaped area of stromal edema

12.7 Investigations

The primary clinical observations used to identify disciform keratitis are the patient's history of recurrent ocular disease and the distinctive slit-lamp examination, to look for anterior chamber inflammation, corneal edema, and KP patterns. Auxiliary diagnostic tests may occasionally be employed to bolster the clinical diagnosis.

12.7.1 Anterior Segment Optical Coherence Tomography (AS-OCT)

This is a noninvasive imaging modality that uses light waves to capture detailed cross-sectional images of the cornea and operates on the principle of low-coherence interferometry. It can help diagnose and monitor disease progression.

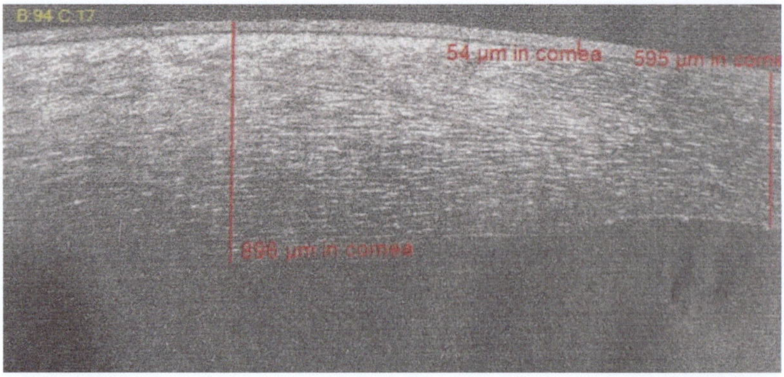

Fig. 12.7 Anterior Segment OCT picture showing the central demarcated area of stromal edema in a case of disciform keratitis with corneal thickness of 696 microns

(a) Detection of stromal edema: AS-OCT can quantify the extent and location of stromal edema, a hallmark of disciform keratitis. The increased corneal thickness can be precisely measured, aiding in early diagnosis (Fig. 12.7).
(b) Visualization of keratic precipitates: AS-OCT can detect keratic precipitates as hyper-reflective spots on the endothelium, confirming the presence of inflammation.
(c) Assessment of Descemet's membrane: Any irregularities or detachment of Descemet's membrane, which can occur in severe cases, are easily visualized with AS-OCT.
(d) Serial imaging for monitoring disease progression: AS-OCT enables longitudinal monitoring of corneal thickness and edema, allowing clinicians to track disease progression and response to treatment.
(e) Response to therapy: Changes in corneal thickness and resolution of keratic precipitates can be objectively assessed, providing insights into the effectiveness of antiviral and anti-inflammatory treatments.

The AS-OCT offers noninvasive, enhanced diagnostic accuracy (by providing objective, quantifiable data on corneal structure), enables early identification of complications such as Descemet's membrane detachment or corneal scarring and can assist in tailoring treatment plans. The limitations of AS-OCT in disciform keratitis are its cost and accessibility, particularly in resource-limited areas and operator dependency as this requires skilled technicians. As, AS-OCT may not effectively image deeper corneal structures in cases of severe edema or scarring due to limited penetration, ultrasound pachymetry may be employed.

12.7.2 Specular Microscopy

This often shows a reduced cell density due to cell loss from virus-induced inflammation. Affected cells may appear enlarged, irregular or with a decreased hexagonality due to swelling and inflammation. In advanced stages, more pronounced cell loss and morphological changes are observed. Corneal thickness variation can be documented using specular microscopy to correlate changes with endothelial morphology. Disease progression can be monitored by regular measurements of changes in cell density and to assess the extent of endothelial damage or worsening cell morphology despite treatment. Severe cases with significant endothelial damage may necessitate consideration of corneal transplantation later.

The technical limitations of specular microscopy are:

(a) Severe corneal edema or lens opacities may affect image quality.
(b) Requires experienced technicians to obtain and interpret high-quality images.
(c) Endothelial cell density and morphology can vary among individuals and may be influenced by other factors, such as age and comorbidities.

12.7.3 In Vivo Confocal Microscopy (IVCM)

It is a noninvasive imaging technology that visualizes corneal cellular components at a microscopic level. IVCM can reveal extensive information regarding corneal endothelium morphology, inflammatory cell infiltration, and viral cytopathic changes in HSV endotheliitis. IVCM observations include hyperreflective endothelial cells, inflammatory cell infiltrates, and viral inclusion bodies, which contribute to diagnosis and surveillance. Endothelial cells exhibited edema and increased intercellular gaps. Inflammatory cells are observed infiltrating the endothelial layer, with the majority of them forming keratic precipitates (KP), either spherical or elliptic, placed between the endothelium by pushing the endothelium aside and resulting in decaying areas between the endothelium.

In CMV infection, giant endothelial cells with nuclei containing a core area of high reflectivity, surrounded by a halo of low reflectivity, may be seen on the corneal endothelium on IVCM.

12.7.4 Laboratory Procedure

To detect viral DNA, laboratory procedures such as polymerase chain reaction (PCR), Nucleic acid amplification tests (NAAT) or viral culture of corneal scrapings or tear fluid may be rarely used. HSV has even been isolated from the aqueous humor from the anterior chamber of patients with HSV endotheliitis.

12.8 Differential Diagnosis

Disc-shaped corneal edema associated with anterior chamber inflammation may result from other causes mentioned in Table 12.2. For a precise diagnosis, a thorough clinical assessment, supplemented by diagnostic tests, is required.

Table 12.2 Differential diagnosis of disciform keratitis

Sr no.	Differential diagnosis	Clinical patterns that may overlap with disciform keratitis
1	VZV endotheliitis	Presents with corneal edema, keratic precipitates, and mild anterior chamber inflammation May lead to significant loss of endothelial cells. May coexist with uveitis. Descemet folds often appear between 4–7 days of onset
2	Adenoviral keratitis	Late stage may present with subepithelial infiltrates, multiple and separated by clear intervals Uninvolved stroma and endothelium
3	CMV keratitis	Can manifest as corneal endotheliitis in immunocompetent individuals. Endotheliitis caused by CMV often presents with linear or coin-shaped KPs Severe and untreated infections can damage the corneal endothelium, causing persistent corneal edema
4	Fuchs endothelial dystrophy	Endothelial coin-shaped lesions with clear spaces in between Lack of any active inflammatory signs Characterized by guttae Presence of generalized corneal edema
5	Interstitial keratitis	The endothelium is unaffected in the early stages but may show decompensation later along with stromal and epithelial edema.
6	Contact lens-induced keratitis	Often presents with peripheral rather than central edema.
7	Schnyder corneal dystrophy	Dominantly inherited corneal dystrophy Bilateral deposition of lipid and/or cholesterol crystals in the superficial to mid stroma Full-thickness corneal involvement is common Prominent corneal arcus, corneal crystals and diffuse corneal haze can be seen in patients by 40 years of age

12.9 Treatment

HSV keratitis has distinct mechanisms of pathogenesis in different corneal layers. Accordingly, the treatment strategy must be targeted for optimal outcomes. The choice of therapeutic intervention is critical depending upon the type of keratitis. Rarely disciform endotheliitis is self-limited and completely resolves even if left untreated. Occasionally, it can significantly impair vision if left untreated. Effective management involves topical corticosteroids, antiviral therapy, and supportive measures to control inflammation, prevent complications, and restore vision.

12.9.1 Medical Management

(a) Topical corticosteroids:
Help control immune reaction, inflammation, vasculitis, and reduce stromal edema, but have to be used with caution and always in conjunction with antiviral therapy to prevent exacerbation of viral replication. The most commonly used topical steroid is Prednisolone Acetate 1%, used four times daily initially and based on clinical response, gradually tapered over several weeks. Another effective option with similar dosing is Dexamethasone 0.1%. Rarely oral corticosteroids may be indicated in selected patients with severe immune response in disciform keratitis.

(b) Antiviral therapy is aimed to reduce viral replication, thereby minimizing the inflammatory response and preventing further damage to the corneal endothelium.
- Oral Acyclovir in dosage of 400 mg five times daily for 7–10 days is prescribed, followed by a maintenance dose of 400 mg twice daily for 1–2 weeks to prevent recurrence. In addition Valacyclovir in dose of 500 mg three times daily; Famciclovir 250 mg three times daily may also be prescribed.
- Topical administration of antivirals like acyclovir eye ointment usually is not needed but may be used in conjunction with oral therapy for local treatment with breakthrough epithelial involvement.

(c) Adjunctive therapies.
- Cycloplegics like Atropine (1%) or Cyclopentolate (2%) two times daily are used to relieve pain from ciliary spasm and prevent synechiae formation.
- Lubricating eye drops can help to maintain corneal hydration and comfort, with concurrent dry eye symptoms.
- Therapeutic/Bandage Contact Lens for protecting the corneal surface, reducing pain, and promoting healing in eyes with ruptured bullae leading to epithelial defects.

12.9.2 Surgical Interventions

Though disciform keratitis responds well to medical management, scarring sequelae might need surgical interventions. Corneal transplantation is indicated in cases of severe scarring or stromal thinning that do not respond to medical therapy [11].

- Penetrating Keratoplasty (PK): Full-thickness corneal transplant.
- Lamellar Keratoplasty: Deep anterior lamellar keratoplasty (DALK) may be preferred over PK for scarring with neovascularization involving the posterior stromal layers.

12.9.3 Management of Complications

A. Secondary glaucoma: Intraocular Pressure (IOP) is controlled by topical beta-blockers (e.g., Timolol), alpha agonists (e.g., Brimonidine), carbonic anhydrase inhibitors (e.g., Dorzolamide) etc. Regular monitoring of IOP measurements and optic nerve assessments are crucial to prevent glaucomatous damage. Topical steroids should be continued as indicated to reduce inflammation and edema and to prevent any associated neovascularization.

B. Stromal and Descemet's scarring: Extensive inflammation, particularly in cases with diffuse endotheliitis, leads to stromal and Descemet's scarring (Fig. 12.8a–e). Particularly with delayed or inappropriate treatment. It is important to aggressively control the inflammation with topical corticosteroids to prevent scarring, neovascularization, and subsequent loss of vision.

C. Corneal decompensation: Endothelial damage because of inflammatory and immunologic insult can lead to corneal decompensation, consequent to permanent endothelial cell loss. It is treated with 5% hypertonic saline in dosing frequency as per severity, in addition to topical steroids and preservative-free ocular surface lubricants. Corneal transplantation may be required in patients with intractable bullous keratopathy causing visual loss.

12.9.4 Follow-Up and Monitoring

- Regular Assessments on Slit-Lamp Examination: To monitor corneal clarity, edema, and presence of keratic precipitates.
- AS-OCT: To measure corneal thickness and detect any structural changes.
- Visual Acuity Testing: To assess improvement in vision and guide treatment adjustments.

12.9.5 Patient Education

- Importance of Adherence: Emphasize the need for strict adherence to antiviral and corticosteroid regimens.
- Recognizing Recurrence: Educate patients on the signs of recurrence, such as redness, pain,

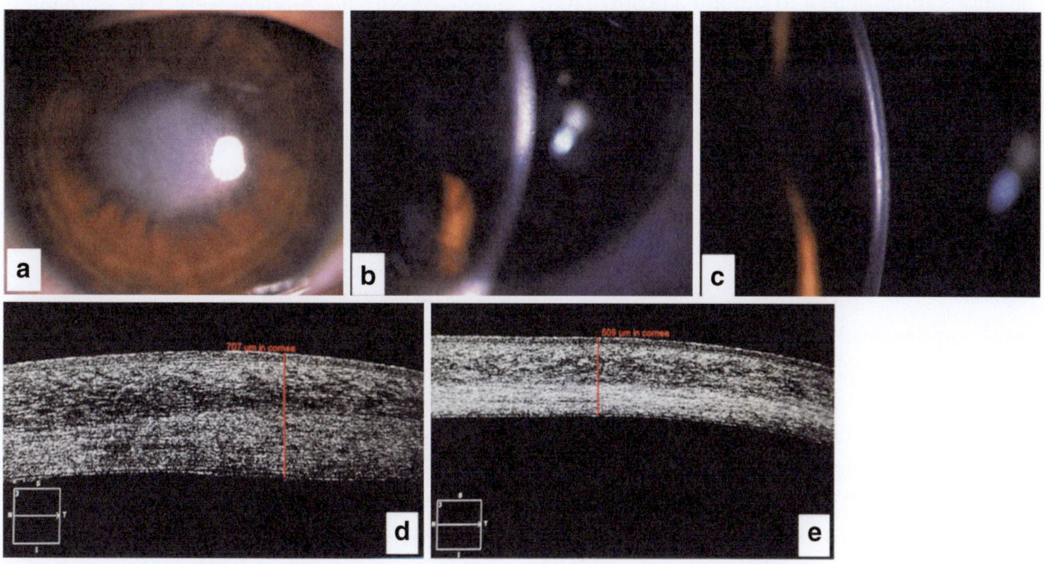

Fig. 12.8 (**a**, **b**) Diffuse and slit image showing disciform keratitis; (**d**) ASOCT image showing central disc-shaped area of stromal edema with corneal thickness of 707 microns; (**c**, **e**) showing post-treatment images with posterior stromal and descemet's scarring

or vision changes, and the need for prompt medical attention.
- Preventive Measures: Advise on general measures to reduce HSV reactivation, such as stress management and avoiding triggers.

12.10 Prevention of Recurrence

The HEDS recurrence rate study has not clearly stated regarding disciform endotheliitis, but indicated that short-course oral treatment during active HSV epithelial keratitis does not prevent subsequent stromal keratitis or iritis [12]. A 12-month regimen of preventive oral acyclovir (400 mg twice a day) dramatically reduced the recurrence risk of stromal involvement. Although the authors of the HEDS study did not recommend acyclovir prophylaxis for more than 12 months, clinical practice recommendations and observations appear to support a positive role for long-term prophylaxis, particularly in patients with a high recurrence rate, corneal thinning at risk of corneal perforation, comorbidities such as atopy, autoimmune diseases or immunocompromised individuals.

12.11 Recent Advances

Novel approaches, such as the multiplex dot hybridization (MDH) assay, the immunochromatographic assay (ICGA, AmpliVue), and the detection of infected cell protein 0 (ICP0) in tears, are also being studied or implemented in clinical practice. The MDH assay is a quick approach that uses a sequence of oligonucleotide probes specific to HSV genes. The MDH assay has significantly higher sensitivity, specificity, positive predictive value (PPV), and negative predictive value (NPV) than real-time PCR. AmpliVue is a commercially accessible immunochromatographic assay and office-based diagnostic test with a 64.7% positive detection rate.

During HSV infection, the infected cell protein 0 (ICP0) is an acute phase protein that contributes significantly to the activation of viral gene expression. ICP0 could be potentially defective in the tears of affected individuals.

One of the potential therapy techniques is to strengthen the patient's immune system against the virus by administering an HSV-1 vaccination. There is currently no licensed vaccination. However, research on the subject is ongoing and the discovery of 15 viral-encoded proteins might prove to be of benefit in formulating the HSV-1 vaccine.

In some cases, when confirming the diagnosis is challenging, the Goldmann-Witmer coefficient (GWC) can be utilized to determine the cause of the current antibodies. The antibody level in the aqueous and/or vitreous fluid is compared to the antibody level in the serum, which is multiplied by total serum globulin. A number greater than 3 implies that the observed antibodies were produced in the eye rather than passively diffusing from the serum. However, because immunocompromised patients produce very few antibodies, the test is of limited use. Combining PCR and GWC analysis can increase diagnostic accuracy.

Some research suggests that ICAM-1 and HLA-DR co-expression play a significant role in the development of immunological responses in HSV keratitis. Increased ICAM-1 expression in leukocytic infiltration areas may govern leukocyte-corneal cell binding, boosting immunological responses and damage by active leukocytes [13].

It has been suggested that anterior chamber associated immune deviation (ACAID) may have a role in HSV-1 endotheliitis. HSV-1 particles discharged into the anterior chamber are collected by indigenous antigen-presenting cells, which then provide an immunogenic signal that activates virus-specific ACAID [4].

Advanced imaging techniques like integration of AS-OCT with other imaging modalities, such as confocal microscopy and ultrasound biomicroscopy, for comprehensive anterior segment evaluation may lead to enhanced diagnosis and monitoring, especially in cases with severe edema. Development of automated algorithms for quantitative analysis of corneal parameters may improve diagnostic accuracy and consistency. Utilizing AS-OCT in remote and telemedicine settings can be envisioned to extend access to specialized care.

12.12 Conclusion

By keeping a high index of clinical suspicion, clinicians can enhance outcomes and quality of life for patients with HSV-associated corneal disorders especially disciform keratitis. Recent advances using multidisciplinary methods that include ophthalmology, immunology, and virology have led to better understanding of the disease. Early detection of disciform keratitis, rapid commencement of topical anti-inflammatory drugs and anti-viral therapy, along with diligent monitoring of treatment response are critical for improving visual outcomes and lowering the risk of sequelae.

Key Points

1. Disciform keratitis, a type of viral keratitis is a potentially severe corneal involvement with vision-threatening implications.
2. Herpes simplex virus (HSV) is the most frequent cause of disciform keratitis, but other viruses such as varicella-zoster virus (VZV), cytomegalovirus (CMV), and adenovirus have also been implicated. The condition primarily affects young adults, significantly impacting their quality of life and vision.
3. Disciform keratitis results from HSV-induced endothelial dysfunction, characterized by disc-shaped corneal edema and keratic precipitates due to anterior chamber inflammation. HSV entry into endothelial cells leads to viral replication and inflammation, impairing corneal clarity and function.
4. Diagnosis is primarily based on clinical examination, but auxiliary tests like anterior segment optical coherence tomography (AS-OCT) and specular microscopy are useful. AS-OCT helps visualize corneal edema, keratic precipitates, and monitor disease progression, while specular microscopy assesses endothelial cell density and morphology.
5. Treatment typically involves topical corticosteroids and antiviral therapy. Topical steroids help reduce inflammation, while antivirals like acyclovir, valacyclovir, and famciclovir manage viral replication. In severe cases, surgical options like corneal transplantation may be necessary.

References

1. Nowińska A. Recent advances in the diagnosis and management of Herpetic Keratitis: infectious eye diseases. IntechOpen; 2021.
2. Wilhelmus KR, Hamill MB, Jones DB. Varicella disciform stromal keratitis. Am J Ophthalmol. 1991;111(5):575–80.
3. Altan-Yaycioglu R, Poyraz S. Bilateral disciform keratitis of presumed adenoviral etiology. Indian J Ophthalmol. 2018 Jan;66(1):132–13.
4. https://eyewiki.aao.org/CMV_Endotheliitis
5. Darougar S, Wishart M, Viswalingam N. Epidemiological and clinical features of primary herpes simplex virus ocular infection. Br J Ophthalmol. 1985;69:2–6.
6. Labetoulle M, Boutolleau D, Burrel S, Haigh O, Rousseau A. Herpes simplex virus, varicella-zoster virus and cytomegalovirus keratitis: facts for the clinician. Ocul Surf. 2023 Apr;28:336–50.
7. Alsarhani WK, Chan CC, Boyd SR, Hasso M, Almeer A, Tan DHS. Monkeypox-associated Disciform Keratitis. Cornea. 2023;42(5):641–4.
8. Song MY, Koh KM, Hwang KY, Kwon YA, Kim KY. Relapsed Disciform Stromal Herpetic Keratitis following mRNA COVID-19 vaccination: a case report. Korean J Ophthalmol. 2022 Feb;36(1):80–2.
9. White ML, Chodosh J. Herpes simplex Virus Keratitis: a treatment guideline. AAO compendium of evidence-based eye care; 2014. Available at: http://www.aao.org/clinical-statement/herpes-simplex-virus-keratitis-treatment-guideline.
10. Borivoje S, Svetlana S, Milan HM, Nela Đ, Olivera MĐ, Filip M, Milenko S, Srbislav P. IL28B genetic variations in patients with recurrent Herpes Simplex Keratitis. Medicina (Kaunas). 2019;55(10):642.
11. CMV, cytomegalovirus, Hsiao CH, Hwang YS, Chuang WY, et al. Prevalence and clinical consequences of cytomegalovirus DNA in the aqueous humour and corneal transplants. Br J Ophthalmol. 2018:bjophthalmol-2018-312196. https://doi.org/10.1136/bjophthalmol-2018-312196.
12. HEDS. Oral acyclovir for herpes simplex virus eye disease: effect on prevention of epithelial keratitis and stromal keratitis. Herpetic Eye Disease Study Group. Arch Ophthalmol. 2000;118:1030–6.
13. Elner VM, Dutt S, Pavilack MA, Sugar A, Foster CS, Elner SG. Intercellular adhesion molecule-1 (ICAM-1) and HLA-DR antigens in herpes keratitis. Ophthalmology. 1992 Sep;99(9):1400–7.

13 Neurotrophic Keratitis

Manpreet Kaur, Siddhartha Rao, Akshaya Balaji, and Jeewan Singh Titiyal

Abstract

Neurotrophic keratopathy refers to degenerative corneal epithelial breakdown resulting from impaired corneal innervation. The loss of sensation during active stages of viral infections such as recurrent HSV or VZV associated with involvement of ophthalmic division of trigeminal nerve leads to degenerative corneal changes considered to be characteristic of neurotrophic keratopathy. This results in non-healing epithelial defects, ulceration, and subsequent perforations. Though corneal innervation may be affected by a variety of etiologies, herpes simplex, and varicella-zoster keratitis are the major causes of neurotrophic keratitis. This chapter provides a detailed overview of post-herpes neurotrophic keratopathy, including its etiopathogenesis, clinical features, investigations, and management.

Keywords

Neurotrophic keratitis · Neurotrophic ulcer · Persistent epithelial defect · Non-healing ulcer

13.1 Introduction

Neurotrophic keratitis is a degenerative disease of the cornea characterized by the breakdown of the corneal epithelium in the absence of desiccation, infection, or trauma [1]. It occurs secondary to loss of corneal sensation, affecting the nerve supply anywhere from the trigeminal nucleus to the corneal nerve endings. It is an orphan disease (ORPHA137596) with an estimated prevalence of less than 5 in 10,000 individuals [2]. Herpes simplex and Varicella-zoster keratitis are the main causes of neurotrophic keratitis and this entity is an important differential for a non-healing epithelial ulcer. Reduced reflex tearing and susceptibility to minor trauma predispose to non-healing epithelial defects, which can eventually progress to stromal lysis and perforation. Early diagnosis is essential, as the epitheliotoxic drugs used in viral epithelial keratitis worsen neurotrophic keratitis. Moreover, post-herpes neurotrophic keratopathy carries a poor prognosis. There are currently no promising treatments available to restore corneal sensitivity making the treatment of neurotrophic keratopathy complex and challenging.

13.2 Etiopathogenesis

The underlying etiopathogenesis of viral neurotrophic keratitis is the loss of corneal sensations caused by herpes simplex virus (HSV) and varicella zoster virus (VZV). Herpes zoster involves

M. Kaur (✉) · S. Rao · A. Balaji · J. S. Titiyal
RP Centre, AIIMS Delhi, New Delhi, India

B. Sharma et al. (eds.), *Viral Keratitis*, https://doi.org/10.1007/978-981-95-3148-6_13

the main trunk of the ophthalmic division of the trigeminal nerve, while herpes simplex predominantly affects the terminal branches [3].

Loss of corneal sensation leading to reduced reflex tear secretion and dry eye was initially believed to be the main pathophysiology of neurotrophic keratitis [4]. This was challenged by Segelman et al. when they demonstrated characteristic findings of neurotrophic keratitis in animal eyes after cutting the trigeminal nerve despite prophylactic tarsorrhaphy [5]. It was then proposed that sensory and autonomic nerves regulate corneal epithelial proliferation via neurotransmitters and trophic factors such as substance P and calcitonin gene-related peptide (CGRP) [6, 7]. Sympathetic stimulation and prostaglandins raise intracellular cAMP, while parasympathetic stimulation increases intracellular cGMP, both of which stimulate epithelial proliferation [8]. Sensory neurons supplying the cornea may directly influence corneal epithelial cell development and integrity. Even if the existing epithelial cells are healthy, any reduction in the proliferation eventually leads to their depletion and subsequent epithelial defects. Impairment of corneal innervation leads to metabolic and morphologic disturbances of the corneal epithelium, leading to persistent epithelial defects. As Thoft described in his well-known 'XYZ' hypothesis, replenishment of corneal epithelial cells occurs by centripetal migration of proliferating limbal cells, which are subsequently shed off at the apex [9]. Hence, the epithelial defect in neurotrophic keratitis typically begins in the centre.

Histopathology reveals reduced epithelial thickness with loss of the surface desquamating layer, and swelling of the remaining cells with depletion of intracellular glycogen. Abnormal basal lamina synthesis impairs epithelial adhesion. There is a loss of surface microvilli, leading to tear film instability, which promotes further epithelial damage.

13.3 Clinical Features

Neurotrophic keratitis presents commonly as recurrent epithelial defect, punctate keratopathy progressing to persistent defect, stromal ulceration, and scarring in long-standing cases (Fig. 13.1a, b). The patients often remain asymptomatic in the early stages due to loss of sensation. However, they can present with symptoms of pain, blurring of vision, and photophobia, especially as the disease severity increases. It is essential to differentiate active viral epithelial keratitis from viral neurotrophic keratitis, as both may be associated with epithelial defect and loss of corneal sensations (Table 13.1).

Morphological appearance of neurotrophic ulcer may vary from surface erosions and lack

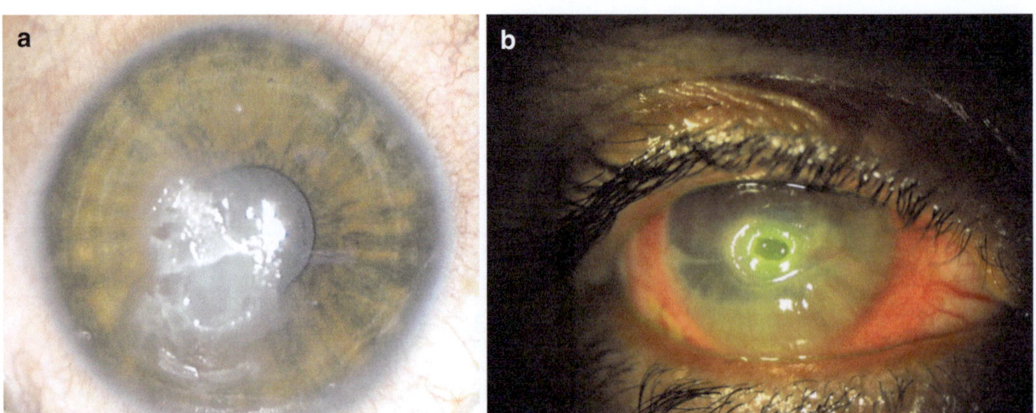

Fig. 13.1 (**a**) Neurotrophic keratitis with persistent epithelial defect showing non-healing margins and surrounding haze. (**b**) Slit-lamp image showing a characteristic central epithelial defect with thinning and rolled out borders stained with Fluorescein with surrounding lustreless cornea and nebulomacular haze

Table 13.1 Differentiating features of viral epithelial keratitis and viral neurotrophic keratitis

	Epithelial keratitis	Neurotrophic keratitis
Appearance	Dendritic or geographic	Round or oval with heaped up borders and boggy epithelium
Staining	Base of dendrite/geographic ulcer stains with fluorescein, and the margins with Rose Bengal	Punctate epithelial keratitis, positive staining with epithelial defect
Location	Any	Interpalpebral area
Etiology	Active infection of epithelium	Nerve damage, epitheliotoxic drugs
Treatment	Topical antivirals	Elimination of epitheliotoxic drugs including antivirals, preservative-free lubricants, growth factors, tarsorrhaphy
Course	Self-resolving in 2 weeks	Chronic, difficult to manage

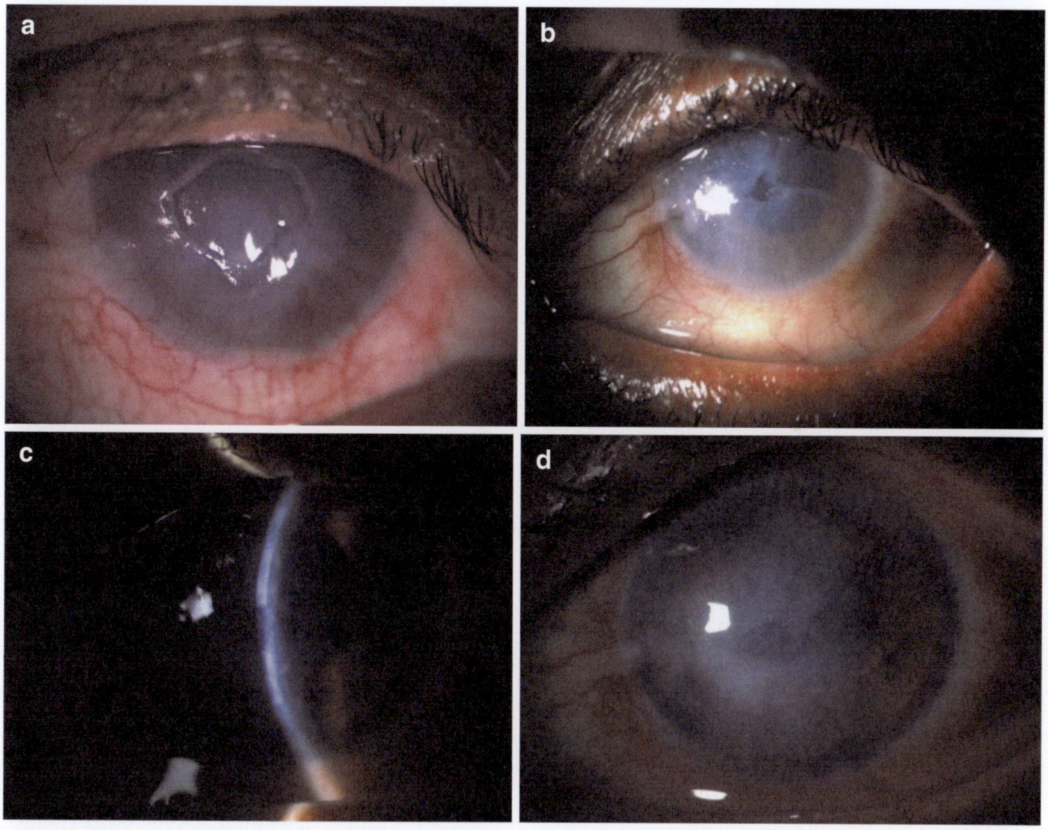

Fig. 13.2 **a–d** Slit-lamp image showing neurotrophic ulcer (**a**) Image showing central circular epithelial defect with smooth and rolled edges. (**b**, **c**) Healing of epithelial defect (**d**) Diffuse surrounding corneal haze suggesting stromal remodelling following epithelial healing.

of corneal lustre in early stages which may progress to persistent epithelial defect. The lesion is typically oval in shape with thickened rolled out borders due to heaped-up epithelium, as opposed to geographic ulcer, which is irregular with scalloped edges. It may progress to stromal ulceration in severe cases with circular configuration, smooth borders, and grey-white opacification (Fig. 13.2a-d). Complications of neurotrophic keratopathy include stromal necrosis, perforation, and secondary bacterial infection with consequent vascularized opacity.

Neurotrophic keratopathy progression occurs in three stages. Some researchers proposed substages.

13.3.1 Staging Proposed by Mackie et al. (1995) [10, 11] (Table 13.2)

(a) Stage I is characterized by punctate epithelial staining and punctate keratopathy, indicating localized areas of epithelial cell damage. There is also evidence of hyperplasia and irregularity in the corneal epithelium, along with superficial neovascularization. This stage is further defined by a decreased tear film break-up time and Rose Bengal staining of the inferior palpebral conjunctiva, highlighting areas of cellular damage or dryness. Gaule spots are noted, representing scattered areas of dried epithelium. Additionally, there is an increase in mucous tear viscosity.
(b) Stage II is characterized by a persistent epithelial defect, typically located on the superior half of the cornea, surrounded by a rim of loose epithelium. The edges of the defect may smoothen and can become loose or roll, leading to further deterioration. There may also be stromal oedema present, indicating swelling within the corneal stroma. An anterior chamber inflammatory reaction is rare but may occur.
(c) Stage III is the most severe form, presenting with a corneal ulcer, where there is a deeper loss of the corneal tissue. There is also stromal melting, a serious condition where the corneal stroma breaks down rapidly, and potentially, perforation of the cornea.

Table 13.2 Classification of neurotrophic ulcer

Mackie Stages	Clinical features
Stage 1	Superficial punctate keratopathy, irregular epithelium, decreased tear breakup time and superficial vascularization
Stage 2	Persistent epithelial defects and folds in Descemet membrane
Stage 3	Stromal melt and ulceration

13.3.2 Staging Proposed by Dua et al. (2018) [12]

(a) Stage I (mild) is characterized by superficial epithelial punctate lesions, alterations in the tear film, and reduced or absent sensitivity in isolated or multiple regions of the cornea.
(b) Stage II (moderate) presents with persistent epithelial defects and may include partial to complete loss of corneal sensation.
(c) Stage III (severe) manifests with stromal involvement, potentially progressing to ulcerations or full-thickness perforations, alongside diminished to entirely absent corneal sensation.

13.3.3 Staging Proposed by Mastropasqua et al. (2019) [13]

(a) Stage I.
  I. Stage IA of neurotrophic keratopathy is identified by a punctate epithelial fluorescein stain, which may occur with or without corneal hypoesthesia. Diagnostic imaging shows that sub-basal nerve fibre density is equal to or greater than 5 μm/mm^2, and total nerve fibres are equal to or greater than 1 μm/mm^2. Anterior-segment optical coherence tomography reveals an irregular epithelial surface, increased epithelial and anterior stromal reflectivity, while stromal thickness and Bowman's layer are preserved.
  II. Stage IB is distinguished by a sub-basal nerve fibre density of less than or equal to 5 μm/mm^2 and total nerve fibres of less than or equal to 1 μm/mm^2.
(b) Stage II.
  I. In Stage IIA, there is an epithelial defect with smooth or rolled edges and corneal hypoesthesia or anaesthesia. The sub-basal nerve fibre density is equal to or greater than 3 μm/mm^2. Optical coherence tomography findings include an interrupted epithelial layer and increased anterior stromal reflectivity, without corneal stroma thinning or ulceration.

II. Stage IIB is characterized by a sub-basal nerve fibre density of less than or equal to 3 μm/mm^2.

(c) Stage III.

I. Stage IIIA presents corneal ulceration with stromal thinning, where the thickness depth is equal to or less than 50%.

II. Stage IIIB is marked by stromal thinning and/or ulceration with a thickness depth of 50% or greater.

Therapeutic approaches are contingent upon the stage of progression [10, 12]. With standard therapy, 60% of cases take longer than 14 days to heal, and approximately 50% heal completely [14].

13.4 Clinical Evaluation

Prior recurrent episodes of blistering, redness, and pain are often associated with viral neurotrophic keratitis. Patient evaluation is directed towards the determination of the primary aetiology of neurotrophic keratopathy, as well as the staging for appropriate management.

A comprehensive ocular and systemic examination is mandatory to evaluate corneal health and rule out ocular and systemic co-morbidities.

13.4.1 Ocular Adnexa and Tear-Film

The eyelid is examined for entropion, ectropion, and lagophthalmos, which can worsen the condition. A careful assessment of the tear film should be done, including the tear meniscus height, tear film break-up time, and Schirmer's test. Reduced reflex tearing can cause aqueous deficiency in the affected as well as the other eye.

13.4.2 Assessment of Corneal Sensations

Assessment of corneal sensation is perhaps the most relevant test for the diagnosis of neurotrophic keratitis. This is done commonly by the cotton wisp method, where a cotton wisp is lightly touched to the central cornea, and then at four quadrants. If the sensation is normal, the patient subjectively feels a touch sensation and a blink reflex is induced. In general, the central, nasal, and temporal cornea is less sensitive than the superior and inferior cornea. An absent blink reflex and no corneal touch sensation are interpreted as complete corneal anaesthesia.

The Cochet-Bonnet esthesiometer measures the depth of corneal anaesthesia [15]. It uses a nylon filament that can be extended from 0 to 6 centimetres to elicit a blink reflex and quantitate the degree of corneal sensitivity loss. Readings of 2 centimetres or less are more likely to develop neurotrophic keratitis [16]. Patchy corneal anaesthesia is a feature of herpes zoster keratitis [3]. Another instrument, less commonly used is the Belmonte non-contact esthesiometer [12]. This is based on the stimulation of three types of neuroreceptors of the cornea, namely thermal, mechanical, and chemical by air puffs of different temperatures, pressures, and concentrations of carbon dioxide. This investigation has the advantage of being less invasive. Another method where 3% hypertonic saline is used to measure corneal sensitivity has also been described.

13.4.3 Slit-Lamp Biomicroscopy

The cornea is examined via slit-lamp biomicroscopy to identify conditions that predispose to reduced corneal sensitivity and to stage the disease. Signs of herpetic keratitis, such as dendrites should be identified. Sectoral iris atrophy is relatively specific for herpes zoster. Dendrites of herpes should not be confused with a healing epithelial defect, which may have a similar shape but is distinguished by the absence of branching and terminal bulbs. The anterior chamber should be examined for the presence of cells, flare, or a sterile hypopyon.

13.5 Investigations

Investigations such as in vivo confocal microscopy have recently been introduced for the visualization and assessment of the corneal nerve plexus at different levels in patients of neurotrophic keratitis. Studies have shown a significant correlation between the reduction in corneal sensation and subepithelial nerve plexus density [17, 18]. Neurotrophic keratitis is also associated with reduced corneal epithelial and endothelial cell density and increased number of hyperreflective keratinocytes compared to controls.

Impression cytology has been used to detect conjuctivalization of the cornea due to limbal stem cell deficiency and epithelial changes related to dry eye [19].

13.6 Management

The management of neurotrophic keratitis is aimed at creating a local environment favourable for corneal healing and preventing progression to stromal lysis and perforation. Concomitant diseases such as limbal stem cell deficiency and eyelid malposition and lagophthalmos accelerate progression of the disease, and require timely correction. No specific medical management exists at present to restore corneal sensation, and surgical approaches such as amniotic membrane graft and conjunctival flaps are often required to prevent progression to stromal melt and perforation. There are several novel therapies, a few recently approved, and a few still in various phases of clinical trials, which may be the future of the management of neurotrophic keratitis.

Early diagnosis and appropriate treatment are the keys to recovery. The patients are often asymptomatic due to corneal anaesthesia, and present late. Timely and adequate management prevents progression to stromal melt and perforation. All epitheliotoxic topical medications should be discontinued [10].

The management of neurotrophic keratitis is based on the stage of the disease (Table 13.3).

Table 13.3 Management of neurotrophic ulcer based on severity

Stages of neurotrophic ulcer	Management options
Stage 1	Use of frequent preservative free lubricant drops and gel. Discontinue epitheliotoxic drugs Night time patching
Stage 2	Topical NSAIDS Topical steroids N-acetylcysteine Medroxy progesterone Oral matrix metalloproteinase inhibitors (doxycycline 100 mg twice a day) Autologous serum and umbilical cord serum Topical preparations of growth factors like insulin, insulin like growth factors, substance -P, Thymosisn beta, and Cenegermin Therapeutic contact lens Multilayered amniotic membrane transplantation Temporary or permanent tarsorraphy
Stage 3	Cyanoacrylate glue with bandage contact lens Penetrating keratoplasty Selective bowman layer transplantation Corneal neurotization Gunderson flap

13.6.1 Medical Management

Stage 1 is characterized by tear film and epithelial abnormalities, and treatment aims to improve epithelial health and transparency and avoid epithelial breakdown. Frequent, preservative-free lubricant drops and gels are the mainstay of management. Soft bandage and scleral contact lenses may be considered, weighing the benefits against the risk of infection [20]. In severe dry eye, punctal plugs may also be considered to improve the ocular surface. Eyelid closure with pressure patching or micropore tape may be used as a temporary measure to protect the cornea and improve the ocular surface.

Stage 2 is characterized by epithelial breakdown and the formation of persistent epithelial defects. As in stage 1, frequent preservative-free lubricants are used to protect the vulnerable epithelium. *Topical steroids* may be used with great caution to reduce ocular inflammation if any, but carry the risk of inhibition of healing and progression to perforation [21]. Topical NSAIDs inhibit healing and should be avoided [22]. An epithelium-friendly *topical antibiotic* such as chloramphenicol is indicated in stages 2 and 3 to prevent superadded infection.

Oral matrix metalloproteinase inhibitors such as doxycycline 100 mg twice a day or tetracycline 250 mg twice a day are useful adjuncts in management, and may prevent stromal lysis [23]. Medroxyprogesterone acetate may be considered. Fastidious care of the anaesthetic cornea is required to prevent progression to epithelial and stromal ulceration.

Different preparations of *growth factors* have been tried with varying success rates. Studies have shown the benefit of substance P, insulin-like growth factor, nerve growth factor, thymosin beta-4, epidermal growth factor, laminin, fibronectin, and albumin, alone or in combination.

The use of 50% *autologous serum, topical platelet-rich plasma*, and *allogenic umbilical cord serum (AUCS)* drops have shown encouraging results in promoting epithelial healing [24, 25].

A few cases progress to stage 3, which comprises of stromal thinning and perforation despite all efforts. Collagenase inhibitors have a role in this stage, and decrease stromal meltdown [26]. Topical cysteine, 20% N-acetyl cysteine, 0.2 mol/L EDTA, and oral tetracyclines have been tried with varying results.

13.6.2 Surgical Management

Surgery is required in advanced cases non-responsive to conservative medical therapy. Lateral or complete *surgical tarsorrhaphy* protects the loosely adherent epithelium from the windshield-wiper effect of the upper eyelid [27]. Tarsorrhaphy can be easily reversed and may be left in place for as long as a year. Alternative measure includes *chemical tarsorrhaphy* with botulinum toxin injection to the levator palpebrae superioris.

Small perforations of less than 2 mm may be managed with *tissue adhesives* such as isobutyl cyanoacrylate glue. They provide tectonic support, create a hypoxic environment that inhibits polymorphonuclear leucocytes, and have a bactericidal action. They also promote neovascularization and serve as a bridge to postpone penetrating keratoplasty, which has high rates of failure when performed in an acutely inflamed eye. An absorbable fibrin sealant patch, TachoSil (Nycomed Pharma, Zurich, Switzerland), with or without amniotic membrane transplant, has also been used successfully to treat noninfective corneal perforation [28].

Another option for cases of neurotrophic keratitis without perforation is a *multilayered amniotic membrane graft (AMG)* (Fig. 13.3) [29, 30]. Multilayered AMG promotes the proliferation of the stromal keratinocytes and helps maintain the stromal thickness once the membrane dissolves. It also inhibits the synthesis of chemotactic factors, reduces inflammation, and secretes growth factors that promote faster epithelial healing.

An almost obsolete, but still useful method for eyes with non-healing ulcers with poor visual prognosis is the *Gunderson flap* [31, 32]. It completely covers the cornea to provide structural support, halt the inflammatory process and improve cosmesis, and is an alternative to evisceration. For small or peripheral ulcers, partial vertical conjunctival flaps may also be used.

Full-thickness corneal transplant, including penetrating keratoplasty and patch grafts are the last resort in large perforations measuring more than 2 mm in diameter [33]. However, the prognosis for graft survival in inflamed eyes is dismal

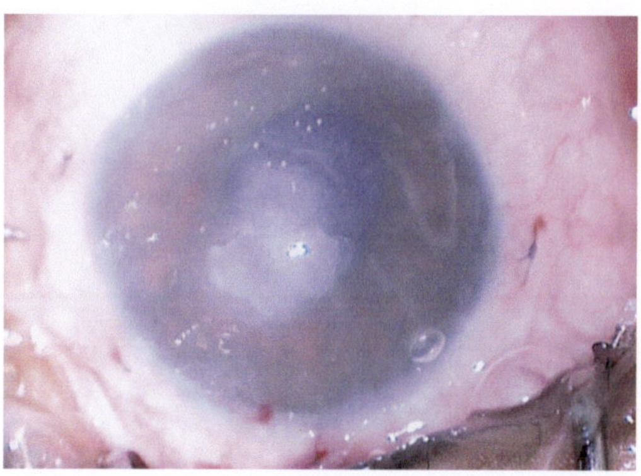

Fig. 13.3 Multilayered AMG in a case of neurotrophic keratitis

[34]. When all else fails, the use of Boston keratoprosthesis has also been described [33].

13.6.3 Regenerative Therapies

Several studies have observed *topical nerve growth factor* therapy to be a promising treatment modality for neurotrophic keratitis [35]. It improves tear and nerve function and stimulates the survival and regeneration of corneal epithelium and nerves. Complete epithelial healing has been observed with some recovery of corneal sensitivity, improvement of visual acuity, and reduced scarring.

Cenegermin 0.02% (Oxervate) is a recombinant human nerve growth factor derived from *Escherichia coli* and is the only FDA-approved treatment for neurotrophic keratitis. It is a propeptide, which is enzymatically cleaved into its active form, nerve growth factor. It binds to a specific, high-affinity tropomyosin receptor kinase A(TrkA) to promote sensory neuron growth, differentiation, and survival via MAPK, RAS, PI3K, Cdc42, and PLC-gamma, and has demonstrated efficacy in all stages of neurotrophic keratitis. It has been shown to significantly increase corneal nerve density, improve corneal sensation and visual acuity, and promote epithelial healing [36–38].

Other agents that have been demonstrated to promote epithelial healing in neurotrophic ulcers include *heparin sulphate-like matrix agent, thymosin beta-4 (a G-actin sequestering molecule), substance P and insulin-like growth factor* [39–41].

Corneal neurotization is a novel technique of reinnervation of the cornea via contralateral supratrochlear and supraorbital nerves, with or without sural nerve transposition, aimed at addressing the root cause of neurotrophic keratopathy, but has shown limited success so far [42].

Etiopathogenesis, clinical features, staging, and treatment of postherpetic neurotrophic keratopathy are summarized in Flow diagram 13.1.

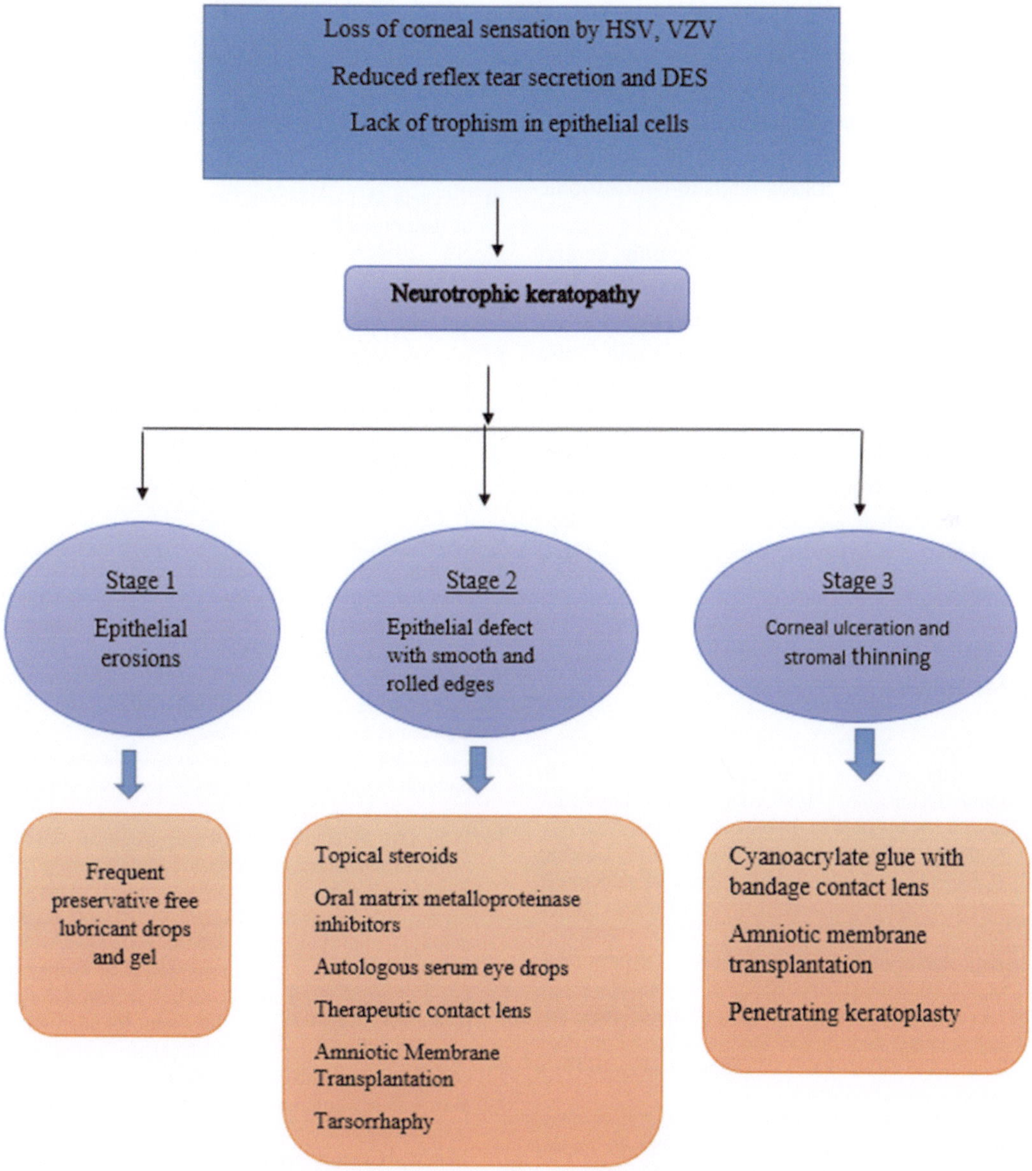

Flow diagram 13.1 Clinical features, staging, and treatment of postherpetic neurotrophic keratopathy

13.7 Conclusion

Viral neurotrophic keratitis may range in severity from recurrent epithelial defect to stromal ulceration and scarring in long-standing cases. A comprehensive ocular and systemic examination is mandatory to evaluate corneal health and rule out ocular and systemic co-morbidities. Neurotrophic keratitis is a challenge to manage due to the paucity of specific treatment modalities. Early diagnosis and appropriate treatment are the keys to recovery. Conservative management should be preferred wherever possible. Penetrating keratoplasty has a poor prognosis due to the high incidence of persistent epithelial defects, infection, melting, and perforation in these cases.

Key Points

1. Neurotrophic keratopathy is a condition that is neither immune nor infective but caused by defective corneal innervation.
2. Impaired corneal nerve supply following HSV and VZV keratitis leads to neurotrophic keratitis.
3. It is characterized by a non-healing central epithelial defect with smooth edges and heaped-up epithelium at the margins.
4. Avoid epitheliotoxic drugs and use preservative-free lubricants in all cases.
5. The degree of nerve damage and corneal sensation loss determines the likelihood of progression to stromal melting and perforation.
6. Proper clinical evaluation and accurate staging of the disease help to follow the staged management.

References

1. Lambiase A, Rama P, Aloe L, Bonini S. Management of neurotrophic keratopathy. Curr Opin Ophthalmol. 1999;10(4):270–6. https://doi.org/10.1097/00055735-199908000-00009.
2. Roth M, Dierse S, Alder J, Holtmann C, Geerling G. Incidence, prevalence, and outcome of moderate to severe neurotrophic keratopathy in a German tertiary referral center from 2013 to 2017. Graefes Arch Clin Exp Ophthalmol. 2022;260(6):1961–73. https://doi.org/10.1007/s00417-021-05535-z.
3. Liesegang TJ. Ocular herpes simplex infection: pathogenesis and current therapy. Mayo Clin Proc. 1988;63(11):1092–105. https://doi.org/10.1016/s0025-6196(12)65504-9.
4. Bonini S, Rama P, Olzi D, Lambiase A. Neurotrophic keratitis. Eye Lond Engl. 2003;17(8):989–95. https://doi.org/10.1038/sj.eye.6700616.
5. Sigelman S, Friedenwald JS. Mitotic and wound-healing activities of the corneal epithelium; effect of sensory denervation. AMA Arch Ophthalmol. 1954;52(1):46–57. https://doi.org/10.1001/archopht.1954.00920050048005.
6. Müller LJ, Marfurt CF, Kruse F, Tervo TMT. Corneal nerves: structure, contents and function. Exp Eye Res. 2003;76(5):521–42. https://doi.org/10.1016/s0014-4835(03)00050-2.
7. Araki-Sasaki K, Aizawa S, Hiramoto M, et al. Substance P-induced cadherin expression and its signal transduction in a cloned human corneal epithelial cell line. J Cell Physiol. 2000;182(2):189–95. https://doi.org/10.1002/(SICI)1097-4652(200002)182:2<189::AID-JCP7>3.0.CO;2-9.
8. Cavanagh HD, Colley AM. The molecular basis of neurotrophic keratitis. Acta Ophthalmol Suppl. 1989;192:115–34. https://doi.org/10.1111/j.1755-3768.1989.tb07103.x.
9. Thoft RA, Friend J. The X, Y, Z hypothesis of corneal epithelial maintenance. Invest Ophthalmol Vis Sci. 1983;24(10):1442–3.
10. Sacchetti M, Lambiase A. Diagnosis and management of neurotrophic keratitis. Clin Ophthalmol Auckl NZ. 2014;8:571–9. https://doi.org/10.2147/OPTH.S45921.
11. Fraunfelder FT, Roy FH. Current ocular therapy 4. Saunders; 1995.
12. Dua HS, Said DG, Messmer EM, et al. Neurotrophic keratopathy. Prog Retin Eye Res. 2018;66:107–31. https://doi.org/10.1016/j.preteyeres.2018.04.003.
13. Mastropasqua L, Massaro-Giordano G, Nubile M, Sacchetti M. Understanding the pathogenesis of neurotrophic keratitis: the role of corneal nerves. J Cell Physiol. 2017;232(4):717–24. https://doi.org/10.1002/jcp.25623.
14. Saad S, Abdelmassih Y, Saad R, et al. Neurotrophic keratitis: frequency, etiologies, clinical management and outcomes. Ocul Surf. 2020;18(2):231–6. https://doi.org/10.1016/j.jtos.2019.11.008.
15. Cochet P, Bonnet R. Corneal esthesiometry. Performance and practical importance. Bull Soc Ophtalmol Fr. 1961;6:541–50.
16. Cobo LM. Corneal complications of herpes zoster ophthalmicus. Prevention and treatment. Cornea. 1988;7(1):50–6.
17. Patel DV, McGhee CNJ. In vivo confocal microscopy of human corneal nerves in health, in ocular and systemic disease, and following corneal surgery: a review. Br J Ophthalmol. 2009;93(7):853–60. https://doi.org/10.1136/bjo.2008.150615.
18. Hamrah P, Cruzat A, Dastjerdi MH, et al. Unilateral herpes zoster ophthalmicus results in bilateral corneal nerve alteration: an in vivo confocal microscopy study. Ophthalmology. 2013;120(1):40–7. https://doi.org/10.1016/j.ophtha.2012.07.036.
19. Sacchetti M, Lambiase A, Cortes M, et al. Clinical and cytological findings in limbal stem cell deficiency. Graefes Arch Clin Exp Ophthalmol. 2005;243(9):870–6. https://doi.org/10.1007/s00417-005-1159-0.
20. Grey F, Carley F, Biswas S, Tromans C. Scleral contact lens management of bilateral exposure and neurotrophic keratopathy. Contact Lens Anterior Eye J Br Contact Lens Assoc. 2012;35(6):288–91. https://doi.org/10.1016/j.clae.2012.07.009.
21. Petroutsos G, Guimaraes R, Giraud JP, Pouliquen Y. Corticosteroids and corneal epithelial wound healing. Br J Ophthalmol. 1982;66(11):705–8. https://doi.org/10.1136/bjo.66.11.705.
22. Hersh PS, Rice BA, Baer JC, et al. Topical nonsteroidal agents and corneal wound healing. Arch Ophthalmol Chic Ill 1960. 1990;108(4):577–83. https://doi.org/10.1001/archopht.1990.01070060125062.

23. Ralph RA. Tetracyclines and the treatment of corneal stromalulceration:areview.Cornea.2000;19(3):274–7. https://doi.org/10.1097/00003226-200005000-00003.
24. Jeng BH, Dupps WJ. Autologous serum 50% eyedrops in the treatment of persistent corneal epithelial defects. Cornea. 2009;28(10):1104–8. https://doi.org/10.1097/ICO.0b013e3181a2a7f6.
25. Yoon KC, You IC, Im SK, Jeong TS, Park YG, Choi J. Application of umbilical cord serum eyedrops for the treatment of neurotrophic keratitis. Ophthalmology. 2007;114(9):1637–42. https://doi.org/10.1016/j.ophtha.2006.12.014.
26. Berman null. Collagenase inhibitors: rationale for their use in treating corneal ulceration. Int Ophthalmol Clin. 1975;15(4):49–66. https://doi.org/10.1097/00004397-197501540-00006.
27. Portnoy SL, Insler MS, Kaufman HE. Surgical management of corneal ulceration and perforation. Surv Ophthalmol. 1989;34(1):47–58. https://doi.org/10.1016/0039-6257(89)90129-x.
28. Grau AE, Durán JA. Treatment of a large corneal perforation with a multilayer of amniotic membrane and TachoSil. Cornea. 2012;31(1):98–100. https://doi.org/10.1097/ICO.0b013e31821f28a2.
29. Kruse FE, Rohrschneider K, Völcker HE. Multilayer amniotic membrane transplantation for reconstruction of deep corneal ulcers. Ophthalmology. 1999;106(8):1504–10.; discussion 1511. https://doi.org/10.1016/S0161-6420(99)90444-X.
30. Khokhar S, Natung T, Sony P, Sharma N, Agarwal N, Vajpayee RB. Amniotic membrane transplantation in refractory neurotrophic corneal ulcers: a randomized, controlled clinical trial. Cornea. 2005;24(6):654–60. https://doi.org/10.1097/01.ico.0000153102.19776.80.
31. Lugo M, Arentsen JJ. Treatment of neurotrophic ulcers with conjunctival flaps. Am J Ophthalmol. 1987;103(5):711–2. https://doi.org/10.1016/s0002-9394(14)74337-5.
32. Buxton JN. Therapeutic conjunctival flaps and tarsorrhaphy. Contact Intraocul Lens Med J. 1981;7(2):150–2.
33. Langston RH, Pavan-Langston D. Penetrating keratoplasty for herpetic keratitis: decision-making and management. Int Ophthalmol Clin. 1975;15(4):125–40. https://doi.org/10.1097/00004397-197501540-00011.
34. Jhanji V, Young AL, Mehta JS, Sharma N, Agarwal T, Vajpayee RB. Management of corneal perforation. Surv Ophthalmol. 2011;56(6):522–38. https://doi.org/10.1016/j.survophthal.2011.06.003.
35. Lambiase A, Rama P, Bonini S, Caprioglio G, Aloe L. Topical treatment with nerve growth factor for corneal neurotrophic ulcers. N Engl J Med. 1998;338(17):1174–80. https://doi.org/10.1056/NEJM199804233381702.
36. Deeks ED, Lamb YN. Cenegermin: a review in neurotrophic keratitis. Drugs. 2020;80(5):489–94. https://doi.org/10.1007/s40265-020-01289-w.
37. Balbuena-Pareja A, Bogen CS, Cox SM, Hamrah P. Effect of recombinant human nerve growth factor treatment on corneal nerve regeneration in patients with neurotrophic keratopathy. Front Neurosci. 2023;17:1210179. https://doi.org/10.3389/fnins.2023.1210179.
38. Pflugfelder SC, Massaro-Giordano M, Perez VL, et al. Topical recombinant human nerve growth factor (Cenegermin) for neurotrophic keratopathy: a multicenter randomized vehicle-controlled pivotal trial. Ophthalmology. 2020;127(1):14–26. https://doi.org/10.1016/j.ophtha.2019.08.020.
39. Aifa A, Gueudry J, Portmann A, Delcampe A, Muraine M. Topical treatment with a new matrix therapy agent (RGTA) for the treatment of corneal neurotrophic ulcers. Invest Ophthalmol Vis Sci. 2012;53(13):8181–5. https://doi.org/10.1167/iovs.12-10476.
40. Dunn SP, Heidemann DG, Chow CYC, et al. Treatment of chronic nonhealing neurotrophic corneal epithelial defects with thymosin beta4. Ann N Y Acad Sci. 2010;1194:199–206. https://doi.org/10.1111/j.1749-6632.2010.05471.x.
41. Yamada N, Matsuda R, Morishige N, et al. Open clinical study of eye-drops containing tetrapeptides derived from substance P and insulin-like growth factor-1 for treatment of persistent corneal epithelial defects associated with neurotrophic keratopathy. Br J Ophthalmol. 2008;92(7):896–900. https://doi.org/10.1136/bjo.2007.130013.
42. Terzis JK, Dryer MM, Bodner BI. Corneal neurotization: a novel solution to neurotrophic keratopathy. Plast Reconstr Surg. 2009;123(1):112–20. https://doi.org/10.1097/PRS.0b013e3181904d3a.

Marginal Keratitis

14

Sridevi Nair and Ayesha Abdul Salam

Abstract

Marginal keratitis is an uncommon form of herpetic keratitis, often caused by herpes simplex virus (HSV) and varicella-zoster virus (VZV). It is characterized by a peripheral corneal infiltrate along the limbus, associated with epithelial changes. The pathogenesis involves an immune-mediated response to viral antigens in the corneal tissue, leading to an inflammatory cascade. Diagnosis is largely clinical, based on slit-lamp examination findings. This chapter provides an overview of the epidemiology, pathophysiology, risk factors, clinical features, differential diagnosis, and management strategies for viral marginal keratitis.

Keywords

Marginal ulcer · keratitis · Pannus

14.1 Introduction

Keratitis is the most common ophthalmic manifestation of Herpes Simplex Virus (HSV). HSV keratitis can manifest in several distinct clinical forms, each defined by distinct pathogenic mechanisms and variable therapeutic responses. Traditionally, HSV keratitis has been classified using morphological descriptors such as dendritic, geographic, immune stromal, disciform, or necrotizing keratitis. However, these descriptions, while visually distinctive, may not reflect the underlying pathogenic mechanisms, leading to diagnostic and therapeutic errors. An alternative and clinically useful approach is to classify HSV keratitis based on the predominantly involved corneal layer—epithelial, stromal, or endothelial. This anatomical classification correlates better with disease pathogenesis and may

S. Nair (✉) · A. A. Salam
Dr R P Centre for Ophthalmic Sciences, AIIMS, New Delhi, India

B. Sharma et al. (eds.), *Viral Keratitis*, https://doi.org/10.1007/978-981-95-3148-6_14

more accurately guide therapeutic decisions [1]. Viral marginal keratitis is a less common but distinct manifestation of HSV epithelial keratitis, characterized by peripheral location and a mixed infectious-immune pathology.

14.2 Epidemiology

While specific incidence rates for the marginal subtype are not isolated in epidemiologic studies, HSV ocular infections in general impose a substantial global burden. Pooled data indicate 1.0 to 1.5 million new ocular HSV cases occur each year worldwide, with about nine million recurrent cases annually [1–3]. Incidence varies by region: in high-income countries, the annual incidence of ocular HSV (new and recurrent) ranges from roughly 4 to 31 per 100,000 people based on studies in the United States and Europe [4–6]. HSV keratitis remains the most common cause of unilateral infectious corneal blindness in developed nations. Studies from India indicate a prevalence of 0.53–7.8% in a hospital-based population [7, 8]. Marginal herpetic keratitis is a less common and clinically underrecognized subtype of HSV epithelial keratitis, with its exact prevalence being poorly documented.

14.3 Pathophysiology

Viral marginal keratitis represents a form of infectious epithelial keratitis caused by active HSV replication. It typically results from reactivation of HSV-1 in the trigeminal ganglion with centrifugal spread of the virus to the cornea. Unlike classic central dendritic ulcers, marginal lesions occur near the limbus. The combination of active viral infection in the peripheral corneal epithelium and the proximity to limbal vasculature triggers a robust immune response. Neutrophils and lymphocytes from limbal vessels infiltrate the cornea and manifest as anterior stromal infiltrates underlying the area of viral ulceration. Thus, the lesion has a dual nature: an infectious epithelial ulcer and an immune-mediated stromal necrosis and degradation [9, 10].

14.4 Risk Factors

A history of previous herpetic keratitis is often present in patients with marginal keratitis. However in some cases, the marginal ulcer may be the initial presentation of ocular HSV infection. Immunocompromised individuals, particularly those with advanced HIV/AIDS, have a predilection for peripheral HSV lesions often with bilateral involvement. These cases often require prolonged therapy and may demonstrate atypical or aggressive features [11]. HSV marginal keratitis has also been reported in patients suffering from autoimmune disorders wherein the systemic immunosuppression has been hypothesized to reactivate the latent HSV [12].

14.5 Clinical Features

HSV marginal keratitis commonly presents as a unilateral, sectoral red eye with peripheral corneal involvement. The marginal ulcer starts as an ulcer due to the breakdown of virus-laden epithelium and is followed by the infiltrate as the disease progresses, although both are usually seen at time of presentation. The disease is characterized by epithelial and superficial stromal infiltration, proximity to limbus, and accompanying vascularization. Patients typically are more symptomatic than those with central dendritic ulcers because of intense inflammation associated with peripheral location. They have symptoms of pain, redness, tearing, and foreign body sensation. Slit-lamp examination typically reveals a marginal epithelial ulcer, which may exhibit the classical dendritic pattern overlying the stromal infiltrate, but in some patients the ulcer may lack the dendritic shape. The lesions usually stain positively with fluorescein and may display terminal bulbs when dendritic in shape. These epithelial defects are frequently associated with underlying anterior stromal infiltrates, indicating a localized immune response. The ulcer is often located adjacent to an area of pronounced limbal conjunctival injection and may have associated new blood vessel at the corneal periphery. Corneal sensations are usually reduced at the site of the marginal lesions [10, 13]. Atypical presentations of viral marginal keratitis resembling peripheral ulcerative keratitis (PUK) has been reported in patients with autoimmune disorders [9, 12]. Peripheral stromal infiltrates and PUK-like picture have been rarely reported in Herpes Zoster Ophthalmicus, but classic viral marginal keratitis remains primarily a manifestation of HSV.

14.6 Diagnosis

The diagnosis of HSV keratitis—including marginal keratitis—is primarily a clinical one, based on history and slit-lamp findings. However, confirmation is useful especially in atypical or peripheral presentations. In practice, it is recommended to initiate treatment for presumed herpetic keratitis if the exam is characteristic, without waiting for lab confirmation. Characteristic features that support a clinical diagnosis of viral marginal keratitis include a unilateral peripheral ulcer with dendritic edges, associated limbal injection, decreased corneal sensation, and history of HSV. In such cases laboratory tests may not be necessary as false-negatives can occur and delays in treatment can worsen outcomes. In atypical or severe cases, or if the ulcer does not respond to initial therapy, diagnostic testing is indicated. Traditional methods include corneal scrapings for viral culture and cytology (e.g. Giemsa or Papanicolaou stains to detect multinucleated giant cells or inclusion bodies). Viral culture has high specificity but moderate sensitivity if the sample is collected early before initiating antivirals. Corneal scraping also helps rule out other infectious aetiologies. Polymerase chain reaction (PCR) assays can detect HSV DNA from cornel scraping, tear film, or anterior chamber fluid. The detection rate with corneal scraping was found to be significantly higher than tear fluid [14]. Studies have also shown PCR to be more sensitive than culture and immunofluorescence assay [15].

In a recent study involving 240 clinically diagnosed cases of herpetic keratitis, tear-film RT-PCR demonstrated an overall sensitivity of 31.6% across all forms of HSK. Notably, the sensitivity reached 97.4% for cases classified as epithelial keratitis [16]. Newer point-of-care tests such as an immunochromatographic HSV antigen detection kit have been developed with moderate sensitivity and high specificity for diagnosing HSV epithelial keratitis but these are not yet widespread [17]. Serology is generally not helpful as most adults will have HSV-1 antibodies. Clinical judgement remains paramount, with lab tests serving to confirm HSV in ambiguous cases or when the response to treatment is poor.

14.7 Differential Diagnosis

The most important differential diagnosis of viral marginal keratitis is staphylococcal marginal keratitis, an immune-mediated condition associated with blepharitis and staphylococcal antigen exposure. With staphylococcal marginal infiltrates, there is a lucid interval between the limbus and the infiltrate with minimal vascularization. Misdiagnosis is critical to avoid, as initiating topical corticosteroids in presumed staphylococcal marginal keratitis without concurrent antiviral coverage, in the presence of HSV, can lead to rapid progression of the ulcer and potentially sight-threatening complications. The lesion progresses centrally with ulceration and subepithelial infiltration. This central progression has the dendritic pattern and can aid in diagnosis.

Table 14.1 Differential diagnosis of marginal Keratitis

Feature	Viral marginal Keratitis	Staphylococcal marginal Keratitis	Autoimmune Peripheral Ulcerative Keratitis (PUK)
Aetiology	HSV-1 epithelial infection with stromal immune component	Type III hypersensitivity to staphylococcal antigens	Immune complex-mediated vasculitis
Location	Peripheral, near limbus	Peripheral, along lid margin (2, 4, 8, and 10 o'clock meridians) where the lid margins are in contact with ocular surface	Peripheral, often crescentic and progressive
Ulcer morphology	Dendritic/non-dendritic/ geographic epithelial ulcer epithelial ulceration followed by stromal infiltration. Progresses often, towards Centre	Typically stromal infiltrates occur first followed by epithelial defect. Progression uncommon, usually peripheral. Lucid interval between the limbus and the infiltrate	Stromal melt with epithelial defect. Usually progresses towards Centre with an overhanging edge.
Progression	Progresses centrally	Spread circumferentially but not centrally	Peripherally can advance centrally
Corneal sensation	Decreased	Normal	Normal or decreased in long-standing cases
Systemic/ ocular association	Viral recurrences	Blepharitis	Rheumatoid arthritis, GPA, SLE
Blepharitis	Not associated with blepharitis	Almost always accompanied by blepharitis	Not associated with blepharitis
Response to steroids	Worsens without antivirals	Rapid improvement	Requires systemic immunosuppression
HSV PCR	Positive	Negative	Negative

Other causes of peripheral ulcerative keratitis (PUK), including autoimmune and collagen vascular diseases, should also be considered in refractory or atypical cases [18]. Table 14.1 details the important features that help differentiate viral marginal keratitis from other peripheral keratitis. Figure 14.1 depicts the clinical spectrum of marginal keratitis.

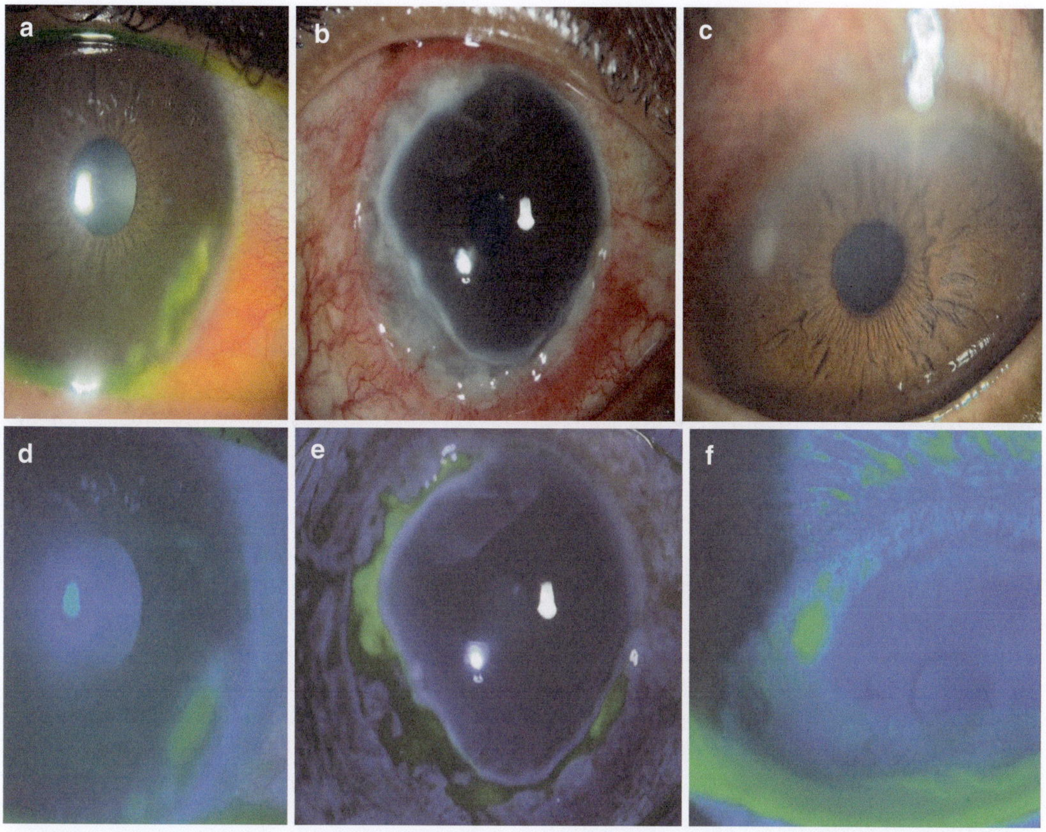

Fig. 14.1 Clinical spectrum of peripheral corneal ulcers. (**a, d**) *Viral marginal keratitis* showing a peripheral dendritiform epithelial ulcer with underlying stromal infiltrate and adjacent limbal injection. (**b**, **e**) *Peripheral ulcerative keratitis (PUK)* with crescentic peripheral stromal thinning and characteristic overhanging ulcer edge.(**c, f**) *Staphylococcal marginal keratitis* presenting with peripheral infiltrates and overlying epithelial defect near the limbus, associated with adjacent conjunctival injection and lucid interval between the infiltrates and limbus

14.8 Treatment

Treatment of viral marginal keratitis, as described in classical literature, requires careful differentiation from other causes of peripheral corneal ulceration and a more nuanced approach than that of central HSV epithelial keratitis. Marginal herpetic ulcers often exhibit a longer clinical course and reduced responsiveness to antiviral therapy alone, likely due to the prominent immune-mediated component resulting from proximity to the limbal vasculature, in addition to viral replication. The treatment must address both the active viral replication and the immune-mediated stromal response, must be aggressive and appropriately prolonged to prevent recurrence or progression [10].

The cornerstone of treatment is antiviral medication to halt HSV replication in the cornea. Topical antivirals are effective in marginal keratitis and agents such as topical acyclovir 3% ointment or ganciclovir 0.15% gel, are prescribed frequently (5×/day) for about 7–14 days or until complete epithelial healing. Oral antivirals such as acyclovir 400 mg (5×/day) or valacyclovir 500 mg (2×/day) or Famciclovir 250 mg (2×/day) are initiated along with topical antivirals for 7–10 days followed by a prophylactic dose that is continued especially when topical steroids are given or in recurrent cases.

Topical corticosteroids are indicated in the presence of significant stromal infiltration or persistent limbal inflammation but must be introduced with caution and always under concurrent antiviral coverage. Close monitoring is essential to prevent complications such as stromal melt or extension of the ulcer into the visual axis. Loteprednol 0.5% or Fluorometholone 0.1% eye drops in tapering doses till the resolution of ulcer is recommended under antiviral cover.

Supportive measures include cycloplegic drops (to reduce pain from ciliary spasm), lubrication, and prophylactic antibiotic ointment (to prevent bacterial superinfection of the ulcer). If a corneal thinning is advanced and perforation is imminent despite medical therapy, surgical interventions such as tissue adhesive or a patch graft may be required as a last resort. Figure 14.2 summarizes the management approach to a case of suspected viral marginal keratitis.

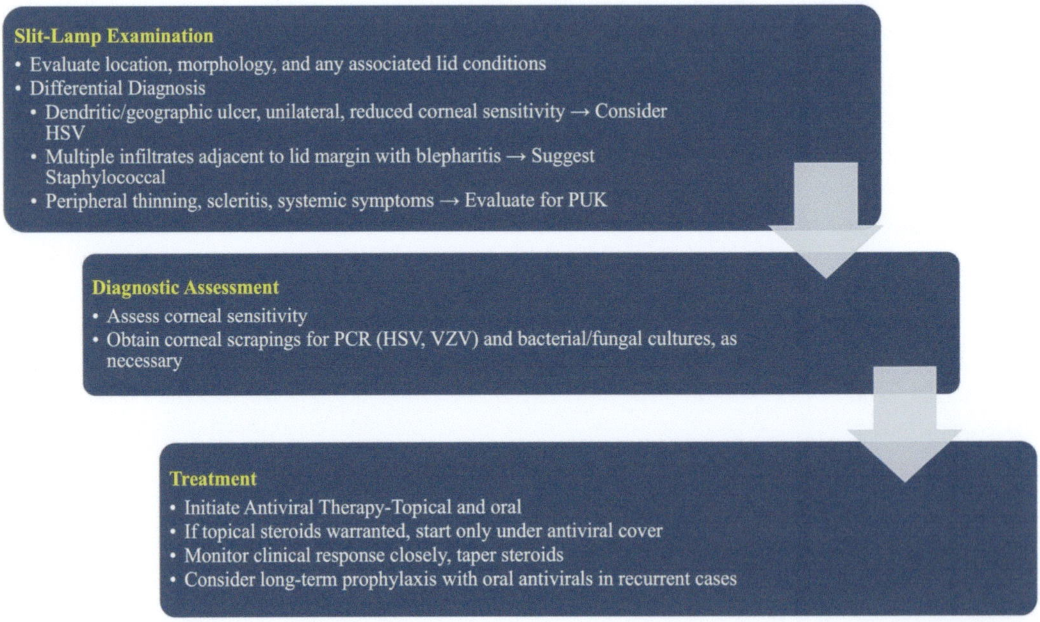

Fig. 14.2 Flowchart outlining the clinical evaluation, diagnosis, and management of viral marginal keratitis

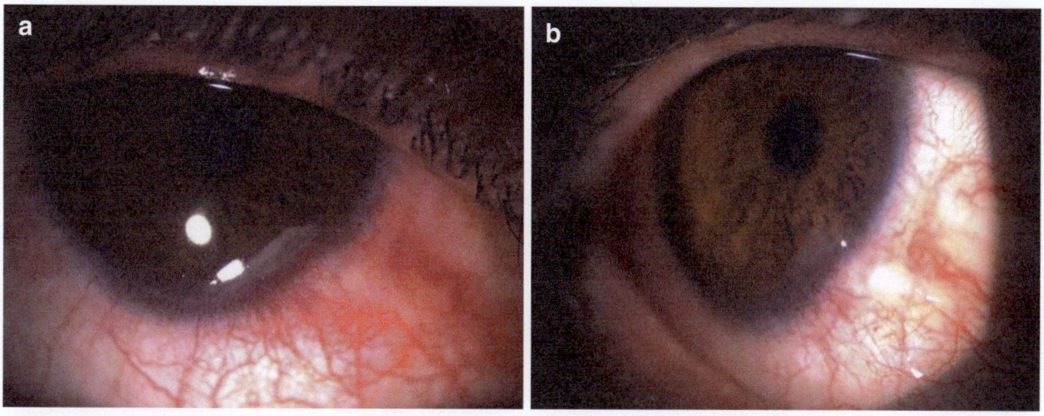

Fig. 14.3 (**a**) Slit-lamp image showing marginal keratitis with peripheral dense stromal infiltration with neovascularization. Note the absence of clear intervening area between lesion and limbus. (**b**). Post-treatment resolution of stromal infiltrates with residual tuft of neo vessels in peripheral cornea

14.9 Prognosis

With prompt and appropriate therapy, most cases of viral marginal keratitis resolve within a few weeks without permanent visual impairment, especially when the lesion is confined to the periphery (Fig. 14.3). However, delayed diagnosis or inappropriate use of corticosteroids can lead to central extension of the ulcer, stromal thinning, or scarring. Recurrences are not uncommon and warrant consideration of long-term antiviral prophylaxis in selected cases.

14.10 Conclusion

Viral marginal keratitis remains a clinically important but often underrecognized variant of HSV keratitis. Its peripheral location, mixed infectious–immune pathogenesis, and potential for misdiagnosis necessitate a high index of suspicion and tailored therapy. Early diagnosis, appropriate use of antivirals, cautious corticosteroid administration under cover, and close follow-up are essential to achieving favourable outcomes. With increasing access to molecular diagnostics and greater awareness of atypical HSV presentations, clinicians are better equipped than ever to manage this nuanced condition effectively and preserve visual function.

Key Points

1. Viral marginal keratitis is caused by an immune-mediated response to replicating viral antigens in the cornea, triggering a local inflammatory reaction.
2. The diagnosis of this entity is clinical with characteristic peripheral corneal epithelial defect followed by an anterior stromal infiltrate without a lucid interval from limbus.
3. Treatment should include topical antiviral along with topical steroid to address both active viral replication and the immune-mediated stromal response.

References

1. Chodosh J, Ung L. Adoption of innovation in Herpes Simplex Virus Keratitis. Cornea. 2020;39(Suppl 1(1)):S7–18.
2. Farooq AV, Shukla D. Herpes simplex epithelial and stromal keratitis: an epidemiologic update. Surv Ophthalmol. 2012 Sep;57(5):448–62.
3. Liesegang TJ. Herpes simplex virus epidemiology and ocular importance. Cornea. 2001 Jan;20(1):1–13.
4. Pepose JS, Keadle TL, Morrison LA. Ocular herpes simplex: changing epidemiology, emerging disease patterns, and the potential of vaccine prevention and therapy. Am J Ophthalmol. 2006 Mar;141(3):547–57.
5. Young RC, Hodge DO, Liesegang TJ, Baratz KH. Incidence, recurrence, and outcomes of herpes simplex virus eye disease in Olmsted County, Minnesota, 1976–2007: the effect of oral anti-

viral prophylaxis. Arch Ophthalmol. 2010 Sep;128(9):1178–83.

6. McCormick I, James C, Welton NJ, Mayaud P, Turner KME, Gottlieb SL, et al. Incidence of herpes simplex virus Keratitis and other ocular disease: global review and estimates. Ophthalmic Epidemiol. 2022 Aug;29(4):353–62.
7. Pramod NP, Rajendran P, Kannan KA, Thyagarajan SP. Herpes simplex keratitis in South India: clinico-virological correlation. Jpn J Ophthalmol. 1999;43(4):303–7.
8. Khurana AK, Gutain HR, Parmar IP. Regional hospital prevalence of viral keratitis. Indian J Ophthalmol. 1984;32(4):205–8.
9. Zaher SS, Sandinha T, Roberts F, Ramaesh K. Herpes simplex keratitis misdiagnosed as rheumatoid arthritis-related peripheral ulcerative keratitis. Cornea. 2005 Nov;24(8):1015–7.
10. Dawson CR. Ocular herpes simplex virus infections. Clin Dermatol. 1984;2(2):56–66.
11. Young TL, Robin JB, Holland GN, Hendricks RL, Paschal JF, Engstrom RE, et al. Herpes simplex keratitis in patients with acquired immune deficiency syndrome. Ophthalmology. 1989 Oct;96(10):1476–9.
12. Praidou A, Androudi S, Kanonidou E, Konidaris V, Alexandridis A, Brazitikos P. Bilateral herpes simplex keratitis presenting as peripheral ulcerative keratitis. Cornea. 2012 May;31(5):570–1.
13. Kekan M, Farooqui JH. Marginal epithelial herpes simplex virus keratitis-There is more than meets the "eye.". J Fr Ophtalmol. 2021 May;44(5):764–5.
14. Acharya M, Dave A, Farooqui JH. Commentary: herpes keratitis: a diagnostic challenge. Indian J Ophthalmol. 2019 Jul;67(7):1046–7.
15. Satpathy G, Mishra AK, Tandon R, Sharma MK, Sharma A, Nayak N, et al. Evaluation of tear samples for herpes simplex virus 1 (HSV) detection in suspected cases of viral keratitis using PCR assay and conventional laboratory diagnostic tools. Br J Ophthalmol. 2011 Mar;95(3):415–8.
16. Hoarau G, Haigh O, Vauloup-Fellous C, Boucher R, Rouquette A, Faure P, et al. Diagnostic performance of real-time quantitative PCR in tear samples in various subtypes of herpes simplex keratitis. J Clin Microbiol. 2023;61(12):e0088523.
17. Inoue Y, Shimomura Y, Fukuda M, Miyazaki D, Ohashi Y, Sasaki H, et al. Multicentre clinical study of the herpes simplex virus immunochromatographic assay kit for the diagnosis of herpetic epithelial keratitis. Br J Ophthalmol. 2013 Sep;97(9):1108–12.
18. Yagci A. Update on peripheral ulcerative keratitis. Clin Ophthalmol. 2012;6:747–54.

Keratouveitis

15

Bhavana Sharma, Parul Mittal,
and Jeewan Singh Titiyal

Abstract

Among the viruses, herpes simplex keratitis is likely the most common ocular condition associated with uveitis. It typically presents as a painful, red eye, accompanied by photophobia and decreased vision. Frequently, patients with HSV stromal keratitis have simultaneous anterior uveitis. Patients with a history of epithelial herpes infection may also develop anterior uveitis, even in the absence of active corneal lesions. Recurrent episodes of anterior uveitis are common, which can complicate to secondary glaucoma and vision loss. This chapter provides a detailed overview of HSV keratouveitis, including its pathogenesis, clinical features, differential diagnosis, investigations, and management.

Keywords

HSV Keratouveitis · hypertensive anterior uveitis · Herpetic iridocyclitis

B. Sharma · P. Mittal
AIIMS Bhopal, Bhopal, Madhya Pradesh, India

J. S. Tityal (✉)
R P Centre, AIIMS Delhi, New Delhi, India

15.1 Introduction

Herpes simplex virus type 1 can cause keratitis associated with anterior uveitis following reactivation in the trigeminal ganglion [1]. Herpes simplex virus (HSV) associated uveitis is a common cause of unilateral keratitis and hypertensive anterior uveitis. Anterior uveitis is more common during reactivation than primary disease. Herpetic anterior uveitis causes approximately 5–10% of uveitis cases [2]. HSV keratouveitis is more common in patients in their 40 s–50 s, affecting both genders equally [1]. Patients may have a history of cold sores or fever blisters. Systemic immunosuppression is associated with a higher risk of HSV reactivation. Keratouveitis and iritis are uncommon manifestations of primary HSV ocular infection. In a study of a large population in the Northern California region of Kaiser Permanente, iritis was the presenting sign in 1% of patients with an initial episode of HSV eye disease [3].

HSV Keratouveitis presents as immune stromal keratitis or endotheliitis, along with iridocyclitis. However, iridocyclitis may occur as an isolated finding as well. Additionally, inflammation of the trabecular meshwork causes trabeculitis, which results in acute elevation of intraocular pressure. Chronic inflammation can lead to secondary glaucoma from inflammatory cells blocking the aqueous outflow pathway. Patients may also present with corneal ghost scarring and concomitant iridocyclitis indicative of previous infectious keratitis.

B. Sharma et al. (eds.), *Viral Keratitis*, https://doi.org/10.1007/978-981-95-3148-6_15

15.2 Pathophysiology

HSV keratouveitis is caused due to live virus replication since viruses have been isolated from the anterior chamber of patients. Primary HSV-1 infection is associated with an immune response mediated by mononuclear inflammatory cells, primarily composed of T cells in addition to plasma cells, macrophages, and natural killer cells. These inflammatory cells, in addition to mediators like MHC-1 and TGF-β1, can downregulate IFN-γ-induced MHC-2 expression, which consequently allows HSV-1 to evade immune detection after reactivation and subsequent keratouveal inflammation [4]. The immunopathology of the development and progression of HSV-induced anterior uveitis is described in the Flow diagram 15.1.

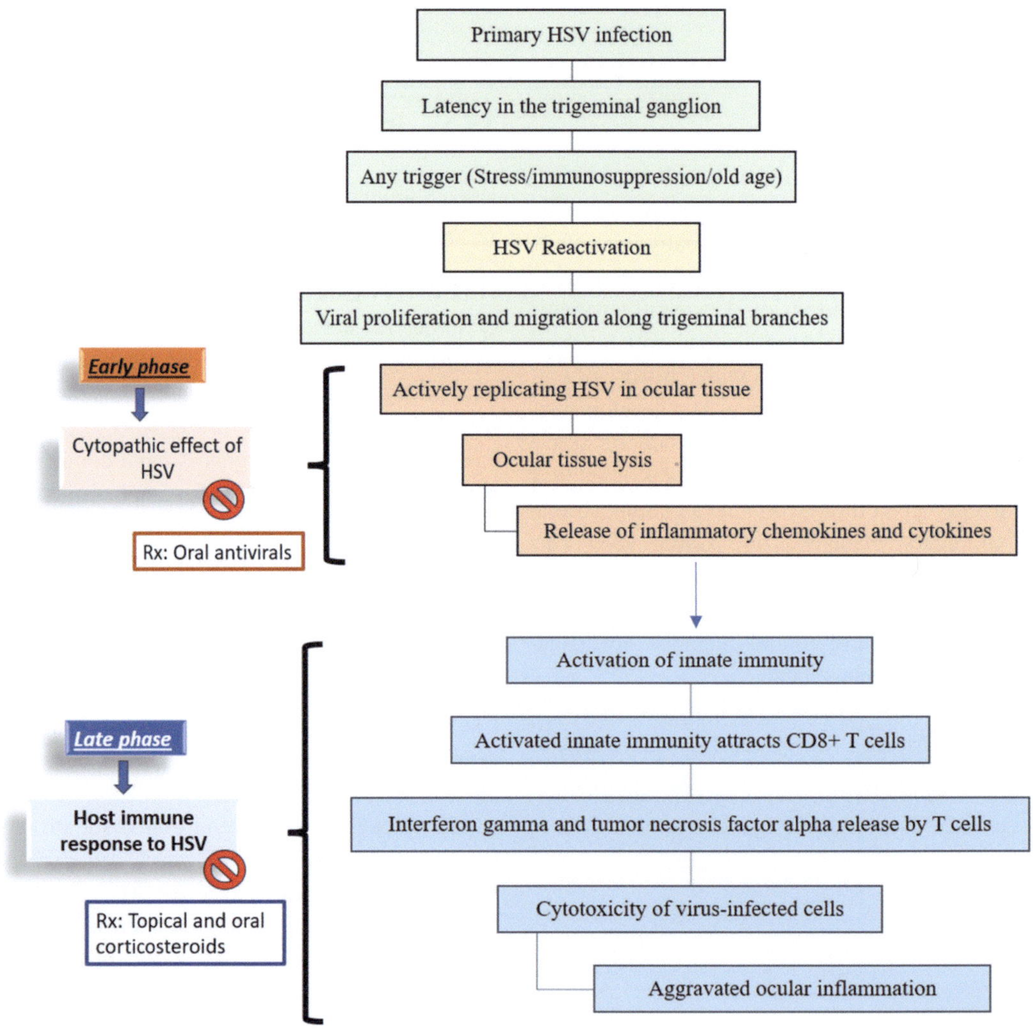

Flow diagram 15.1 Immunopathology of Herpes Simplex anterior uveitis

15.3 Clinical Features

15.3.1 Symptoms

In patients with keratouveitis, pain, photophobia, and decreased vision are seen because of keratitis and corneal oedema. Additionally, patients present with signs and symptoms typical of iridocyclitis, including blurring or diminution of vision, redness, photophobia, pain, and watering [5]. If there is an accompanying high IOP, headache, eye pain, and coloured haloes due to corneal oedema may be seen. However, in cases with significant damage to the fifth cranial nerve, from prior episodes of HSV, the patient may not have significant pain.

15.3.2 Signs

Patients present with keratitis and iritis with features comprising of epithelial and/or stromal oedema, stromal keratitis, keratic precipitates, endotheliitis, along with iridocyclitis [6, 7]. Keratic precipitates can be granulomatous, non-granulomatous (Fig. 15.1a), or stellate. They are usually seen as a cluster on the endothelial surface, underlying a localized corneal oedema (Figs. 15.2 and 15.3). Furthermore, they can be seen in the inferior one-third of the cornea (Fig. 15.1b, c) or diffusely distributed as stellate KP. The presence of patchy iris transillumination defects is an important diagnostic feature (Fig. 15.4); however, the absence of transillumination defects does not rule it out. Slit-lamp examination reveals fine KP, anterior chamber pigment dispersion and cells/flare of varying severity. Sectoral iris atrophy due to ischemic necrosis of the iris stroma may be seen [8]. Chronic cases may develop posterior synechiae in addition to hyphema and fibrinous exudate in the anterior chamber. Other features comprise corneal hypoesthesia and concomitant raised IOP [9].

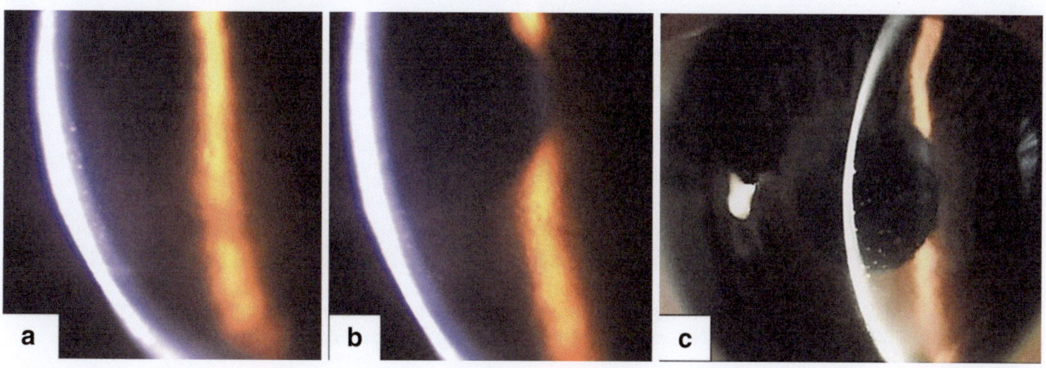

Fig. 15.1 (**a, b**) Slit-lamp image showing (**a**) medium-sized keratic precipitates. (**b**, **c**) Inferior distribution in Arlt's triangle

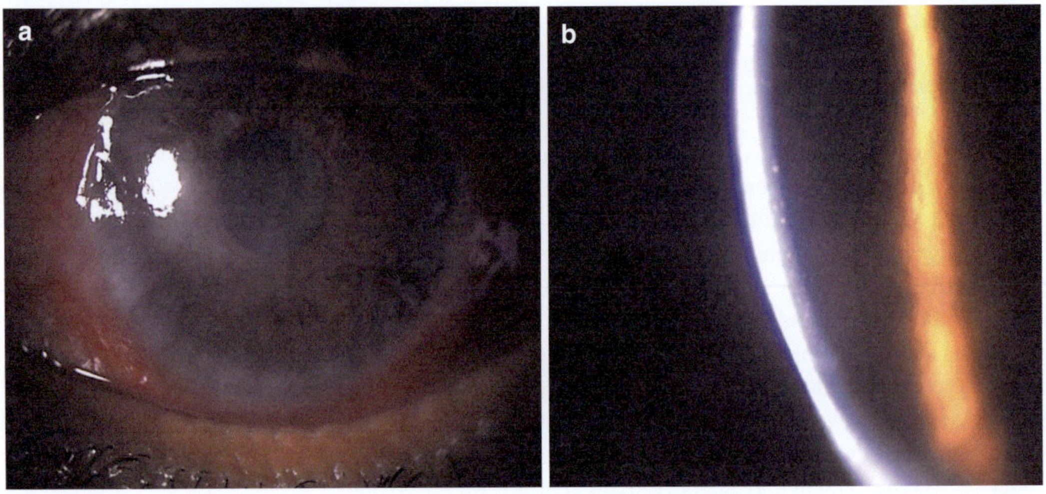

Fig. 15.2 (**a, b**) Slit-lamp image showing HSV keratouveitis with stromal infiltrates and oedema, uveal pigment dispersion, and keratic precipitates

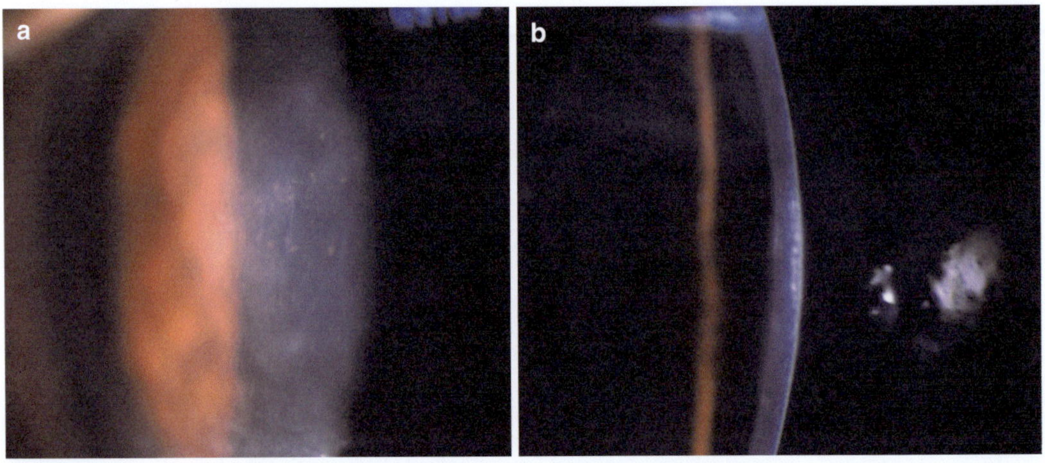

Fig. 15.3 (**a, b**) HSV keratouveitis showing stromal infiltrates, oedema, and uveal pigment dispersion over involved area. (**b**) Slit beam depicts stromal oedema and subepithelial scarring in corneal decompensation

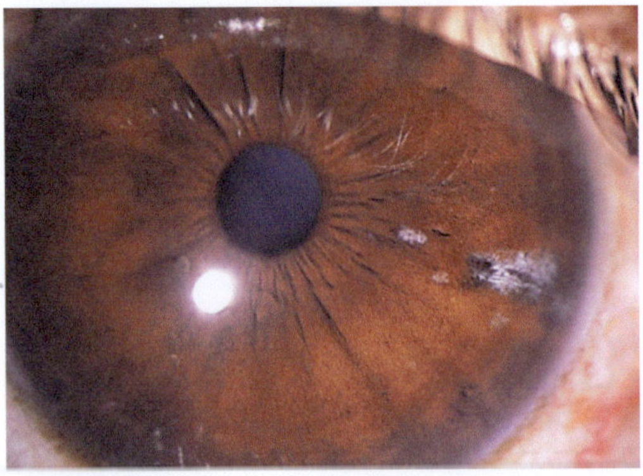

Fig. 15.4 Slit-lamp image showing patchy iris atrophy in a case of HSV keratouveitis

15.4 Differential Diagnosis

The disease entity should be differentiated from Fuchs heterochromic iridocyclitis, Posner–Schlossman syndrome, CMV, and VZV-induced uveitis. The potential diagnosis of Posner-Schlossman syndrome needs to be carefully considered, especially when clinical exam findings demonstrate episodes of anterior chamber cell with extremely elevated IOP, with quiescence and normal IOP in between episodes. Some studies have suggested HSV as a possible infectious etiology for Posner-Schlossman syndrome, although cytomegalovirus is also implicated. Fine, stellate KPs along with mild anterior chamber cells are also associated with Fuchs heterochromic iridocyclitis (FHI), and there has been evidence to suggest that HSV (and other infectious etiologies) may potentially cause FHI. In FHI, there may be prominent iris and angle vessels visible due to iris atrophy. The differentiating features are described in Table 15.1.

Table 15.1 Differential diagnosis of HSV anterior uveitis [10, 11]

Clinical features	HSV anterior uveitis	VZV anterior uveitis	CMV anterior uveitis	Fuchs heterochromic iridocyclitis	Posner-Schlossman syndrome
Onset & severity	Acute, recurrent, severe	Acute	Acute	Chronic & mild	Acute, recurrent, mild
Symptoms	Painful red eye, blurred vision, photophobia	Same as HSV	Same as HSV	Usually, asymptomatic	Blurred vision, photophobia, coloured haloes
Laterality	Unilateral > bilateral	Unilateral	Unilateral	Unilateral	Unilateral
Keratic precipitates (KPs)	Diffuse medium-large mutton fat KPs, sometimes stellate	Same as HSV	Focal small ring or coin-shaped KPs, Circinate pattern	Diffuse fine, stellate KPs	Small white KPs inferiorly
Iris findings	Small patchy iris atrophy (round or scalloped)	Sectoral > patchy iris atrophy	Diffuse iris atrophy	Radial transillumination defects, iris heterochromia	May have iris atrophy and thinning
Posterior synechiae	Present	Present	Rare	Absent	Absent
IOP	High	High	High	Can be normal or high	Markedly high but transient
Other features	Prior episode or active HSV keratitis Candy—cane hypopyon	Periorbital HZO lesions, pigmentation, or scars	Endothelitis with reduction in endothelial cells	No ciliary injection Prominent iris and angle vessels	No ciliary injection Depigmentation of trabecular area

15.5 Diagnosis

Clinical diagnosis aided by detailed slit-lamp evaluation remains the most important diagnostic modality. However, viral culture is advised for definitive diagnosis. Specimen should be subjected to culture in the early course of the disease to ensure viral adequacy. Viral isolates may then be identified as HSV-1 or HSV-2 [12, 13]. Cytologic examination of specimens stained with Giemsa or Wright stains showing multinucleated giant cells may be seen; however, this is a nonspecific test as giant cells may be seen in both VZV and HSV. Intranuclear inclusion bodies are considered more specific for herpesviruses [14]. The Herpchek, Virogen-latex agglutination, enzyme immunofiltration, and the 1-h enzyme-linked immunoassay can detect HSV antigen in cell culture and direct specimens [15]. Polymerase chain reaction (PCR) is another specific test for confirmation of viral DNA polymerase and viral thymidine kinase. The sample is taken from anterior chamber tap with a high sensitivity (91.3%) and specificity (98.8) [16]. Immunoblotting and enzyme-linked immunosorbent assay are other tests that can be employed for diagnosis.

15.6 Complications

Secondary open angle type glaucoma is a common complication of HSV iritis and can serve as a diagnostic hallmark. The IOP is high in the range of 50–60 mm Hg during an episode of acute iritis. This is to trabeculitis, as well as inflammatory cells clogging the trabecular meshwork. The mainstay of treatment is control of inflammation by topical/systemic steroids in addition to systemic antiviral drugs. Antiglaucoma therapy is required to control intraocular pressure, however, for a short duration till resolution of inflammation and IOP. Chronic and episodes of inflammation may cause peripheral anterior synechiae (PAS) leading to secondary angle closure type of glaucoma. Posterior synechiae may form in long standing cases [1]. Spontaneous hyphema can occur as well as layers of hyphema mixed with hypopyon, known as a candy-cane hypopyon is a characteristic involvement seen in HSV.

15.7 Management

Immune-mediated inflammation in HSV keratouveitis requires corticosteroids as the mainstay of treatment. Prednisolone 1% or Dexamethasone 0.1% eye drop in 6–8 times dosing per day can be given as per disease severity. In more severe cases, oral corticosteroids 1 mg/kg body weight may be given. Antiviral cover in the form of oral acyclovir, 400 mg five times a day, is used in addition to topical corticosteroids for control of infection. Steroids are recommended for slow tapering and may require long-term, low-dose topical corticosteroid therapy to control chronic inflammation.

IOP-lowering medications are required to control the inflammation-induced intraocular pressure rise. Both oral carbonic anhydrase inhibitors, topical beta-blockers, and alpha-adrenergic agonists can be prescribed; however, prostaglandin analogues are to be avoided in view of rebound inflammation. The pressure rise typically responds well to topical corticosteroids. Cycloplegic agents are to be used to decrease symptoms of photophobia and break posterior synechiae. Topical antiviral agents are of limited use in the treatment of HSV iritis, since these agents do not penetrate well into the anterior chamber with additional risk of surface toxicity.

Systemic antiviral agents, such as acyclovir, famciclovir, or valacyclovir, achieve optimum concentration in AC with rapid resolution of iritis. Systemic acyclovir, 400 mg five times per day for 1–2 weeks, followed by a maintenance dose of 400 mg three times for 2–4 weeks is the standard regimen. Valacyclovir, 1000 mg three times per day; famciclovir, 250 mg three times per day can also be given. Adequacy of renal function should be ensured during prolonged treatment of more than 4 weeks.

Long-term, low-dose, systemic antiviral therapy may be beneficial for some patients in order to decrease the frequency of recurrences of iritis. Oral doses for prophylaxis for ocular herpes simplex disease are acyclovir, 400 mg twice per day, or valacyclovir, 500–1000 mg daily.

15.8 Conclusion

HSV keratouveitis represents a significant cause of ocular morbidity, which, if untreated, can result in chronic inflammation, vision impairment, corneal scarring, and secondary glaucoma. Early diagnosis and prompt management are essential in preventing long-term visual sequelae. Antiviral therapy plays a key role in controlling the viral replication, while corticosteroids, when used judiciously, help to manage inflammation. However, challenges remain in addressing recurrent episodes and the potential for long-term complications.

Key Points

1. HSV is the most common cause of viral keratouveitis, and it can occur with or without active corneal lesions.
2. The characteristic clinical findings include a unilateral painful red eye with diffusely distributed KPs, anterior chamber cells, flare, and patchy iris atrophy.
3. HSV keratouveitis is one of the causes of hypertensive anterior uveitis.
4. Treatment includes oral acyclovir and topical corticosteroids to combat viral replication and immune-mediated inflammation during the early and late phases of the disease pathogenesis.
5. Recurrence can be minimized by prophylactic acyclovir (especially in high-risk cases).

References

1. Chan NSW, Chee SP. Demystifying viral anterior uveitis: a review. Clin Experiment Ophthalmol. 2019;47:320–33.
2. Rathinam SR, Namperumalsamy P. Global variation and pattern changes in epidemiology of uveitis. Indian J Ophthalmol. 2007;55:173–83.
3. Gritz DC, Wong IG. Incidence and prevalence of uveitis in Northern California; the Northern California epidemiology of uveitis study. Ophthalmology. 2004;111:491–500. discussion 500
4. Greenan E, Gallagher S, Khalil R, Murphy CC, Ní Gabhann-Dromgoole J. Advancing our understanding of corneal herpes simplex virus-1 immune evasion mechanisms and future therapeutics. Viruses. 2021;13(9):1856. https://doi.org/10.3390/v13091856. PMID: 34578437; PMCID: PMC8473450.
5. Azher TN, Yin XT, Tajfirouz D, Huang AJ, Stuart PM. Herpes simplex keratitis: challenges in diagnosis and clinical management. Clin Ophthalmol. 2017;11:185–91. https://doi.org/10.2147/OPTH.S80475. PMID: 28176902; PMCID: PMC5261835.
6. Sundmacher R. A clinico-virologic classification of herpetic anterior segment diseases with special reference to intraocular herpes. In: Sundmacher R, editor. Herpetische Augenerkrankungen [Internet]. Munich: J.F. Bergmann-Verlag; 1981. p. 203–10. [cited 2025 Apr 5] Available from: http://link.springer.com/10.1007/978-3-642-80499-1_34.
7. Ahonen R, Vannas A. Clinical comparison between herpes simplex and herpes zoster ocular infections. In: Maudgal PC, Missotten L, editors. Herpetic Eye Diseases [Internet]. Dordrecht: Springer; 1985. p. 389–94. ([cited 2025 Apr 5] Henkes HE, editor. Documenta Ophthalmologica Proceedings Series; vol. 44). Available from: http://link.springer.com/10.1007/978-94-009-5518-9_52.
8. Sun Y, Ji Y. A literature review on Fuchs uveitis syndrome: An update. Surv Ophthalmol. 2020;65(2):133–43. https://doi.org/10.1016/j.survophthal.2019.10.003. Epub 2019 Oct 14. PMID: 31622627.
9. Kardeş E, Bozkurt K, Sezgin Akçay Bİ, Ünlü C, Aydoğan Gezginaslan T, Ergin A. Clinical features and prognosis of herpetic anterior uveitis. Turk J Ophthalmol. 2016;46(3):109–13. https://doi.org/10.4274/tjo.92053. Epub 2016 Jun 6. PMID: 27800272; PMCID: PMC5076292.
10. Terada Y, Kaburaki T, Takase H, Goto H, Nakano S, Inoue Y, et al. Distinguishing features of anterior uveitis caused by herpes simplex virus, varicella-zoster virus, and cytomegalovirus. Am J Ophthalmol. 2021;227:191–200.
11. Sakai JI, Usui Y, Suzuki J, Kezuka T, Goto H. Clinical features of anterior uveitis caused by three different herpes viruses. Int Ophthalmol. 2019;39:2785–95.
12. Pavan-Langston D. Major ocular viral infections. In: Antiviral agents and viral diseases of man. New York: Raven Press; 1990. p. 183–233.
13. Athmanathan S, Bandlapally SR, Rao GN. Collection of corneal impression cytology directly on a sterile glass slide for the detection of viral antigen: an inexpensive and simple technique for the diagnosis of HSV epithelial keratitis – a pilot study. BMC Ophthalmol. 2001;1:3.
14. Kaplowitz LG, Baker D, Gelb L, Blythe J, Hale R, Frost P, et al. Prolonged continuous acyclovir treatment of normal adults with frequently recurring genital herpes simplex virus infection. The Acyclovir Study Group. JAMA. 1991;265:747–51.
15. Tullo AB. Herpes simplex Keratitis. Semin Ophthalmol. 1986;1:213–20.
16. Sugita S, Ogawa M, Shimizu N, Morio T, Ohguro N, Nakai K, et al. Use of a comprehensive polymerase chain reaction system for diagnosis of ocular infectious diseases. Ophthalmology. 2013;120:1761–8.

Section II

Herpes Zoster Eye Disease

Herpes Zoster Ophthalmicus

16

Amit Gupta, Anchal Thakur, and Fazal Mohd Khan

Abstract

Herpes Zoster Ophthalmicus (HZO) is a reactivation of the Varicella Zoster Virus (VZV) in the ophthalmic division (V1) of the trigeminal nerve, affecting the skin and ocular structures. It commonly occurs in older adults and immunocompromised individuals, presenting with a painful unilateral skin rash, often accompanied by ocular complications such as conjunctivitis, keratitis, uveitis, and glaucoma. Hutchinson's sign, indicating nasociliary nerve involvement, is a key predictor of severe ocular involvement. The pathophysiology involves viral reactivation from its latent state in sensory ganglia, leading to neural inflammation and damage, which contributes to post-herpetic neuralgia (PHN). Diagnosis is primarily clinical, with laboratory confirmation in atypical or immunosuppressed cases. Early antiviral therapy within 72 h of symptom onset reduces severity and complications. Topical antivirals, corticosteroids, and intraocular pressure management are essential for ocular involvement. Surgical interventions may be required for corneal complications and non-healing ulcers. Despite treatment, HZO can lead to long-term complications, including chronic ocular inflammation, vision loss, and post-herpetic neuralgia. Preventive measures such as vaccination in high-risk populations can significantly reduce disease incidence and severity.

Keywords

Herpes Zoster Ophthalmicus (HZO) · Varicella Zoster virus (VZV) · Trigeminal nerve · Post-herpetic neuralgia

16.1 Introduction

Varicella Zoster virus, also known as Human Alphaherpes virus 3, is one of the herpes virus commonly known as shingles, which can infect humans. The primary disease is the chicken pox which is caused by the same virus; however, after resolution of chicken pox, in approximately 20% of infected individuals virus becomes latent, in the dorsal root or cerebral ganglia with reactivation at a later time and development of herpes zoster (HZ) [1, 2]. Herpes Zoster Ophthalmicus is defined as reactivation of VZV (Varicella Zoster) in the ophthalmic division of the trigeminal nerve (V_1). It is characterized by a unilateral painful skin rash over the eye and ocular adnexa in one or more dermatome distributions of the trigeminal nerve and represents 10–20% of all zoster cases [3, 4]. Infection acquired from contact with patient of HZO causes the classical infec-

A. Gupta (✉) · A. Thakur
Advanced Eye Centre, PGIMER, Chandigarh, India

F. M. Khan
AIIMS Bhopal, Bhopal, India

B. Sharma et al. (eds.), *Viral Keratitis*, https://doi.org/10.1007/978-981-95-3148-6_16

tious "chicken pox" and not HZ. HZO occurs typically in older adults but can present at any age as a result of decreased immunity [2].

It can affect any age group with variable outcome; however, immunosuppressed individuals particularly have a complicated course. The ocular manifestations occur over wide distribution of trigeminal nerve including forehead, eyelids, conjunctiva, cornea, and other structures of anterior and posterior segment. The typical rash is the commonest manifestation of varicella, which, however, heals without scarring [2].

16.2 Incidence

HZO is considered a disease of increasing senescence, incidence being common in 6th to 9th decade. The relative incidence (incidence rate) of HZO in the general population in the world is reported as 1.4–15.9% (0.31–0.35 per 1000 person-years) [5, 6]. Higher incidence is also observed in people with lower immunity levels, or after major surgery, trauma, or radiation. This is to the tune of 10% in HIV and 3.2–11.3% in patients with haematological malignancies [7, 8]. Although, this disease was previously viewed as primarily a disease of the "West" although it has increasingly been reported in India over the last two decades. A recent observational study from India (1752 diagnosed HZO patients) has documented the prevalence rate of 0.058% (95%CI: ±0.0006%) or 58/100,000 population [9].

16.3 Pathophysiology

The virus reactivates from its latent state in the sensory neural ganglion as a result of decrease in immunity, multiplies within the nerve cells, and releases virions from the cells that are transported via the axons to the skin that the ganglion supplies [10]. The local immune response at the tissue level causes inflammation, in the form of skin vesicles or ocular inflammation depending on the tissues affected. Nerve involvement in the form of perineuritis causes intense pain along the nerve distribution.

Studies conducted by Rowbotham et al. propose that the peripheral sensory fibres do not die, but rather sustain axonal damage that gives rise to hyperexcitability, marked by spontaneous firing, exaggerated neural impulses in response to stimuli, and lower excitation threshold [11, 12]. Fewer axons in the affected dermatome or unchecked inflammatory response at the neuronal level leads to the development of pain. Paresthesia and segmental pain at the area supplied by trigeminal nerve may be seen before the onset of rash.

16.4 Risk Factors

Virulence of VZV and the immune status of the host are main factors in the development of HZO. The incidence and severity of herpes zoster increases with advancing age and in debilitating illnesses. An immunocompromised patient is more likely to have a prolonged illness, with systemic complications like myelitis and vasculopathy. The risk of herpes zoster is greater in men with HIV than in men without HIV [6]. One study showed that racial factors may play a role since elderly black patients were one fourth as likely as elderly white patients to develop herpes zoster [7].

16.5 Clinical Presentation

HZO exhibits a prodromal phase of fever, malaise, headache, and eye pain prior to the eruption of the skin rash, with severe pain in the distribution of the trigeminal nerve. The patient may describe heaviness over eyes, tearing, redness, or decreasing vision.

Zoster manifests as a painful vesicular dermatitis localized to a single dermatomal distribution on the thorax or face. In the initial period (2–3 days), there is maculopapular rash, followed by vesicles and then pustules. The classical "Hutchinson sign" is described when there is involvement of the tip of the nose, indicating the nasociliary branch involvement and much higher risk of ocular manifestations (Fig. 16.1a, b). The

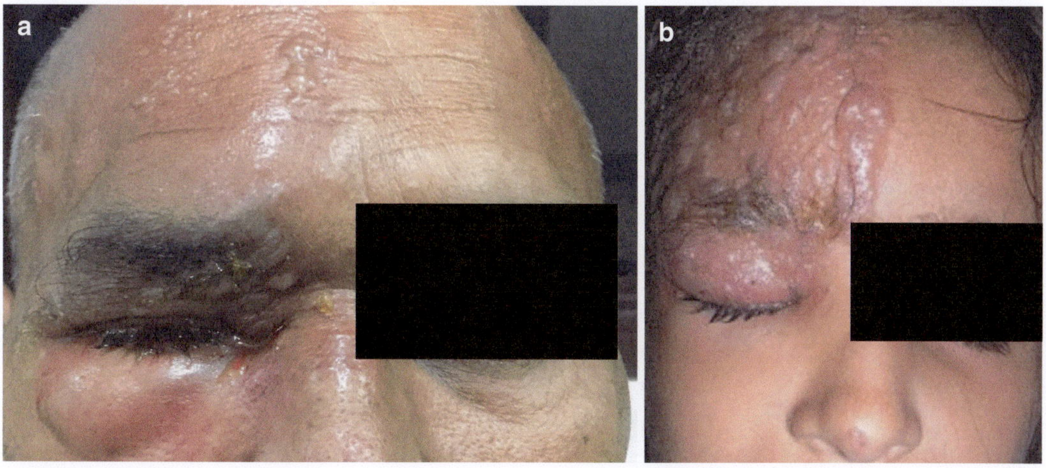

Fig. 16.1 (**a**) Herpes zoster skin vesicular eruption with classical involvement of tip of the nose (Hutchinson sign). (**b**) Herpes zoster skin vesicular eruption with classical involvement of the tip of nose (Hutchinson sign) in a 8-year-old immunocompetent patient

skin vesicles continue to form over 3–4 days eventually lasting 6–7 days, following which there is crust formation. Depending on the depth of dermal involvement and the presence of a secondary bacterial infection, healing of the skin lesions vary from skin scars or slight pigmentation to significant scar contracture with eyelid margins deformation and consequently development of trichiasis, ectropion, entropion, or even lagophthalmos [13, 14]. Unlike Varicella (Chicken pox), HZO skin vesicles are all in same phase at any time and often heal with scarring (Fig. 16.2).

In atypical cases of HZ sine herpete patients show variable symptoms, such as pain over dermatomal distribution, fever, constitutional symptoms, or neuralgia, however with minimal rash over the involved dermatomal area, which makes clinical diagnosis difficult (Fig. 16.3). The misdiagnosis or delayed diagnosis of sine herpete and consequent delayed antiviral treatment may lead to severe sequelae.

The pain decreases as the lesions resolve but the neuralgia can be present for months together [15]. The severity of pain ranges from mild to incapacitating. Patients complain of a prodrome of fever, malaise, redness, and increased sensation in the involved dermatome [16]. Paresthesia and segmental pain at the area supplied by trigeminal nerve may be noted before the onset of rash.

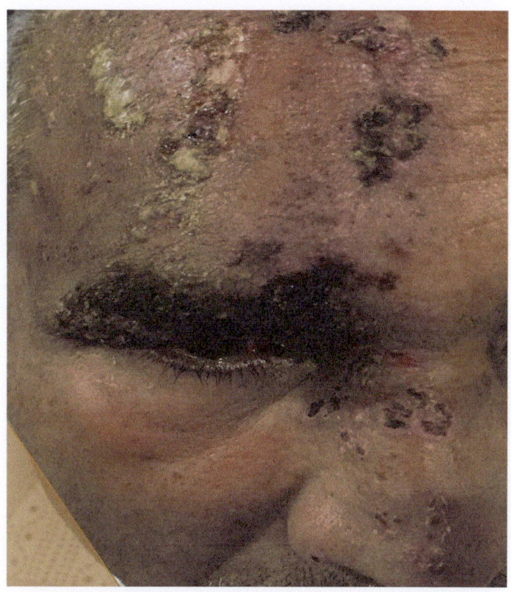

Fig. 16.2 A patient with Herpes Zoster Ophthalmicus on day 10 shows crusting and scab formation, indicating evolution of the disease and possible secondary bacterial infection of the skin lesions on the left part of the forehead

16.5.1 Ocular

Herpes zoster can have ocular involvement as listed in Table 16.1.

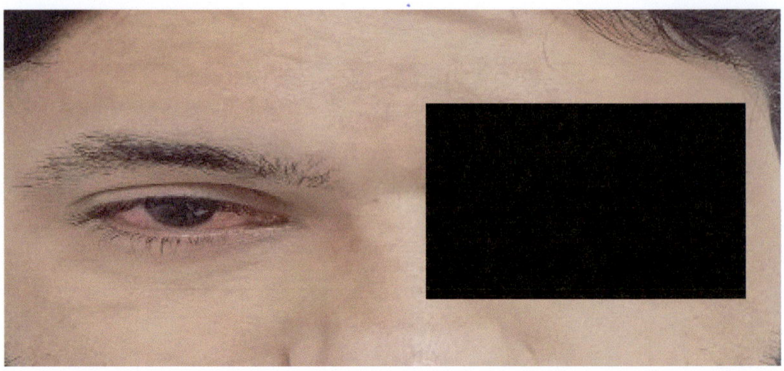

Fig. 16.3 Herpes Zoster sine herpete with minimal rash and acute conjunctivitis

Table 16.1 showing ocular involvement in HZO

Orbit	Orbital apex syndrome
Lid and adnexa	Blepharitis—secondary infection with *Staphylococcus aureus* Vesicular lid eruption Cicatricial entropion with or without trichiasis Cicatricial ectropion Canaliculitis Ptosis Dacryoadenitis
Conjunctiva	Hyperemic follicular conjunctivitis (rare) Papillary conjunctivitis Petechial haemorrhagic conjunctivitis Vesicular conjunctivitis Conjunctival edema Cicatricial conjunctival changes
Cornea (65% of HZO patients)	Acute epithelial keratitis Coarse punctate keratitis "Pseudodendritic" keratitis ("zoster dendrites") Mucous plaques/Nummular anterior stromal keratitis Interstitial keratitis Fascicular vascularizing keratitis Serpiginous ulceration Disciform keratitis Corneal hypesthesia or anaesthesia; Neurotrophic keratitis, Corneal scars Calcific band keratopathy Lipid keratopathy Peripheral corneal ulceration
Sclera and Episclera	Scleritis Episcleritis
Anterior Chamber Angle	Glaucoma, secondary to trabeculitis or attendant steroids
Pupil	Adie's tonic pupil, Horner's syndrome
Uvea	Iritis Sectoral iris atrophy Iridocyclitis, occasionally "plastic" with hypopyon Anterior segment necrosis Choroiditis Panuveitis
Lens	Cataract, secondary to inflammation or attendant steroids
Vitreous and Retina	Retinitis or neuroretinitis Macular oedema Retinal vasculitis (Perivasculitis, arteritis and thrombophlebitis) Retinal detachment, exudative or rhegmatogenous Acute retinal necrosis (ARN) Progressive outer retinal necrosis (PORN)

Table 16.1 (continued)

Orbit	Orbital apex syndrome
Optic Nerve	Optic neuritis Retrobulbar neuritis Optic atrophy Papillitis and papilledema Neuroretinitis (papilledema and macular star)
Extraocular Muscles	Extraocular muscle palsies (ophthalmoplegia), myositis Ptosis Diplopia Exophthalmos Proptosis

16.6 Differential Diagnosis

HZO presents with characteristic clinical feature. However, other conditions that create vesicular rashes without severe pain comprise of contact dermatitis and vaccinia dermatitis. Differential diagnosis for ocular lesions are recurrent erosions, other infectious and non-infectious keratitis, corneal melts, and PUK. Additionally, other infectious and non-infectious entities of anterior and posterior segment can exhibit ocular inflammation in the aqueous, vitreous, optic nerve, retina, and choroid.

16.7 Diagnosis

The diagnosis of HZO is mainly a clinical diagnosis based on the characteristic signs and symptoms. However, laboratory testing may be warranted in immune suppressed individuals or with atypical features. Test samples are taken to detect herpetic viral antigen or nucleic acid from vesicular fluid or corneal samples.

The Tzanck smear is used to confirm multinucleated giant cells and the characteristic acidophilic intranuclear inclusions in material scraped from the cornea or the base of a vesicle. The giant cells are due to epithelial cell fusion that is mediated by viral glycoproteins.

Immunofluorescence, polymerase chain reaction, and ELISA are other sensitive tests which can detect small amount of viral particles. Fluorescent-antibody-to-membrane antigen test (FAMA) is the most reliable test for VZV-specific antibodies.

16.8 Complications

Zoster skin manifestations involving the deep dermis can result in lagophthalmos, lid scarring, ectropion, and entropion. Severe disease, immunosuppressed state, or inappropriate treatment can cause scleritis, secondary glaucoma, optic neuritis, retinitis, and choroiditis. The following ocular complications can be seen:

1. Lid scarring
2. Uveitis
3. Scleritis
4. Ocular motor palsies
5. Secondary glaucoma
6. Acute retinal necrosis (ARN)
7. Ptosis

16.9 Post-Herpetic Neuralgia (PHN)

The most common complication which can develop from months to years after the resolution of herpes zoster is the development of post-herpetic neuralgia seen in 13%–15% of patients with zoster. It is seen in 36.6% of patients over the age of 60 and in 47.5% over the age of 70 [17]. Factors that increase the likelihood of developing PHN include increasing age and intense initial symptoms. Both peripheral and central pathophysiological mechanisms contribute to PHN pain. Some PHN patients have abnormal sensitization of unmyelinated cutaneous nociceptor while some patients have pain associated with small fibre deafferentation. In such patients, pain and temperature sensation are profoundly impaired but light moving mechanical stimuli can often produce severe pains [11, 12].

16.10 Management

16.10.1 Medical Management

Early initiation of antiviral treatment, pain management, and prevention of HZO with the use of vaccination are the mainstays of management. Treatment is aimed at accelerating healing, limiting severity and duration of pain, reducing complications, and avoiding disseminated disease. Antiviral treatment reduces the risk of chronic ocular complications by 20% to 30%. Initiation of early antiviral therapy (especially within the first three days of symptoms) has a favourable effect on post-herpetic neuralgia [18, 19]. It does not prevent post-herpetic neuralgia but reduces the duration of the pain by about 50%.

Acyclovir works by interfering with viral thymidine kinase and DNA polymerase resulting in viral DNA chain termination. Valacyclovir is a prodrug of acyclovir and produces serum acyclovir levels three to five times high. Famciclovir is a prodrug and has a similar mechanism of action.

Acyclovir (800 mg 5 times a day for 7–10 days), valacyclovir (1 g 3 times a day for 7 days), and famciclovir (500 mg orally three times a day for seven days) should be started preferably within 72 h of appearance of rash [18, 20–23]]. Oral antivirals shorten the duration of illness by accelerating cutaneous healing and decreasing the formation of new lesion.

Intravenous acyclovir is reserved for immunosuppressed individuals at a dose of 15 to 20 mg/kg per day in adults and up to 30 mg/kg per day in patients with disseminated zoster.

Treatment with intravenous acyclovir is effective at avoiding the complication of disseminated infection [22]. Antivirals have to be given for 7–10 days, which can be extended in case of complications. Systemic antiviral treatment is summarized as

- For immunocompetent individuals (Single agent):
  - Acyclovir 800 mg orally five times per day for at least 7 days
  - Valacyclovir 1000 mg orally every eight hours for at least 7 days
  - Famciclovir 500 mg orally three times per day for at least 7 days
- For immunocompromised individuals:
  - Acyclovir 10 mg/kg of ideal body weight (IBW) intravenously (IV) every eight hours for at least 7 days
  - Foscarnet 90 mg/kg IV every 12 h (typically reserved for severe or acyclovir-resistant disease)

Supportive treatment comprising of analgesics and anti-inflammatory drugs like Diclofenac 50 mg TID, tramadol hydrochloride 50 mg BID gabapentin (150–300 mg/day) can be used for pain relief depending on the severity of symptoms. Raised IOP is to be managed by Acetazolamide 250 mg 8 hourly till normalization of pressure.

For post-herpetic neuralgia Tricyclic antidepressants 10–25 mg orally QID or Amitriptyline 25 mg BD-QID is prescribed. Pregabalin 150 mg/day in divided doses may alleviate pain due to acute herpetic neuralgia. The other drugs used are Cimetidine and lidocaine 5% topical patches.

Topical therapy is intended to control viral replication, ocular surface restoration and lubrication. Acyclovir 3% eye ointment or Ganciclovir .15% ointment used 3–5 times a day are added in ocular involvement till healing of epithelial lesions and to prevent complications. Preservative-free artificial tears or gels for ocular surface lubrication in addition to cycloplegics are prescribed. Other adjunct therapies, such as antibiotics, topical or systemic corticosteroids, and corneal epithelial debridement, are considered on a case-by-case basis.

Topical steroids like Loteprednol .5% and Dexamethasone .1% are used to control inflammation and immune reactions such as keratouveitis, disciform keratitis, sclerokeratitis, interstitial keratitis, episcleritis, and trabeculitis. However topical corticosteroids should be used with caution as they predispose to chronicity and recurrences. Systemic corticosteroids in conjunction with antivirals are indicated for vitritis, retinitis, optic neuritis, and acute retinal necrosis [24, 25]. Inflammatory glaucoma is treated with topical corticosteroids and aqueous suppressants like timolol, brimonidine, and dorzolamide.

Given the elderly age group and immune senescence patients are to be monitored every 3–12 months for late sequelae like glaucoma, cataract, corneal scarring, and retinochoroidal manifestations.

16.10.2 Surgical Management

Surgical treatment is mainly required for non-healing corneal defects, corneal scarring, melting, and perforation. Conjunctival flap, amniotic membrane transplantation, or tarsorrhaphy is effective in non-healing corneal epithelial defect and exposure keratopathy. For small perforations, glue adhesives and bandage contact lens can be considered in addition to corneal patch graft. Larger perforations might require penetrating keratoplasty. Deep anterior lamellar keratoplasty (DALK) is considered in anterior scarring consecutive to stromal keratitis. It is important that transplantation procedures are delayed till complete resolution of tissue inflammation. Depending on the type of surgery performed, the patient should be closely monitored for disease reactivation which is commonly associated after surgical procedures. Prophylaxis with antiviral therapy is recommended for prevention of recurrences and complications.

16.11 Conclusion

Herpes Zoster Ophthalmicus (HZO) is a significant ophthalmic and systemic disease resulting from the reactivation of Varicella Zoster Virus (VZV) in the ophthalmic division of the trigeminal nerve. It primarily affects older adults and immunocompromised individuals, leading to a spectrum of ocular and neurological complications, including keratitis, uveitis, glaucoma, and post-herpetic neuralgia (PHN). Early antiviral therapy within 72 h of symptom onset reduces severity and complications Pain management and ocular treatment, including topical antivirals, corticosteroids, and intraocular pressure control, play a vital role in minimizing long-term sequelae. In cases of severe corneal involvement or structural damage, surgical interventions such as keratoplasty or amniotic membrane transplantation may be required. Despite advancements in treatment, HZO can lead to chronic pain, visual impairment, and recurrences, necessitating long-term monitoring and management. Early diagnosis, prompt intervention, and preventive strategies are key to minimizing morbidity and preserving ocular health in affected individuals.

Key Points

1. HZO is caused by the reactivation of Varicella Zoster Virus (VZV) in the ophthalmic division (V1) of the trigeminal nerve and common in older adults with higher risk in immunosuppressed individuals.
2. Clinical diagnosis is mainly based on symptoms. Laboratory tests (Tzanck smear, PCR, ELISA) can confirm VZV in atypical cases.
3. Early antiviral therapy within 72 h is crucial in reducing disease severity, preventing complications, and improving outcomes.
4. Vaccination against VZV in high-risk populations remains the most effective preventive measure, significantly reducing the incidence and severity of HZO.

References

1. Arffa RC. Viral diseases. In: Arffa RC, Grayson M, editors. Grayson's diseases of the cornea. 4th ed. St. Louis: Mosby; 1997.
2. Dahmiwal S, Priyanka JNCSR, Singh K, Siddiqui SA, Sharma B. Changing age pattern and diverse outcomes of herpes zoster ophthalmicus: exploring the temporal trend, decrease in incident age and influence of treatment strategies. Int Ophthalmol. 2024;44(1):443 https://doi.org/10.1007/s10792-024-03369-2.
3. Liesegang TJ. Herpes zoster virus infection. Curr opin Ophthalmol. 2004;15:531–6.

4. Litt J, Cunningham AL, Arnalich-Montiel F, Parikh R. Herpes zoster ophthalmicus: presentation, complications, treatment, and prevention. Infect Dis Ther. 2024;13(7):1439–59.
5. Kawai K, Gebremeskel BG, Acosta CJ. Systematic review of incidence and complications of herpes zoster: towards a global perspective. BMJ Open. 2014;4(6):e004833.
6. Kong CL, Thompson RR, Porco TC, Kim E, Acharya NR. Incidence rate of herpes zoster ophthalmicus: a retrospective cohort study from 1994 through 2018. Ophthalmology. 2020;127(3):324–30.
7. Schmader K, George LK, Burchett BM, Pieper CF, Hamilton JD. Racial differences in the occurrence of herpes zoster. J Infect Dis. 1995;171(3):701–4.
8. Giannelos N, Curran D, Nguyen C, Kagia C, Vroom N, Vroling H. The incidence of herpes zoster complications: a systematic literature review. Infect Dis Ther. 2024;13(7):1461–86.
9. Rathi A, Das AV, Ramappa M. Clinical and demographic profile of herpes zoster ophthalmicus: a hospital-based study of 1752 Indian patients. Indian J Ophthalmol. 2024;72(Suppl 4):S645–9.
10. Zerboni L, Sen N, Oliver SL, Arvin AM. Molecular mechanisms of varicella zoster virus pathogenesis. Nat Rev Microbiol. 2014;12(3):197–210.
11. Rowbotham MC, Fields HL. Post-herpetic neuralgia: the relation of pain complaint, sensory disturbance, and skin temperature. Pain. 1989;39(2):129–44.
12. Fields HL, Rowbotham M, Baron R. Postherpetic neuralgia: irritable nociceptors and deafferentation. Neurobiol Dis. 1998;5(4):209–27.
13. Goh CL, Khoo L. A retrospective study of the clinical presentation and outcome of herpes zoster in a tertiary dermatology outpatient referral clinic. Int J Dermatol. 1997;36:667–72.
14. Cobo M, Foulks GN, Liesegang T, Lass J, Sutphin J, Wilhelmus K, et al. Observations on the natural history of herpes zoster ophthalmicus. Curr Eye Res. 1987;6:195–9.
15. Harding SP, Lipton JR, Wells JC. Natural history of herpes zoster ophthalmicus: predictors of posther-petic neuralgia and ocular involvement. Br J Ophthalmol. 1987;71:353–8.
16. Lee SM, Han J, Yang CM, Choi CY, Khoramnia R, Chung TY, Lim DH. Chronic and recurrent herpes zoster ophthalmicus. Medicina (Kaunas). 2021;57(10):999.
17. Womack LW, Liesegang TJ. Complications of herpes zoster ophthalmicus. Arch Ophthalmol. 1983;101:42–5.
18. Morton P, Thomson AN. Oral acyclovir in the treatment of herpes zoster in general practice. N Z Med J. 1989;102:93–5.
19. Huff JC, Bean B, Balfour HH Jr, Laskin OL, Connor JD, Corey L, et al. Therapy of herpes zoster with oral acyclovir. Am J Med. 1988;85:84–9.
20. McGill J, Chapman C, Mahakasingam M. Acyclovir therapy in herpes zoster infection A practical guide. Trans Ophthalmol Soc U K. 1983;103(Pt 1):111–4.
21. Tyring SK. Efficacy of famciclovir in the treatment of herpes zoster. Semin Dermatol. 1996;15(2 Suppl 1):27–31.
22. Balfour HH Jr. Varicella zoster virus infections in immunocompromised hosts. A review of the natural history and management. Am J Med. 1988;85(2A):68–73.
23. Schuster AK, Harder BC, Schlichtenbrede FC, Jarczok MN, Tesarz J. Valacyclovir versus acyclovir for the treatment of herpes zoster ophthalmicus in immunocompetent patients. Cochrane Database Syst Rev. 2016;11(11):CD011503.
24. Wood MJ, Johnson RW, McKendrick MW, Taylor J, Mandal BK, Crooks J. A randomized trial of acyclovir for 7 days or 21 days with and without prednisolone for treatment of acute herpes zoster. N Engl J Med. 1994;330(13):896–900.
25. Khadamy J, Khademi P, Baharypour S. Accelerated recovery: the role of oral steroid in the management of herpes zoster ophthalmicus-related ophthalmoplegia. Cureus. 2023;15(12):e50553.

17 Herpes Zoster Keratitis

Jeewan Singh Titiyal, Neeti Gupta, and Bhavana Sharma

Abstract

Herpes zoster ophthalmicus (HZO) is a significant manifestation of varicella-zoster virus (VZV) reactivation that affects the ophthalmic branch of the trigeminal nerve. This condition presents with dermatological and ophthalmic complications, including keratitis, uveitis, and neurotrophic keratopathy, which can lead to permanent vision impairment. Understanding the epidemiology, clinical features, and treatment strategies for HZO is essential for effective management and prevention of long-term complications. Introduction of recombinant zoster vaccine has significantly reduced the incidence of HZO. This chapter provides an overview of the pathophysiology, diagnosis, treatment, and prevention of HZO, supported by recent research.

Keywords

Herpes zoster · Herpes zoster ophthalmicus · Varicella-zoster virus · Herpes zoster keratitis · Post-herpetic neuralgia

J. S. Titiyal (✉)
R P Centre, AIIMS Delhi, Delhi, India

N. Gupta
AIIMS Rishikesh, Rishikesh, Uttarakhand, India

B. Sharma
AIIMS Bhopal, Bhopal, Madhya Pradesh, India

17.1 Introduction

Herpes Zoster (HZ) infection is caused by localized reactivation of varicella zoster virus (VZV), resulting in painful rash in a dermatomal distribution in patients who had previously suffered chickenpox or varicella. Herpes Zoster Ophthalmicus (HZO) is a manifestation of herpes zoster (shingles) when the reactivated varicella-zoster virus affects the ophthalmic branch of the trigeminal nerve. It accounts for approximately 10–20% of all herpes zoster cases, with 20–70% developing ocular findings. A recent report suggests a figure of 7.9% cases of HZO [1]. It poses a significant risk for ocular complications, including vision-threatening conditions.

17.2 Etiology

HZO is caused by the reactivation of VZV in the trigeminal ganglion, particularly affecting the ophthalmic branch (V1). The exact triggers for reactivation are not entirely understood but include immunosuppression, aging, stress, and chronic illnesses [2]. The frontal branch, which innervates the skin of the forehead and upper eyelid, is most frequently involved in HZO. The strongest predictor of ocular inflammation and corneal anaesthesia is involvement of both branches of the nasociliary nerve.

B. Sharma et al. (eds.), *Viral Keratitis*, https://doi.org/10.1007/978-981-95-3148-6_17

17.3 Epidemiology

Global incidence of HZO varies subject to demographic and environmental conditions. Approximately one million new HZ cases occur annually in the U.S, with 10–20% involving HZO. The lifetime risk of developing HZO is 10–30% [2]. HZO is more common in older adults, but incidence in younger individuals is rising [3]. Immunosuppression, malignancies, and autoimmune diseases increase susceptibility to HZ infection. Although immunocompromised individuals are more susceptible, recent trends reflect that more than 90% of patients with HZ infection are not immunosuppressed [4]. Other risk factors are physical or mental stress, renal diseases, prolonged illness, debilitated states, and heart failure. Recent articles report the use of statins to be a predisposing factor for developing HZ with a dose-dependent risk [5].

17.4 Pathophysiology

After primary infection, VZV establishes latency in the dorsal root ganglia or cranial nerve ganglia. Upon reactivation, the virus travels along sensory nerves to the skin and ocular tissues, leading to inflammation, necrosis, and secondary immune-mediated damage. Unlike chickenpox, shingles spreads by direct contact with fluids in the vesicles of the acute rash to a person with no history of chicken pox infection or VZV vaccination.

17.5 Clinical Features

The disease heralds with a prodromal phase with fever, malaise, headache, and unilateral burning pain along the ophthalmic nerve distribution which often precedes the rash. Maculopapular rash evolving into vesicular lesions, often respecting the midline, appears after the prodromal phase. The ophthalmic division is most commonly affected in herpes zoster out of the three divisions of the trigeminal nerve. Vesicles on the tip of the nose, indicating nasociliary nerve involvement and increased risk of ocular complications is known as *Hutchinson's sign*. It is classically associated with ocular involvement, although it is present in less than a quarter of patients with HZO [6]. The frontal nerve is the most commonly affected of the three branches of the ophthalmic nerve. Ocular involvement may occur early or present within 1 month after the onset of rash. The most common ocular findings of HZO are conjunctivitis, uveitis, and keratitis [7].

17.5.1 Acute Phase

HZO-induced inflammation can cause hyperemia, both papillary and follicular reaction, and pseudo-membrane formation in extensive involvement. Vesicular eruptions with subsequent rupture and scarring may also be seen in severe cases with formation of symblepharon and punctal scarring. HZO can cause inflammation of the episclera and sclera, leading to episcleritis, anterior scleritis, or posterior scleritis. In the acute phase, episcleritis is typically seen, while scleritis is seen in chronic cases. It is usually perilimbal with diffuse or nodular appearance [8]. Resultant scleral thinning and staphyloma formation can occur as a result of chronic scarring [9]. HZO involves the cornea in multiple forms with varied presentations. Corneal manifestations occur in about two-thirds of patients with ocular HZO. From anterior to posterior layers, it can cause punctate epithelial keratitis, pseudodendrites, anterior stromal infiltrates, sclerosing keratitis, keratouveitis, serpiginous keratopathy, and neurotrophic keratitis.

(a) **Punctate epithelial keratitis**:
It is seen as multiple, elevated, coarse punctate epithelial keratitis with swollen epithelial cells. They are usually focal, peripherally located, small sized which stain with rose Bengal. VZV has been isolated from these lesions [10] (Fig. 17.1).

(b) **Pseudodendrites**:
Psuedodendrites are considered to be the hallmark of VZV infection seen within 1st week of HZO. They are heaped up epithe-

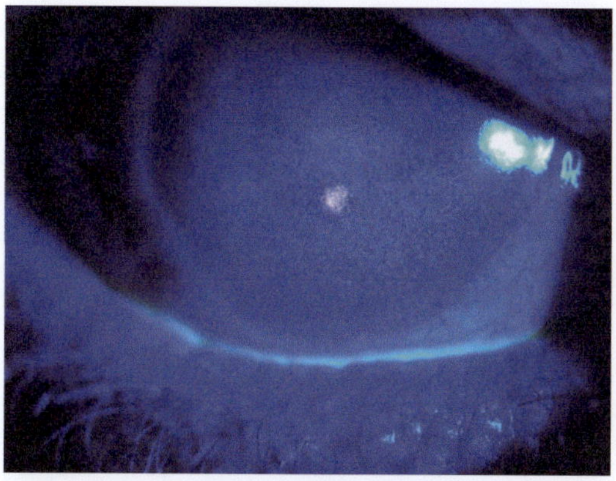

Fig. 17.1 HZ epithelial keratitis showing multiple superficial punctate epithelial erosions

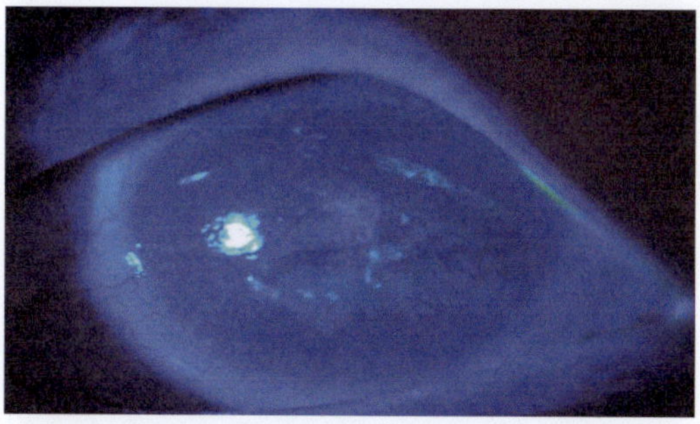

Fig. 17.2 Fluorescein-stained corneal epithelium under cobalt blue illumination showing pseudodendrites with characteristic elevated, stuck-on appearance

lium with branching pattern and a stuck-on appearance (Fig. 17.2). Unlike HSV dendrites, they are not true epithelial defects and lack central ulceration. Usual presentation is multiple elevated epithelial lesions with surrounding oedema in a dendritic or stellate formation. These lesions are peripherally located and differ from herpes simplex viral dendrites in that they are raised above the surface and superficially placed, lack terminal end bulbs and central ulceration hence stain minimally with fluorescein and rose Bengal. VZV has been isolated from these lesions [10, 11]. The microscopic examination reveals multinucleated giant cells and intranuclear inclusion bodies [12].

(c) **Stromal Keratitis**:
Immune infiltrates appear almost always after the epithelial lesion heals and leave behind a scar or area of thinning. Stromal keratitis is caused due to direct viral involvement or stromal reaction to viral antigens from spill-over epithelial keratitis. It is characterized by the presence of stromal infiltrates and oedema in the anterior or mid stroma, which is frequently a contiguous involvement from an epithelial lesion and underlies the area involved (Fig. 17.3a). Anterior stromal keratitis is often observed first during the second week manifesting as subepithelial nummular infiltrates in the stroma. These infiltrates are immune-mediated response to viral antigens. Lesions heal by neovascularization and/corneal scarring.
Deep stromal keratitis can manifest as necrotizing or non-necrotizing type several months after the infection. The lesions heal by the formation of stromal opacities (Fig. 17.3b, c).

(d) **Sclerosing keratitis**:
Stromal keratitis consequent to VZV scleritis is seen as peripheral variable-sized triangular or tongue-shaped dense stromal infiltrates as an extension of contiguous scleritis (Fig. 17.4a, b). Lesions heal by formation of stromal opacity with or without vascularization, stromal thinning, or peripheral furrowing of the cornea (Fig. 17.4c).

(e) **Mucous plaque keratopathy**:
The VZV mucous plaque keratitis is caused by immune-mediated inflammation, adhesion of mucous plaques to inflamed epithelium, or direct viral invasion [11, 13]. Mucous plaques present as a delayed manifestation several months after HZO in cases with previous epithelial keratitis. They are clinically seen as variable-sized, elevated, coarse, grey-white filamentary branching lesions on the surface of edematous epithelial cells, which lack terminal end bulbs and stain sparingly with fluorescein and rose Bengal (Fig. 17.5a, b).

(f) **Disciform keratitis**:
VZV disciform keratitis presents with a lesion similar to HSV. Disc-shaped area of stromal infiltrate and oedema which is present in the central or paracentral area with

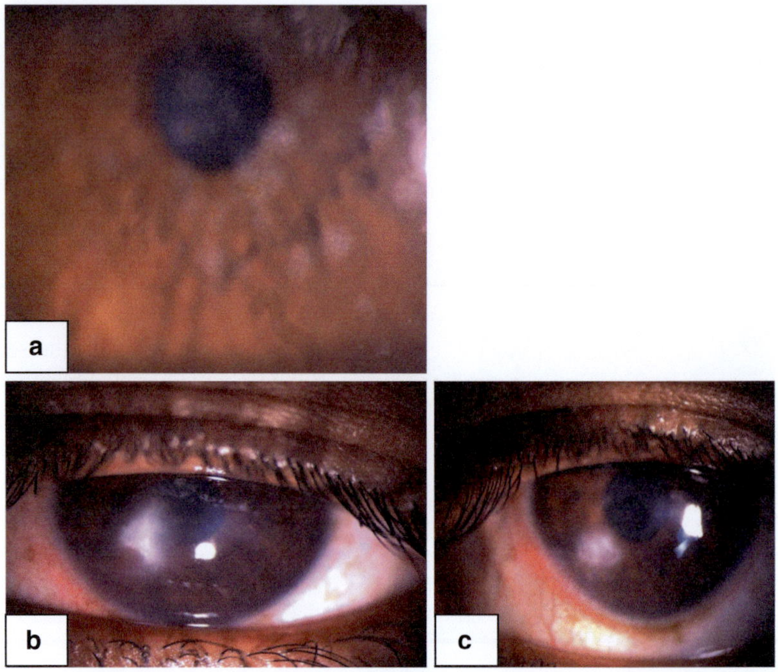

Fig. 17.3 (**a**) Slit-lamp image showing HZ nummular keratitis as multiple coin-shaped, granular anterior stromal opacities in the central and paracentral cornea. (**b**) HZ stromal keratitis with dense stromal infiltrates and neovascularization. (**c**) Post-treatment image showing leucomatous corneal opacity with sectoral vascularization

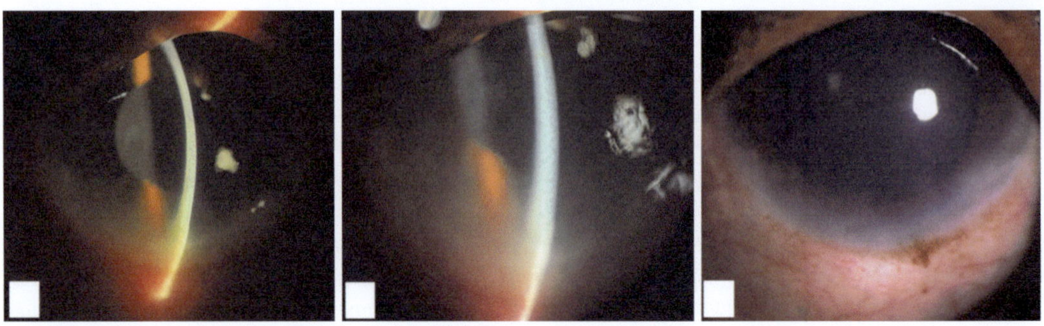

Fig. 17.4 (**a** and **b**) Showing peripheral tongue-shaped dense stromal infiltrates as an extension of contiguous scleritis. (**c**) Post-treatment image showing healing sclerosing keratitis

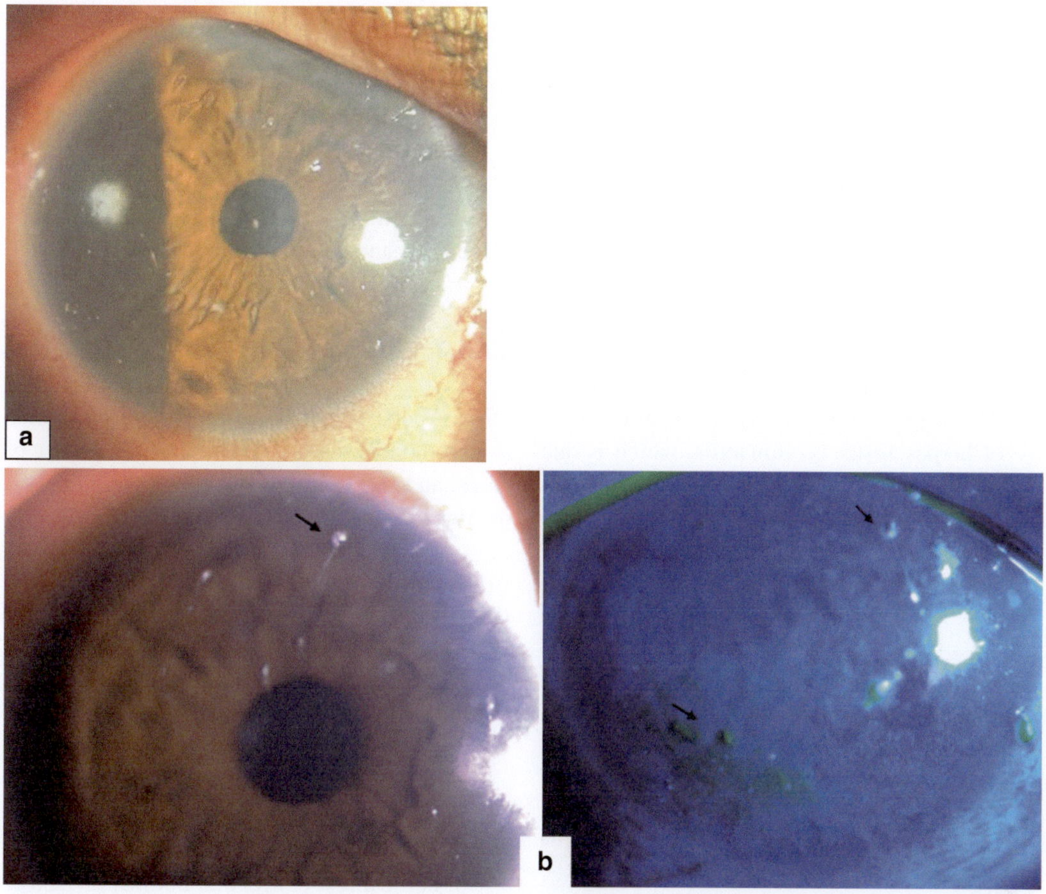

Fig. 17.5 (**a** and **b**) Mucous plaque keratopathy showing elevated, filamentary branching lesions over epithelium

Fig. 17.6 Diffuse and slit image showing disc-shaped area of central stromal oedema with an intact overlying epithelium

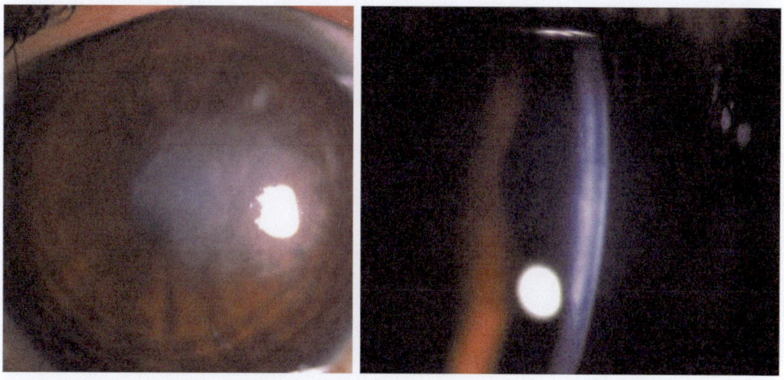

intact overlying epithelium (Fig. 17.6). The degree of AC reaction may be variable and may present as hypopyon or hyphema. Cornea can show multiple areas of oedema in a relatively quiescent eye. It is caused either due to direct VZV infection of the endothelium or an immune mediated reaction to viral antigen in the corneal stroma [14]. Wessely's immune ring formation can be seen reflective of antigenic response with deposition of antigen–antibody complex.

(g) **Keratouveitis**:
VZV can cause inflammation of the Descemet endothelial complex and anterior uveal tissue, leading to keratouveitis. This is caused either by direct viral invasion of the endothelium or immune reaction to viral antigens. Disease heralds with the onset of descemet folds, endothelitis, a cluster of fresh keratic precipitates with overlying stromal edema. In severe cases, stromal oedema may result in contiguous epithelial involvement and epithelial oedema and bullae. Sectoral iris stromal atrophy is characteristic of herpes zoster keratouveitis, which is due to ischemia caused by the occlusive vasculitis (Fig. 17.7). Associated uveitis is manifested as the presence of cells and flare, iritis, and ciliary tenderness. Secondary glaucoma can be seen in severe involvement and trabeculitis

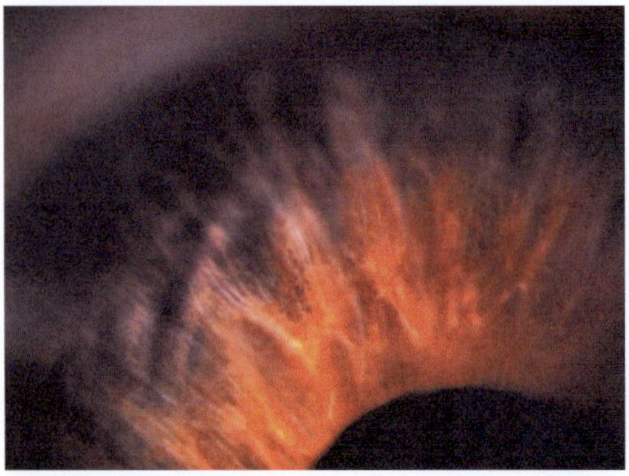

Fig. 17.7 HZ keratouveitis showing sectoral iris stromal atrophy

(h) **Corneal decompensation** (Fig. 17.8a, b)
HZO-induced corneal decompensation is seen in severe involvement, which may result in bullous keratopathy. Probable mechanism is inflammation or an immune mechanism induced endothelial damage or direct viral affection. It can also occur subsequent to uveitis and a secondary rise of IOP.

17.5.2 Chronic Phase

Disease persisting for 3 or more months is termed as chronic eye disease. It occurs in a quarter of cases, and recurrent eye diseases develop in one quarter for more than 5 years [15].

(a) **Neurotropic Keratitis**:
(b) HZ is the most common cause of NK occurring in 12.8% of HZ keratitis [16]. It is defined as a disease related to alterations in corneal nerves leading to impairment in sensory and trophic functions with consequent breakdown of corneal epithelium, affecting the health and integrity of the tear film, epithelium, and stroma. The initial sign is a lack of corneal lustre, irregular corneal surface or mild coarse superficial punctate keratitis. Over time, a haze develops with epithelial oedema resulting in oval punched out epithelial ulcers with rolled out edges due to heaped up epithelial cells (Fig. 17.9a). It may complicate secondary infections, thinning and perforations, or fibrovascular scarring (Fig. 17.9b). The etiology is attributed to

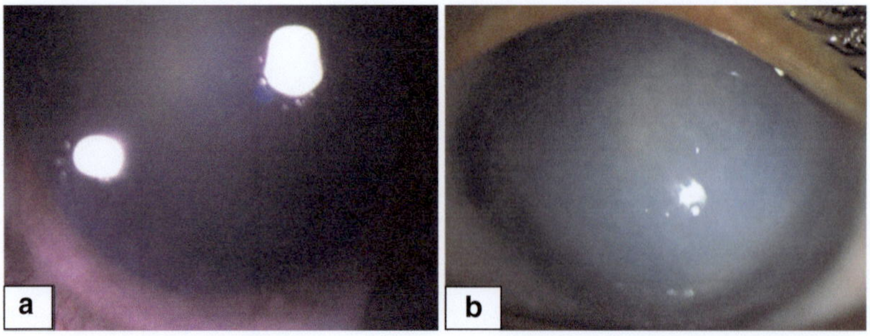

Fig. 17.8 (**a**) Image showing corneal oedema, stromal haze with diffusely scattered keratic precipitates, anterior chamber reaction, and mild injection of episclera after HZO. (**b**) Corneal decompensation in a case of chronic HZO Keratitis

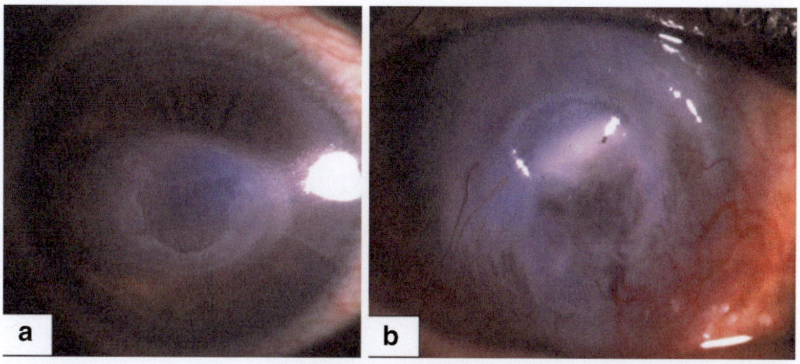

Fig. 17.9 (**a**) HZO-induced neurotropic keratitis showing central circular epithelial defect with rounded irregular margins and underlying stromal opacification. (**b**) HZ neurotrophic keratitis with corneal melt

nerve damage, compromised trophic functions of the ocular surface with resultant decrease of tear secretion and impaired epithelial healing due to ongoing inflammation and surface toxicity of topical medications [11, 17].

(c) **Metaherpetic/trophic ulcer**:
Metaherpetic ulcer is seen as a chronic involvement of the ocular surface because of impaired trophic mechanisms. It is usually seen after non-healing epithelial ulcers due to ongoing inflammation, impairment of neural functions, surface toxicity of antiviral drugs, and dry eye. They are seen as grey white epithelial or superficial stromal ulcers with elevated borders that exhibit reverse staining (Fig. 17.10).

(d) **Lipid keratopathy**:
VZV-induced severe corneal inflammation results in vascularized corneal scar, leading to lipid deposition through the encroaching vessels. The yellowish white circular, variable-sized lesion is usually paracentral and in proximity to tuft of blood vessels (Fig. 17.11). Studies have reported persistence of VZV in the involved area. The mainstay of treatment is control of inflammation and elimination of feeder vessels by diathermy or argon laser photocoagulation of the inciting blood vessels. Intrastromal anti-VEGF agents have been described as an effective therapeutic option for destroying neovessels.

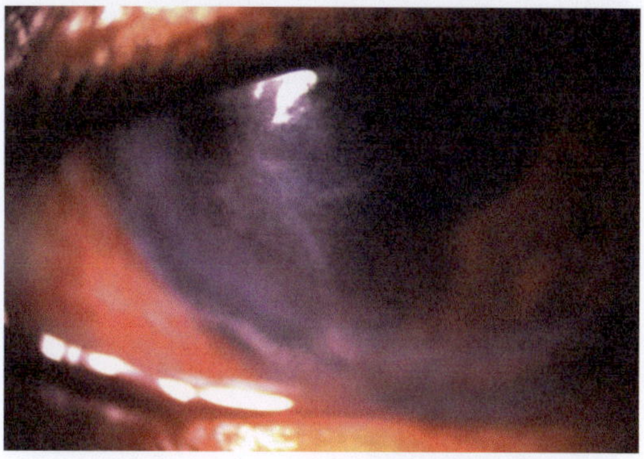

Fig. 17.10 Slit-lamp image showing HZ metaherpetic ulcer with persistent non-healing epithelial defect

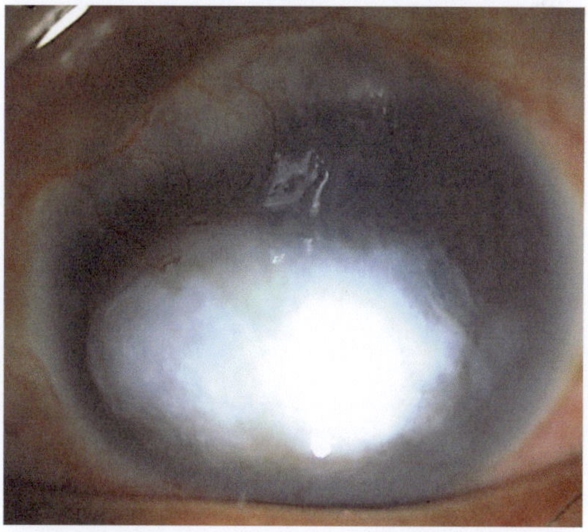

Fig. 17.11 Lipid keratopathy showing white circular lesion with proximity to tuft of blood vessels

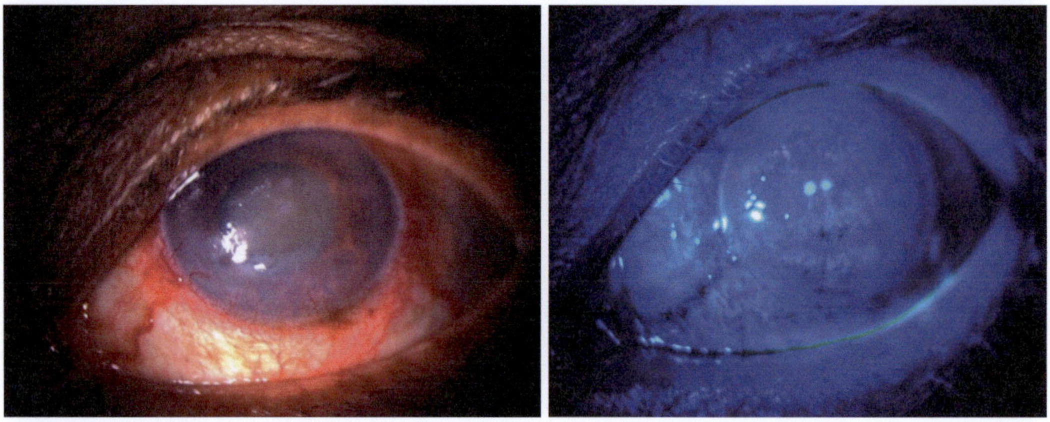

Fig. 17.12 Slit-lamp image showing HZO-induced vascularized corneal opacity with surface erosions and bad ocular surface

(e) **Corneal opacity**:
More than 10% of the patients of HZO develop moderate to severe vision loss due to scarring [18] (Fig. 17.12).

17.6 Diagnosis

Careful clinical examination is the mainstay of diagnosis. It is based on characteristic rash and ocular involvement. Slit-lamp examination is done to assess corneal and anterior segment involvement, for assessing the severity, treatment, and follow-up. In atypical cases, PCR or direct immunofluorescence is recommended for definitive VZV diagnosis.

17.7 Differential Diagnosis

The differential diagnosis of Herpes zoster keratitis has been described in Table 17.1.

Table 17.1 Showing differential diagnosis of Herpes Zoster Keratitis

Herpes Zoster Keratitis	Differential diagnosis
Pseudodendrite	**Herpes Simplex Keratitis**: *True dendrites*: linear ulcer with dichotomous branching, terminal bulbs, and swollen borders with intraepithelial cell infiltration
HZ Stromal Keratitis	**Acute bacterial keratitis**: *Adnexal signs*: Eyelid oedema, blepharospasm, matting of lashes, purulent discharge *Anterior segment* shows conjunctival chemosis, circumcorneal congestion, epithelial defect, stromal oedema, stromal infiltrate, Descemet membrane folds, endothelial plaque, hypopyon, and ischemic pupil
Herpes zoster ophthalmicus	**Contact dermatitis**: Itchy rash following contact with an irritant substance *Acute*: vesicles or pustules with oedema, oozing, crusting, tenderness *Subacute*: crusting, and hyperpigmentation *Chronic*: Lichenification **Toxic epidermal necrolysis**: History of drug intake (antibiotics, antiepileptics, NSAIDS) Ill-defined erythematous macular rash and bullae, which then coalesce to form sheet-like blisters The vesicular eruption is typically preceded by pain

17.8 Complications

Secondary superinfection by bacterial or fungal pathogens due to compromised ocular surface and inappropriate treatment can cause ensuing complications. Corneal complications include secondary infectious keratitis, ulceration with hypopyon, keratolysis, and corneal perforation. The stromal keratitis may heal, leaving a scar, or if the infection reaches deeper layers, may lead to corneal perforation. Secondary glaucoma may be due to inflammation of the trabecular meshwork in cases of keratouveitis or in steroid responders.

17.9 Treatment

During the acute phase of HZV keratitis, systemic antiviral, along with adjuvant therapy is recommended for management as per the clinical involvement. Oral Valacylovir 1000 mg 3 times/day or Acyclovir 800 mg 5 times/day or Famciclovir 500 mg 3 times/day, within 72 h of rash onset, is started to reduce severity and complications and should be continued for 7 to 10 days. Topical antivirals like Gancyclovir .15% or Acyclovir 3% ointment 3–5 times per day are recommended in cases with epithelial and stromal involvement. Additionally, artificial tears for ocular surface restoration and cycloplegics to prevent ciliary spasm and synechiae formation are prescribed. Anti-glaucoma medication is recommended in keratouveitis with high intraocular pressures. Topical steroids are restricted for usage in immune-related keratitis and uveitis, along with systemic and topical antiviral agents. Specific treatment of various types of corneal involvement is described in Table 17.2

Treatment of corneal involvement in the chronic phase mainly involves restoration of ocular surface and prevention of further complications. The mainstay of treatment of neurotropic keratitis remains frequent lubrication and removal of epitheliotoxic drugs [19]. Surgical treatment with amniotic membrane transplants and tarsoraphy may help in the healing of the ulcers and decrease the exposed surface area. Punctal occlusion for preservation of tears, Tenon's patch graft for small perforations and tectonic keratoplasty are other options. Newer treatment modalities are Recombinant nerve growth factor (cenegermin 0.002%) eye drops and corneal neurotization [20, 21].

Table 17.2 Treatment of different types of HZO keratitis

Keratitis type	Pathophysiological mechanism	Treatment
Viral conjunctivitis	Inflammatory reaction/direct viral invasion	Artificial tears, Topical steroids
Punctate epithelial keratitis	Direct viral invasion	Topical antiviral/oral antivirals; Artificial tears; Cycloplegics
Pseudodendrite	Direct viral invasion	Topical antiviral/oral antivirals; Artificial tears; Cycloplegics
Stromal keratitis	Immune mediated	Oral antivirals along with topical steroids
Keratouveitis	Immune mediated	Oral antivirals along with topical steroids
Lipid keratopathy	intra- and extracellular lipid deposition	Obliteration of feeder vessels; Topical steroids
Mucous plaques	Inflamed ocular surface	Artificial tears; Topical steroids; 2% Acetyl cysteine drops

17.10 Conclusion

HZO remains a significant ophthalmic and systemic challenge, especially in ageing populations. Given the recent trend of a decrease in incident age at which patients with HZO are diagnosed, it is prudent to mitigate predisposing factors, initiate prompt treatment, and avoidance of steroids in the early phase of the disease. Long-term prevention strategies, particularly vaccination, are critical in reducing disease burden.

Key Points

1. Herpes zoster ophthalmicus (HZO) can cause corneal involvement in varied forms.
2. Approximately 10–20% of herpes zoster cases involve the ophthalmic nerve division, with 20–70% developing ocular findings.
3. HZO is frequently associated with chronic ocular involvement in addition to acute manifestations.
4. The mainstay of treatment is systemic antiviral agents for 7–14 days.

References

1. Kong CL, Thompson RR, Porco TC, Kim E, Acharya NR. Incidence rate of herpes zoster ophthalmicus: a retrospective cohort study from 1994 through 2018. Ophthalmology. 2020;127(3):324–30.
2. Barry Lee W. Herpes Zoster Keratitis. In: Krachmer J, Mannis M, Holland E, editors. Cornea: fundamentals, diagnosis and management. 4th ed. Edinburgh/London/New York/Oxford/Philadelphia/St. Louis/Sydney/Toronto: Elsevier; 2017.
3. Dahmiwal S, Priyanka, Jain NC, Rajamathangi S, Singh K, Siddiqui SA, Sharma B. Changing age pattern and diverse outcomes of herpes zoster ophthalmicus: exploring the temporal trend, decrease in incident age and influence of treatment strategies. Int Ophthalmol. 2024;44(1):443.
4. Kawai K, Yawn BP, Wollan P, Harpaz R. Increasing incidence of herpes zoster over a 60-year period from a population-based study. Clin Infect Dis. 2016;63(2):221–6.
5. Zuin M, Rigatelli G, L'Erario R, Zuliani G, Bilato C, Roncon L. Herpes zoster infection and statins: which implications in clinical practice? Eur J Clin Microbiol Infect Dis. 2019;38(1):93–9.
6. Szeto SK, Chan TC, Wong RL, Ng AL, Li EY, Jhanji V. Prevalence of ocular manifestations and visual outcomes in patients with herpes zoster ophthalmicus. Cornea. 2017;36(3):338–42.
7. Li JY. Herpes zoster ophthalmicus: acute keratitis. Curr Opin Ophthalmol. 2018;29(4):328–33.
8. Naumann G, Gass JDM, Font RL. Histopathology of herpes zoster ophthalmicus. Am J Ophthalmol. 1968;65:533–41.
9. Penman GG. Scleritis as a sequel of herpes ophthalmicus. Br J Ophthalmol. 1931;15:585–8.
10. Pavan-Langston D, McCulley JP. Herpes zoster dendritic keratitis. Arch Ophthalmol. 1973;89:25–9.
11. Liesegang TJ. Corneal complications from herpes zoster ophthalmicus. Ophthalmology. 1985;92:316–24.
12. Pavan-Langston D, Yamamoto S, Dunkel EC. Delayed herpes zoster pseudodendrites. Arch Ophthalmol. 1995;113:1381–835.
13. Marsh RJ, Cooper M. Ophthalmic zoster: mucous plaque keratitis. Br J Ophthalmol. 1987;71(725–728):35.
14. Yu DD, Lemp MA, Mathers WD, Espy M, White T. Detection of varicella-zoster virus DNA in disciform keratitis using polymerase chain reaction. Arch Ophthalmol. 1993;111(2):167–8.

15. Tran KD, Falcone MM, Choi DS, Goldhardt R, Karp CL, Davis JL, Galor A. Epidemiology of herpes zoster ophthalmicus: recurrence and chronicity. Ophthalmology. 2016;123(7):1469–75.
16. Dworkin RH, Johnson RW, Breuer J, Gnann JW, Levin MJ, Backonja M, et al. Recommendations for the management of herpes zoster. Clin Infect Dis. 2007;44(Suppl 1):S1–26.
17. Mackie IA. Role of the corneal nerves in destructive disease of the cornea. Trans Ophthalmol Soc U K. 1978;98:343–7.
18. Niederer RL, Meyer JJ, Liu K, Danesh-Meyer HV. Herpes zoster ophthalmicus clinical presentation and risk factors for loss of vision. Am J Ophthalmol. 2021;226:83–9.
19. Cohen EJ, Jeng BH. Herpes zoster: a brief definitive review. Cornea. 2021;40(8):943–9.
20. Pflugfelder SC, Massaro-Giordano M, Perez VL, Hamrah P, Deng SX, Espandar L, et al. Topical recombinant human nerve growth factor (cenegermin) for neurotrophic keratopathy: a multicenter randomized vehicle-controlled pivotal trial. Ophthalmology. 2020;127(1):14–26.
21. Park JK, Charlson ES, Leyngold I, Kossler AL. Corneal neurotization: a review of pathophysiology and outcomes. Ophthalmic Plast Reconstr Surg. 2020;36(5):431–7.

Herpes Zoster Keratouveitis

18

Sunita Chaurasia

Abstract

Herpes zoster ophthalmicus (HZO) is a consequence of reactivation of varicella zoster virus in the ophthalmic or the first division (V1) of the trigeminal nerve. The varicella zoster virus residing in the trigeminal ganglion gets reactivated causing involvement of the skin, ocular tissues and the adnexa leading to a significant visual morbidity. Keratouveitis can occur in both the acute and chronic phase of the disease. The diagnosis can be made easily on clinical history and examination. Management is based on the severity of the clinical presentation. This chapter is focused on the clinical features and management guidelines of keratouveitis in various stages of HZO.

Keywords

Herpes zoster ophthalmicus · Keratitis · Keratouveitis · Endotheliitis

18.1 Introduction

Reactivation of varicellazoster virus residing in trigeminal ganglion causes lesions of skin, ocular tissues and adnexa leading to visual morbidity. Ocular involvement in acute HZO can occur as eyelid lesions/vesicles, conjunctivitis, episcleritis, keratitis, uveitis, scleritis, trabeculitis, optic neuritis, retinal vasculitis, giant cell arteritis, retinopathy and cranial nerve defects [1, 2]. The acute disease is followed by a subacute and chronic stage lasting up to years after the initial episode, which can lead to vision-threatening sequelae and complications. Corneal involvement along with anterior uveitis characterized by keratouveitis is a significant cause of visual impairment in such cases [3, 4].

18.2 Epidemiology and Pathophysiological Mechanisms

HZO is seen in 4–20% of those with HZ [5, 6]. Approximately 50% of patients with HZO develop ocular disease, of which up to 25 % develop chronic or recurrent disease [7]. The most frequent ocular manifestations in acute HZO are conjunctivitis (57%) and anterior uveitis (18%). Keratitis is a common presentation, with an incidence that varies by subtype, including stromal (7%), epithelial (5%) and endothelial (1.2%) [8]. Uveitis tends to accompany most forms of keratitis, but it is especially frequent and difficult to manage in herpes zoster keratouveitis. Up to 40% of patients with HZO may develop recurrent anterior uveitis [9].

S. Chaurasia (✉)
L V Prasad Eye Institute,
Hyderabad, Telangana, India
e-mail: sunita@lvpei.org

B. Sharma et al. (eds.), *Viral Keratitis*, https://doi.org/10.1007/978-981-95-3148-6_18

The ocular manifestations occur due to interplay of several pathogenic mechanisms, which include active viral replication, inflammatory and immune reaction, neuronal and vascular inflammation and secondary degenerative changes [10]. In the early course of the disease, the active virus replication can cause epithelial keratitis with or without involvement of the anterior segment. In the later course of the disease, an inflammatory response to the HZ virus can cause immune stromal keratitis, endothelial disease, anterior uveitis and secondary glaucoma. Vascular and neural inflammation leads to a disturbed ocular surface, corneal anaesthesia, impaired healing with secondary changes. Various complications can occur in the chronic recurrent course of the disease such as ulceration, neurotrophic keratitis and corneal scarring.

18.3 Risk Factors

The specific risk factors for HZO remain uncertain, and the general risk factors for HZ can also be applied to HZO [7]. Although most cases of HZO occur in immunocompetent individuals, severe manifestations of HZO are associated with immunosuppression. The presence of less common manifestations such as acute retinal necrosis, orbital apex syndrome and panuveitis has been shown to be significantly associated with immunosuppression and diabetes [6]. Some studies found an increased risk of HZ after COVID-19 infection and after COVID-19 vaccination [11–13].

Herpes zoster can recur following an initial episode [13]. The cumulative recurrence risk in HZO varies widely between studies and reported to range between 7.1% to 52.6% during the follow-up period [14, 15]. A study from the US reported a cumulative recurrence risk of 8% after 1 year that increased to 31% after 6 years [16]. The risk factors identified with HZO recurrence included keratouveitis, ocular hypertension and chronic HZO. Recurrence of ocular HZ presents commonly as immune stromal keratitis, keratouveitis and secondary glaucoma. The recurrence of HZO following cataract surgery was observed to vary from 25% to 40.4% [17, 18].

18.4 Characterization of HZ Keratouveitis

Corneal manifestations occur in about two-thirds of patients with ocular disease related to different mechanisms with varying clinical features, which is described in detail in previous chapter. Keratouveitis is described as active corneal inflammation which is associated with anterior chamber inflammation of varying severity. Figure 18.1a–f shows the clinical spectrum of keratouveitis at various stages of the disease. The clinical features are dependent on the virulence of organism, and the immune response of the host.

18.4.1 Endothelitis

Occurs because of direct viral invasion of the endothelium along with an immune reaction varying from mild disciform keratitis to more severe granulomatous inflammatory reaction which can occur as early as 1 week of the disease onset to several months later. Clinical signs comprise of stromal oedema overlying keratic precipitates, folds in Descemet's membrane and anterior uveitis. Four morphological patterns of endothelitis have been described—linear, sectorial, disciform and diffuse. Severe and diffuse endothelitis can eventually result in loss of endothelial cells, corneal decompensation and persistent oedema. Delayed treatment can be a cause of deep vascularization, progressive stromal thinning and subsequent scarring.

18.4.2 Anterior Uveitis

This may present as isolated manifestation or in combination with keratitis as described above (keratouveitis). The inflammation can be granulomatous or non-granulomatous with a chronic

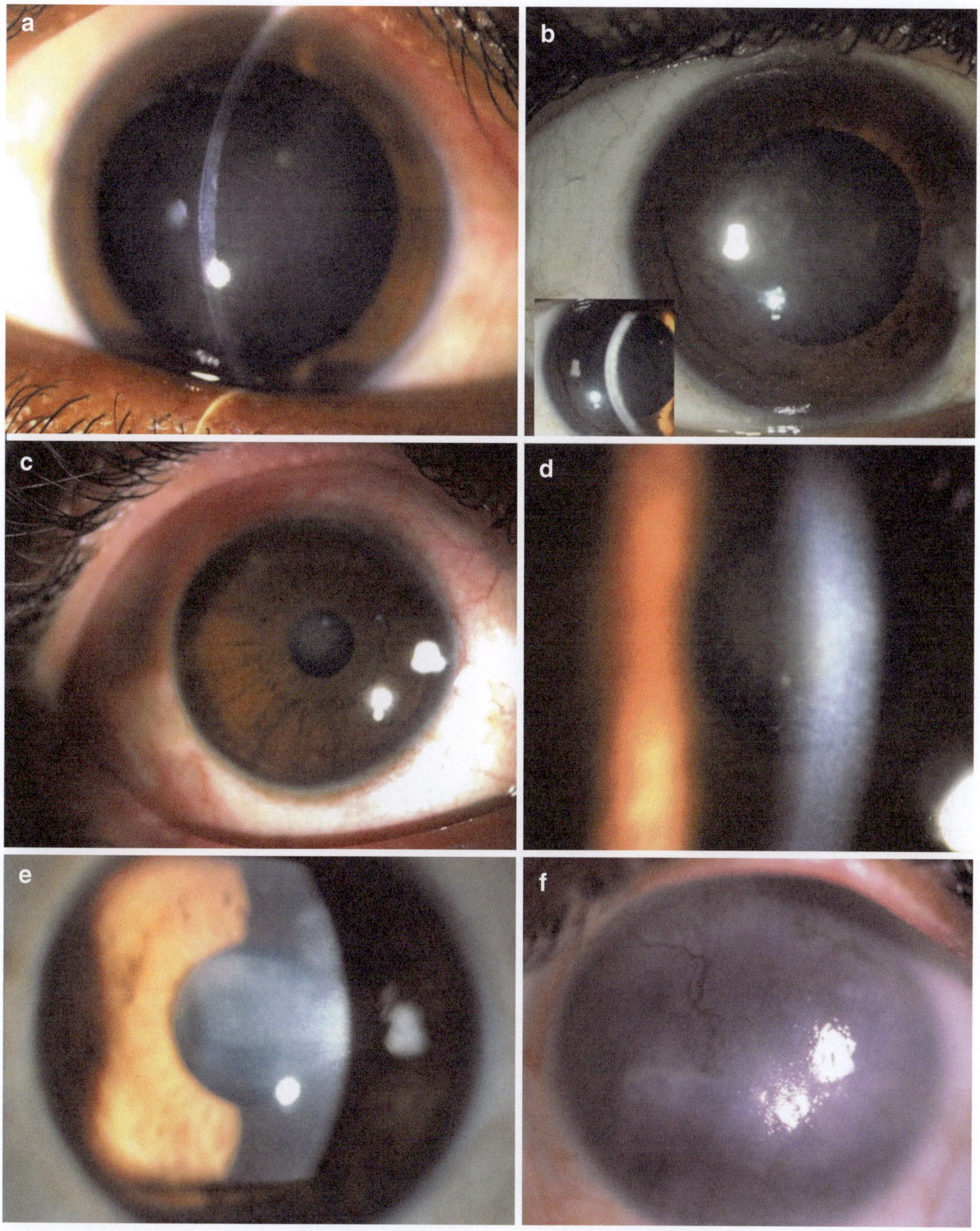

Fig. 18.1 (**a**–**f**) Keratouveitis at various time intervals after acute HZO: (**a**) Slit lamp photograph of a patient showing DM folds, keratic precipitates at 1 month of HZO; (**b**) Localised endothelitis; (**c** and **d**) Keratouveitis at 2 months after HZO showing central corneal haze, keratic precipitates, and an area of epithelial lesion at subacute stage; (**e**) Immune stromal keratouveitis at 2 years after the acute disease; (**f**) Vascularised corneal scar following recurrent episodes of immune stromal keratitis

course. The onset is typically seen 2–4 weeks after the onset of HZO, though some cases may show delayed presentation as well. Clinical features comprise of intense photophobia, ciliary injection, aqueous cells and flare, keratic precipitates, oedema, posterior synechiae and hypopyon or hyphaema in severe cases.When the anterior chamber reaction is intense, consecutive secondary glaucoma ensues due to inflammatory exudates like cellular debris, iris pigment or blood blocking the trabecular meshwork, inflammation of trabecular meshwork or ischemic vasculitis of ciliary body in addition to pupillary block glaucoma from posterior synechiae. Secondary glaucoma is reported to be seen in 56% of patients with HZO [19]. Ongoing inflammation in chronic uveitis can lead to pathognomic sectoral iris atrophy due to occlusive vasculitis from chronic uveitis (Fig. 18.2). On slit lamp it is seen as transillumination defects in retro-illumination mode. While anterior segment angiography demonstrates occlusion of iris vasculature with sectoral iris atrophy and iris pigment epithelial loss [20]. Other signs are presence of posterior synechiae, festooned pupil and complicated cataract (Fig. 18.3a, b). In advanced cases continuing chronic inflammation can cause spill over involvement of ciliary body which can lead to ciliary body hyposecretion, hypotony, cyclitic membrane and atrophic/phthisis bulbi.

18.4.3 Posterior Uveitis

HZO may result in acute retinal necrosis, which may initially begin with anterior uveitis and keratic precipitates (Fig. 18.4a, b). Acute retinal necrosis progresses as patches of peripheral retinitis that coalesce rapidly, accompanied by occlusive vasculitis and vitreous inflammation. The acute phase of retinal necrosis may persist for few months and can lead to retinal detachments within 3 weeks to 5 months of onset. The immunocompromised individuals are at particular risk of progressive outer retinal necrosis.

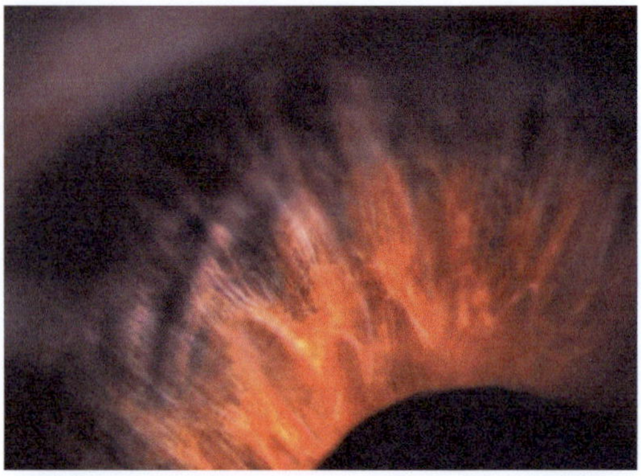

Fig. 18.2 HZ keratouveitis showing sectoral iris stromal atrophy

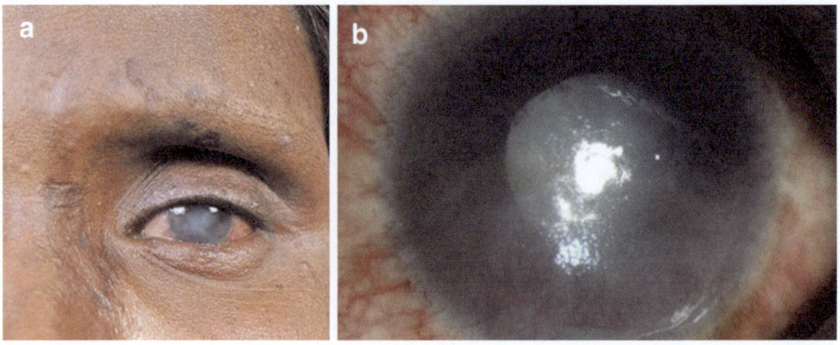

Fig. 18.3 (**a** and **b**) Keratouveitis with severe vascularization and Complicated cataract with hypotony at 2 months after acute HZO

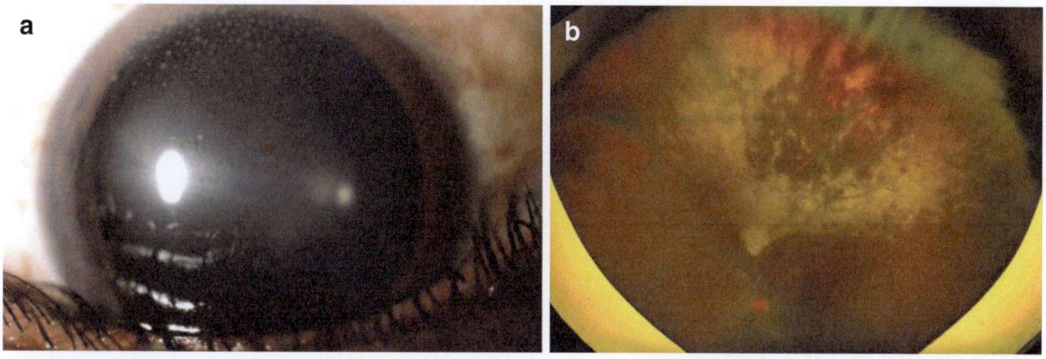

Fig. 18.4 (**a** and **b**) Anterior Uveitis and Acute Retinal Necrosis in the same patient

18.5 Differential Diagnosis

Keratouveitis can occur in any stage of HZO. The condition may be difficult to diagnose in the prodromal stage as the clinical symptoms overlap with the constitutional symptoms of any other viral disease. The ocular symptoms in the chronic and sequelae stage may also sometimes pose difficulties in the situations where the previous history of blistering skin eruptions in unavailable. The differential diagnosis depending on the clinical picture and stage of the disease are following:

18.5.1 Neuralgic Pain

In the initial phase of the disease when pain is the only predominant symptom, other conditions such as cluster and migraine headaches need to be ruled out.

18.5.2 Ocular Features Without Skin Rash (Herpes Zoster Sine Herpte)

In the presence of eyelid swelling, excoriation and conjunctivitis, pre-septal and orbital cellulitis must be differentiated. In eyes with corneal lesions such as pseudodendrities and superficial punctate erosions, possibility of Acanthmoeba keratitis should be made and ruled out.

18.5.3 Rash

A vesicular rash in a dermatomal pattern is suggestive of HZO, other differentials such as contact dermatitis, impetigo and primary herpes simplex virus (HSV) infection should be ruled out.

18.5.4 Keratouveitis in Healed Stage

The presence of posterior synechiae, old keratic precipitates with atrophic iris patches are more commonly due to HZO, however other causes of viral keratitis with anterior uveitis should be differentiated. The associated non-ocular and constitutional symptoms in the acute stage of the disease and the history of the systemic status helps in formulating an accurate diagnosis of keratouveitis. Keratouveitis may be caused by several other viruses such as herpes viruses, cytomegalovirus, Epstein- Barr virus, rubella virus, chikungunya virus and mumps virus. HSV keratouveitis is a close differential as overlapping features with HZ keratouveitis are common. The anterior uveitis of HZ tends to be chronic when compared to HSV infection which is acute and recurrent. CMV keratouveitis presents with conspicuous anterior segment involvement such as corneal oedema, coin shaped keratic precipitates, anterior chamber inflammation with or without raised intraocular pressure [21]. Relapses of keratouveitis can occur in CMV infection and endothelial imaging reveals an owl's- eye morphology that is characteristic of CMV infection. It is important to differentiate this infection as topical steroids may lead to worsening of the uveitis associated with CMV and does not respond to oral acyclovir.

18.6 Management

18.6.1 Acute Stage of HZO with Keratouveitis

Management in acute stage of the disease with corneal involvement is the same as for HZO, typically with systemic Acyclovir/Valacyclovir/Famciclovir. The oral treatment should be initiated promptly, ideally within 72 h from the onset of the rash [22]. Although the effectiveness of antiviral treatment beyond 72 h is not clearly established, systemic treatment may have a role in deterring the ongoing viral replication till the duration the rash looks active. Commonly, oral acyclovir is prescribed on a dosage of 800 mg five times daily for 1–2 weeks, until the healing of the skin rash [23]. Famciclovir in a dose of 500 mg three times daily and Valacyclovir 1000 mg three times daily are the other alternatives to acyclovir. Topical treatment acyclovir 0.3% or ganciclovir 0.15% gel five times daily can be used additionally for managing active keratitis [24].

Patients without anterior segment involvement can be followed up at 2–3 weeks after the onset of the acute disease, while those with presence of concomitant corneal/anterior segment involvement should be reviewed early within 1–2 weeks based on the severity of the initial disease. The subsequent follow-up may be every 2–6 months thereafter to monitor for delayed sequelae of the disease [7].

18.6.2 Subacute and Chronic Stage of the Disease

Corneal involvement after the resolution of acute infective phase of the disease usually occurs due to vasculitis and inflammatory causes. Topical steroids either Prednisolone acetate 1% or Loteprednol etabonate 4–6 times per day accompanied by ointment at night, works to suppress the inflammatory reaction and remains the mainstay of treatment in immune-related corneal and anterior segment diseases such as endothelitis, keratouveitis, limbitis, sclerokeratitis and peripheral ulcerative keratitis. In severe cases, oral corticosteroids are recommended as anti-inflammatory agents.

Corneal oedema should be treated with 5% NaCl drops 4–8 times per day with or without 6% NaCl ointment at night depending on the severity of oedema. Adjunctive treatment with ocular surface lubricants and cycloplegic drops should be supplemented as deemed necessary.

Antiglaucoma medications like systemic carbonic anhydrase inhibitors 250 mg 8 hourly, topical Beta blockers, Alpha agonists in BD dosing should be administered to decrease the intraocular pressure. Prostaglandin analogues may be best avoided in the management of raised intraocular pressure.

18.6.3 Management of Complications

Recurrent keratouveitis can lead to complicated cataract and secondary glaucoma. Elevated IOP usually occurs secondary to zoster-induced trabeculitis. However, it may also occur due to obstruction of the trabecular meshwork from the inflammatory cell and protein debris or from the formation of synechiae as a consequence of extensive intraocular inflammation. Surgical management of glaucoma may be needed in cases of raised intraocular pressures not responding to anti glaucoma medications. Ideally, inflammation should be controlled for as long as safely possible prior to glaucoma surgery to optimize a favourable outcome in these high-risk eyes. Perioperative corticosteroid therapy provided topically, orally, or as a sub-Tenon injection together with intraoperative mitomycin C and postoperative 5-flourouracil is advised.

Persistent corneal oedema following repeat episodes of endothelitis and corneal scarring because of chronic relapsing nature of the stromal disease will necessitate keratoplasty. Endothelial dysfunction can be managed with endothelial keratoplasty; however, stromal scarring necessitates penetrating keratoplasty. The success of penetrating keratoplasty is limited in eyes with severely anaesthetic cornea. Corneal neurotization may be needed prior to penetrating keratoplasty in select eyes to improve the success of keratoplasty and graft survival.

People with previous HZO keratitis or uveitis are more likely to develop cataract because of their age, exposure to inflammation, and topical steroid use; they are predisposed to surgical complications and the risk for recurrent inflammation. Hence, careful patient selection, detailed informed consent, a long period of disease quiescence before cataract surgery (minimum 6 months; ideally 1 year), and consideration of oral antiviral therapy in those with a history of multiple disease recurrences is essential. An increased risk for recurrence is associated with shorter periods of quiescence and a greater number of recurrences before surgery. Hydrophobic acrylic IOLs are well tolerated in uveitic eyes and reduce the rate of posterior synechiae formation. Heparin surface modified IOLs (HSM-IOLs) may be associated with a reduced rate of postoperative uveitis. Angulated, sharp square optic edge IOL haptics help to reduce the amount of contact between the iris and the optic and decreases the chance of PCO formation [25, 26].

It is generally recommended to plan any surgical intervention after an adequate period of quiescence, ideally one year or a minimum of 6 months). Recurrences of ocular inflammation have been reported after cataract surgery [27]. Hence, it is worthwhile to consider perioperative antiviral prophylaxis. The Zoster Eye Disease Study (ZEDS) is currently underway in the United States to understand the role of antiviral therapy in the treatment and prevention of chronic/recurrent HZO.

18.7 Conclusion

The severity of keratouveitis in association with HZO can range from mild to severe. The diagnosis is made on clinical examination. The degree of severity of involvement should be ascertained and prompt treatment should be instituted.

Key Points

1. Varicella zoster virus reactivation may lead to a myriad of ocular complications including but not limited to keratitis, uveitis, retinal vasculitis and optic neuritis. Keratouveitis continues to be a major cause of visual impairment in HZO.
2. Immunosuppression, diabetes, cataract surgery and COVID-19 infection/vaccination increase the risk of severe and recurrent HZO.
3. Recurrent HZO may be complicated by cataract formation, secondary glaucoma and corneal scarring.
4. Treatment of HZO depends on the stage of the disease; acute stages are treated primarily with antivirals while subacute and chronic stages warrant corticosteroids and antiglaucoma medications to manage inflammation and secondary IOP spike. Surgery may be considered for severe corneal scarring.

References

1. Dahmiwal S, Priyanka, Jain NC, et al. Changing age pattern and diverse outcomes of herpes zoster ophthalmicus: exploring the temporal trend, decrease in incident age and influence of treatment strategies. Int Ophthalmol. 2024;44(1):443.
2. Liesegang TJ. Herpes zoster ophthalmicus natural history, risk factors, clinical presentation, and morbidity. Ophthalmology. 2008;115(Suppl 2):S3–12.
3. Liesegang TJ. Corneal complications from herpes zoster ophthalmicus. Ophthalmology. 1985;92(3):316–24.
4. Curran D, Callegaro A, Fahrbach K, et al. Metaregression of herpes zoster incidence worldwide. Infect Dis Ther. 2022;11(1):389–403.

5. Kong CL, Thompson RR, Porco TC, Kim E, Acharya NR. Incidence rate of herpes zoster ophthalmicus: a retrospective cohort study from 1994 through 2018. Ophthalmology. 2020;127(3):324–30.
6. Dmitriev AA, Odden J, Mora-Boellstorff D, et al. Herpes zoster ophthalmicus: frequency and risk factors for developing uncommon ocular manifestations. Can J Ophthalmol. 2024;59(3):201–7.
7. Litt J, Cunningham AL, Arnalich-Montiel F, et al. Herpes Zoster Ophthalmicus: Presentation, Complications, Treatment, and Prevention. Infect Dis Ther. 2024;13(7):1439–59.
8. Szeto SK, Chan TC, Wong RL, et al. Prevalence of ocular manifestations and visual outcomes in patients with herpes zoster ophthalmicus. Cornea. 2017;36:338–42.
9. Womack LW, Liesegang TJ. Complications of herpes zoster ophthalmicus. Arch Ophthalmol. 1983;101:42–5.
10. Niederer RL, Meyer JJ, Liu K, Danesh-Meyer HV. Herpes zoster ophthalmicus clinical presentation and risk factors for loss of vision. Am J Ophthalmol. 2021;226:83–9.
11. Akpandak I, Sechrist SJ, Miller DC, Sun Y, Arnold BF, Kelly JD, Acharya NR. Risk of herpes zoster ophthalmicus after COVID-19 vaccination in a large US Health Care Claims Database. Am J Ophthalmol. 2024;258:139–44.
12. Bhavsar A, Lonnet G, Wang C, et al. Increased risk of herpes zoster in adults ≥50 years old diagnosed with COVID-19 in the United States. Open Forum. Infect Dis. 2022;9(5):ofac118.
13. Parikh R, Spence O, Giannelos N, et al. Herpes zoster recurrence: a narrative review of the literature. Dermatol Ther (Heidelb). 2024;14(3):569–92.
14. Yawn B, Wollan P, Sauver J, Butterfield L. Herpes zoster eye complications: rates and trends. Mayo Clin Proc. 2013;88(6):562–70.
15. Lee S, Han J, Yang C, Choi C, Khoramnia R, Chung T, et al. Chronic and recurrent herpes zoster ophthalmicus. Medicina (Kaunas). 2021;57(10):999.
16. Tran K, Falcone M, Choi D, Goldhardt R, Karp C, Davis J, et al. Epidemiology of herpes zoster ophthalmicus: recurrence and chronicity. Ophthalmology. 2016;123(7):1469–75.
17. Lu L, McGhee C, Sims J, Niederer R. High rate of recurrence of herpes zoster-related ocular disease after phacoemulsification cataract surgery. J Cataract Refract Surg. 2019;45(6):810–5.
18. He Y, Melo FR, Kron-Gray M, Musch D, Soong H. Outcomes of cataract surgery in eyes with previous herpes zoster ophthalmicus. J Cataract Refract Surg. 2015;41(4):771–7.
19. Thean JH, Hall AJ, Stawell RJ. Uveitis in herpes zoster ophthalmicus. Clin Experiment Ophthalmol. 2001;29:406–10.
20. Marsh RJ, Easty DL, Jone BR. Iritis and iris atrophy in herpes zoster ophthalmicus. Am J Ophthalmol. 1974;78:255–61.
21. Kim M, Chun YS, Moon NJ, Kim KW. Clinical factors associated with the early reduction of corneal sensitivity in herpes zoster ophthalmicus. Korean J Ophthalmol. 2022;36(2):147–53.
22. Katherine SBH, Ngim YS, Juliana J, Ramli N. Herpes zoster keratouveitis with hypopyon and hyphema. Taiwan J Ophthalmol. 2020;10(1):54–7.
23. Koizumi N, Inatomi T, Suzuki T, et al. Japan Corneal Endotheliitis Study Group. Clinical features and management of cytomegalovirus corneal endotheliitis: analysis of 106 cases from the Japan corneal endotheliitis study. Br J Ophthalmol. 2015;99(1):54–8.
24. Rathi A, Das AV, Ramappa M. Clinical and demographic profile of herpes zoster ophthalmicus: a hospital-based study of 1752 Indian patients. Indian J Ophthalmol. 2024;72(Suppl 4):S645–9. https://doi.org/10.4103/IJO.IJO_2634_23.
25. Leung TG, Lindsley K, Kuo IC. Types of intraocular lenses for cataract surgery in eyes with uveitis. Cochrane Database Syst Rev. 2014;3:CD007284.
26. Kim WS, Kim KH. Uveitis cataract. In: Challenges in cataract surgery; 2016. p. 11–6.
27. Lu LM, McGhee CNJ, Sims JL, Niederer RL. High rate of recurrence of herpes zoster-related ocular disease after phacoemulsification cataract surgery. J Cataract Refract Surg. 2019;45(6):810–5.

19 Other Ocular Affections

Amber Amar Bhayana, Ronnie Abhishek, Mudit Tyagi, and Brijesh Takkar

Abstract

Viruses impact the posterior segment of the eye in various ways. They can present as acute emergencies with sudden onset vision loss and features of retinitis, as well as painful anterior uveitis. They can present simultaneously with active systemic viral infections as well in immune-deficiency states. Variably, these may also be detected as intrauterine or congenital infections with retinal manifestations. Rarely, as in cases with Herpetic Zoster, overlapping presentation may also be noted together with corneal, orbital and neuro-ophthalmic disease. This chapter summarizes uveo-retinal manifestations of viral infections along with their management in brief.

Keywords

Retinitis · Retinal necrosis · Keratouveitis · Virus

A. A. Bhayana
GNEC, Maulana Azad Medical College, Delhi, India

R. Abhishek · M. Tyagi · B. Takkar (✉)
L V Prasad Eye Institute,
Hyderabad, Telangana, India

19.1 Anterior Manifestations

19.1.1 Herpetic Keratouveitis

Herpetic uveitis or keratouveitis is an anterior chamber manifestation of reactivation of the virus from trigeminal nucleus, primary infection being a very rare cause [1]. Subjects affected are usually over 60 years of age, though younger population may be involved. HSV-1 is the most common causative virus among the family, others being HSV-2, VZV and CMV. Reactivation occurs following a stressor like fever, cold sore, blisters or rarely immunosuppression [2].

Eye involvement is usually unilateral and presents as painful diminution of vision due to ciliary spasm with ciliary congestion. Patient presents with small to medium-sized KPs (keratic precipitates), some of the fresh KPs may be pigmented with elevated intraocular pressures due to trabeculitis, which may be episodic [3]. Patchy iris atrophy with corneal hypoesthesia indicates the diagnosis. Fuch's uveitis syndrome forms a close differential with similar features of diffuse stellate keratic precipitates with subtle or absent heterochromia without posterior synechiae and has been mainly associated with viral infections [4]. Anterior chamber cells and accompanying trabeculitis are associated with significant ocular hypertension as opposed to other uveitis where accompanying cyclitis/cyclitic membranes usually causes hypotony. Incidence of corneal

B. Sharma et al. (eds.), *Viral Keratitis*, https://doi.org/10.1007/978-981-95-3148-6_19

involvement in HSV ranges from 33–41% and can present as active keratitis (epithelial, stromal, interstitial and disciform), old corneal scar, endotheliitis and reduced corneal sensation [3]. Though the condition is generally diagnosed clinically, anterior chamber tap for polymerase chain reaction for viral DNA is the definitive diagnostic modality.

Treatment is oral acyclovir 400 mg 5 times a day for 2–3 weeks followed by two times a day for maintenance along with topical steroids to control the inflammation and cycloplegics to reduce the pain and prevent posterior synechiae. Alternatively, valacyclovir, a prodrug with better bioavailability may be used 500 mg three times a day for 4 weeks followed by 500 mg twice a day for maintenance [5]. Accompanying/preceding episode of shingles/zoster dermatitis point towards VZV being the cause which requires double the oral dose of acyclovir (800 mg five times a day). Topical antivirals due to poor penetrance have no role for anterior uveitis except in CMV anterior uveitis where topical 2% ganciclovir is considered useful [6]. Systemic steroids are thought to further enhance immunosuppression and should be avoided.

19.1.2 Viral Scleritis

For viral scleritis, the most common causes include VZV, HSV-1, Ebstein Barr virus and rarely cytomegalovirus. Zoster is the most common among them and presents clinically as nodular scleritis or sclerouveitis [7]. Recurrent episodes, associated uveitis, associated corneal opacities, corneal hypoesthesia and history of herpes/zoster infection with pigmented skin scars are clinical clues to the scleritis being of viral etiology which otherwise is difficult to differentiate from immunological nodular scleritis [8]. Topical steroids may mask the pain in such cases, but the organism proliferates underneath, warranting systemic antivirals. In fact, early relief followed by relapse while on topical steroids is another sign of an infectious etiology.

Clinically appearing as ulcer like nodule with intense congestion, the lesions heal with scleral atrophy with uveal tissue show, with chances of staphyloma formation and poor healing/wound closure if later operated upon for other indications like cataract.

19.2 Posterior Manifestations of Infective Retinitis

19.2.1 Acute Retinal Necrosis

ARN or acute retinal necrosis is a type of necrotizing retinitis caused by Herpes family virus (HSV1, HSV2, VZV, CMV and EBV) in both immunocompetent and immunosuppressed individuals [9]. VZV is a common cause of ARN followed by HSV1 and HSV2 even though HSV2 is the major cause in children [9, 10].

Pathophysiology of Retinitis

The pathophysiology of retinitis is partly like keratitis. Primary infection or more commonly reactivation after laying dormant in the dorsal root ganglion, allows the virus to invade the retinal tissue and cause direct toxic effect to the cells and immune mediated damage ultimately leading to necrosis [11]. Occlusive retinal vasculitis is a hallmark feature which exponentiates damage and necrosis.

ARN is also known to present with pigmented KPs which may be either granulomatous or non-granulomatous, raised intraocular pressure and sometimes with anterior scleritis [12]. In acute stages ARN presents as patchy retinitis; usually starts peripherally and then progresses to become increasingly confluent while advancing more towards the posterior pole [13]. Retinal arteries are commonly affected, and it causes occlusive retinal vasculitis leading to localized retinal ischemia and non-perfusion (Fig. 19.1). Occlusive vasculitis progresses beyond the area of retinitis [14]. The lesions heal with pigmentation and RPE hypertrophy. The risk of fellow eye involvement is high in the first three months [15]. The necrotic retinal tissue often becomes thin and forms atrophic holes/tears at junction of normal and diseased retina which can cause rhegmatogenous detachments. Diagnostic criteria for ARN

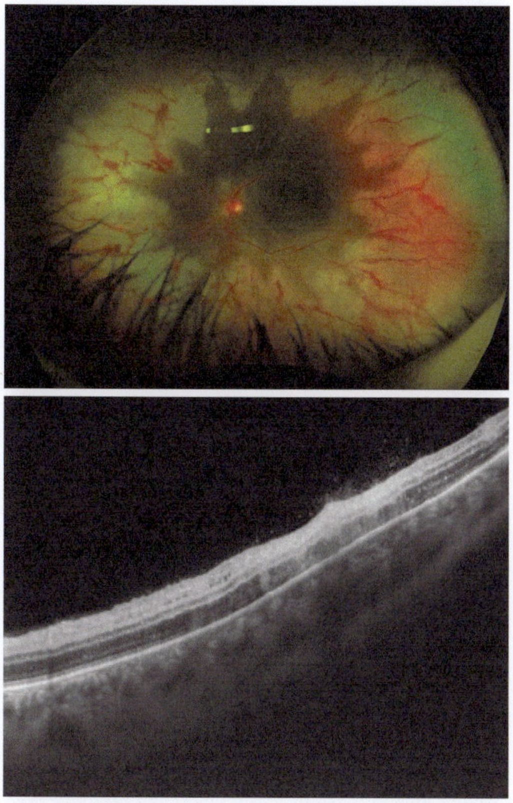

Fig. 19.1 Ultra-widefield fundus photography showing acute retinal necrosis. Circumferential peripheral confluent retinitis patches are seen with relative sparing of the posterior pole. Peri-vascular haemorrhages and vascular sheathing suggest obliterative inflammatory changes of vessels. Optical coherence tomography shows accompanying vitritis, inflammatory changes in the entire retinal thickness, more so on in the inner retinal layers with choroidal congestion

by American Uveitis Society in 1994 included (1): one or more foci of retinitis in the peripheral retina, (2) progression in the absence of antiviral therapy, (3) circumferential spread, (4) occlusive arteriolitis and (5) Vitritis and anterior chamber reaction [16]. OCT may show inner as well as a pan-retinal hyperreflectivity with signs of retinal necrosis. Acute stages involve thickening of the retinal tissue with fluid and exudates in the intraretinal or subretinal space. The layers become disorganized as the disease advances. As the inflammation subsides, thinning and atrophy may ensue with possible hyporeflective spaces signifying tissue loss. qPCR gives definitive evidence of viruses in aqueous and vitreous samples with sensitivity of 70–90% and specificity of 100%. Even though it is commonly a unilateral condition, bilateral retinal necrosis is known too [17]. Antiviral treatment is known to reduce the risk of developing bilateral ARN [18].

Treatment involves battling the virus acutely and managing the late sequelae. Antiviral therapy involves oral/intravenous antiviral agents. The various antiviral regimens followed are mentioned below:

1. Intravenous acyclovir 13 mg/kg/dose divided 8 h for 7 days followed by oral acyclovir 800 mg five times a day for 3–4 months
2. Oral valaciclovir 1–2 g 8 h for induction for 3 weeks followed by slow taper over 3–4 months
3. Intravitreal foscarnet 2.4 mg/0.1 ml as an adjunct in macular-threatening retinitis
4. Intravitreal ganciclovir 200–2000 µg/0.1 ml as an adjunct in macular- or nerve-threatening disease.

19.2.2 Progressive Outer Retinal Necrosis

PORN is a similar spectrum viral retinitis seen in immunocompromised individuals with CD4 counts <50–100. The most common cause is reactivation of indolent VZV with intraretinal spread followed by HSV1 and HSV2. A hallmark feature is minimal anterior chamber reaction and vitritis due to immunocompromised status unlike ARN which has marked vitritis. Also PORN has a propensity to involve the posterior pole and then spread to periphery. Perivascular sparing can cause the fundus to have a cracked mud appearance late in the disease [19]. Imaging and management is similar as in ARN with poor visual outcomes. The degree of inflammation in ARN and PORN depends on immune state of the individual and may vary within a single episode of eye infection.

19.2.3 Cytomegalovirus (CMV) Retinitis

Cytomegalovirus is a double stranded virus of herpesviridae family, predominantly affecting the immunocompromised patients with CD4 counts below 50 cells/mm^3 [20]. HIV being the most common association, a latent virus in immunocompetent individuals can reactive when immunity is compromised due to any reason [21]. CMV Retinitis is known to present clinically in three different forms: (a) Fulminant form where the retinitis presents with multiple haemorrhages (b) Indolent granular form in which the vascular endothelium is affected initially with multiple small retinitis lesions (c) Frosted branch angitis like clinical picture which is a rare form [14]. One can recognize CMV retinitis from its white borders and the central clearing (retinal atrophy) (Fig. 19.2). Cavernous retinitis is prominent feature on OCT where there is bridging of retinal tissue having preponderance to retinal detachment [22].

In HIV individuals it is of utmost importance to start the anti-retroviral treatment (HAART) to stop the progression of the retinitis and to avoid fellow eye involvement. Oral valganciclovir is started at 900 mg dose of two times per day for first 3 weeks as an induction dose followed by the maintenance dose of 450 mg two times till the CD4 counts rises to more than 200 for minimum three consecutive months and upon resolution of retinitis [23] (Table 19.1). Intravenous Foscarnet inhibits DNA replication. Cidofovir is given in patients with resistance for ganciclovir. Intravitreal ganciclovir injections are given biweekly until response is seen followed by weekly injections.

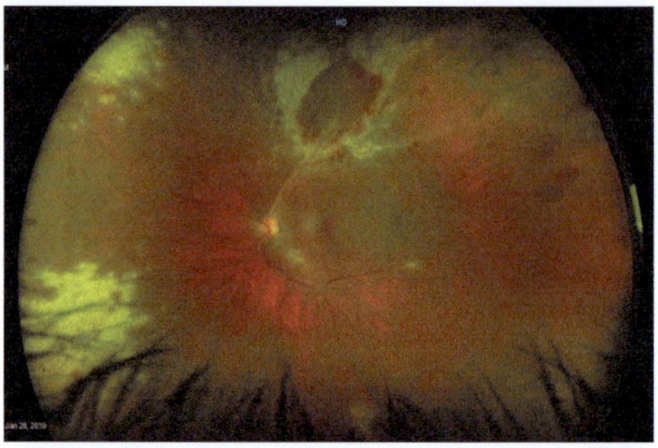

Fig. 19.2 Ultra-widefield fundus photograph of a subject with CMV retinitis showing lesions in the supero-nasal and infero-nasal quadrants and also along the superior vascular arcade. Lesions can be closer to posterior pole when compared to acute retinal necrosis. Coexisting retinitis and haemorrhages in sectoral configuration can presume pizza pie like appearance. Rest of the retina and vitreous may be considerably quiet due to coexisting immunocompromised status and poor inflammatory response

Table 19.1 Showing differences between Herpetic and CMV retinitis

Herpes simplex retinitis	CMV retinitis
Seen in immunocompetent/immunocompromised	Seen usually in immunocompromised classically when CD4 counts <50/microlitre
Commences as peripheral retinitis patches which coalesce to form peripheral continuous thick annular bands of tissue necrosis	Involves posterior pole earlier
Specific—obliterative endarteritis	Specific—Pizza pie appearance due to haemorrhages
Intense vitritis is usually present due to immune system being usually competent	Vitritis is lacking due immunosuppression
Treatment—Acyclovir/valacyclovir	Treatment- Ganciclovir/Valganciclovir
OCT features—Vitritis, pan retinal inflammation and hyper-reflectivity corresponding to yellow retinitis lesions, intraretinal oedema in outer nuclear layer, disorganization of retinal layers during active inflammation, subretinal fluid in occasional cases Lesions heal with retinal thinning and disappearance of retinal hyperreflectivity as inflammation resolves	OCT features—common features—for peripheral CMV lesions with propensity to involve ellipsoid zone and photoreceptor layers. Macular lesions addedly involve PVD, ERM, vitreomacular adhesion and traction lesions

19.3 Congenital and Intrauterine Infections (Table 19.2)

19.3.1 Rubella

Rubella virus is an RNA virus of the Togaviridae family and one of the common causes of congenital infectious oculopathies. The transmission of infection from the maternal placenta is maximum in the first trimester and decreases as the pregnancy progresses [24]. The teratogenic probabilities are maximum during first trimester infection and reduce later as the immunological status of the fetus matures. Systemic manifestations include sensorineural deafness, heart defects, microcephaly and intellectual disability [25]. Ocular manifestations of the newborn include corneal opacities (feature of healed keratitis/keratouveitis/glaucomatous changes), patches of iris atrophy, poorly dilating pupil with posterior synechiae (marker of intrauterine uveitis), total or membranous cataract, salt and pepper retinopathy (due to retinal pigment epithelium changes) [26]. Glaucoma may occur due to angle development anomalies or may be uveitis/lens induced. Microphthalmos may be seen accompanying general growth retardation. Antenatal diagnosis is mainly by detecting IgM in maternal serum or serially increasing IgG titers. Post-natal IgG in the baby's serum is of little value as it reflects old maternal transmitted antibodies [27]. Treatment is aimed at managing complications like cataract, while the disease itself is a self-limiting intrauterine episode, the sequelae being debilitating. Rarely, some of these patients may develop neovascular membranes originating from the choroid during follow up [28].

Table 19.2 Showing intrauterine infections and associated ocular features

Ocular features	Rubella	Cytomegalovirus	Herpes	Measles/SSPE	Zika virus
Microphthalmos	Yes	Yes	Yes	Phthisis bulbi	
Iris atrophy	Yes		Yes		
Cataract	Yes	Yes	Yes	Yes	
Cornea	Opacities		Keratitis	Scarring	
Chorioretinitis	Yes	Full-thickness retinitis lesions	Uncommon	Necrotizing	
Chorioretinal atrophy		Nummular chorioretinal scars		Chorioretinal scars in longstanding	Cluster (polar bear tracks), non-macular, colobomatous atrophy
Pigmentary changes	Salt pepper retinopathy			Multifocal placoid pigment epitheliopathy	Macular and peripheral pigmentary mottling
Optic neuritis			Yes	Yes	
Optic nerve pallor				Yes	Yes
Optic nerve hypoplasia		Atrophy		Atrophy	Yes
Cortical blindness		Yes		Yes	Yes
Coloboma		Retina and optic nerve	Pseudocoloboma of retina- choroid and optic nerve		Iris coloboma, colobomatous atrophy
Glaucoma	Yes, well decribed				
Strabismus	Yes	Yes	Yes		

19.3.2 Cytomegalovirus

CMV is the most common cause of maternally transmitted congenital infections which may occur pre-natally (from maternal infection/reactivation causing acute viremia), perinatally (during birth from maternal secretions) and postnatally from breast milk [29]. Systemic features include microcephaly with intracranial calcification, growth retardation, deafness. Ocular signs include microphthalmos, cataracts, healed chorioretinal scars, optic nerve atrophy and developmental anomalies and coloboma like lesions in retina and of optic nerve [29]. Post-natal infections can present with CMV retinitis just like in adults warranting intravitreal and systemic antivirals.

19.3.3 Herpesvirus

80–90% of neonatal HSV infections occur during the perinatal period because of aspiration of infected fluids or direct contact to mucosal surfaces. Systemic and ocular complications are similar. Microphthalmia, complicated cataracts, iris atrophy, healed uveitic lesions and pseudocolobomas of retina-choroid and optic nerves are the usual observations [30]. Acute perinatal infections are managed with systemic antivirals with renal function test monitoring.

19.3.4 Measles Virus

Measles virus can cause encephalitis typically in children [31]. Ophthalmological findings manifest few weeks to a few years before the neurological manifestations [32]. Different ocular manifestations are summarized in the table below, typically associated with subacute sclerosing pan-enchaphelitis. Cortical and neuro-ophthalmic manifestations may or may not accompany these.

Chorioretinitis with macular involvement is characteristic [33]. Necrotizing chorioretinitis is characterized by dilated tortuous veins, retinal haemorrhages with subretinal exudates and retinal and macular pigmentary changes [34]. In long-standing cases a healed retinal scar with well-defined borders around the central retinal atrophy is seen. Findings of disc oedema, whitish retinal lesions and retinal vasculitis have also been described. The OCT findings from a singular case showed the primary involvement of the plexiform layers on SD-OCT which may indicate that measles viruses are concentrated at synapses in the retina. As the infection spreads, necrosis progresses with increased inner reflectivity, hyporeflective cystoid spaces and necrosis of inner retinal layers. Further non-intervened course would lead to the outer retinal layers necrosis, outer hyper-reflective dots with moth-eaten appearance [35]. Therapy is on the lines of measles encephalitis.

19.3.5 Zika Virus

Pregnant women are susceptible to ZIKV during all trimesters of pregnancy and maternal-foetal transmission has been confirmed [36]. Pregnant women who contract ZIKV have a risk of preterm birth, miscarriage and a congenital Zika syndrome that consists of intrauterine growth retardation, microcephaly, brain, auditory, skeletal and ocular abnormalities [37]. Animal model studies suggest that, before the blood-retinal barrier and host immunity are well developed, ZIKV may enter the retinal tissue and infect susceptible cellular populations [38]. Though cortical impairment is more common, classic retinal signs include well-circumscribed atrophy and pigment mottling at the macula [39]. OCT findings are known to corroborate with the retinal signs. Other signs include optic nerve pallor, increased cup to disc ratio and optic nerve hypoplasia with double ring sign. Peripheral pigmentary changes and cluster atrophic changes (polar bear tracks) and uveal colobomas are also described [40]. Neuro ophthalmic manifestations may also occur.

19.4 Other Viral Infections with Inflammatory Sequalae

19.4.1 Dengue Virus

Dengue fever-related ocular involvement is known to be inflammatory, with signs of both vasculitis and chorioretinitis [41]. Fundus findings include venous and arteriolar sheathing with haemorrhages and leakage from both arterioles and venules on angiography. Yellow submacular dots are also described along with microvascular occlusions [42]. Foveolitis may lead to significant irreversible central scotoma [43]. Steroids and anti-inflammatory agents are treatment options but should be administered carefully in view of possible viremia and hypocoagulative state [44].

19.4.2 Chickungunya Virus

Chikungunya fever (CHIKV) is an emerging mosquito borne disease [45]. Diagnosis chiefly relies on serology [46]. Ophthalmic manifestations may be unilateral or bilateral. Retinitis presents between 2 and 4 weeks after febrile period of systemic disease [47]. Anterior uveitis can have pigmented KPs and ocular hypertension controlled by topical and systemic corticosteroids [48]. Posteriorly, it typically presents as unifocal or multifocal retinitis or retinochoroiditis accompanied by vitritis and iritis [49]. Patchy retinal whitening at the posterior pole round vascular arcades with haemorrhages and oedema is known. OCT has demonstrated inner retinal layer thickening and hyper-reflectivity with posterior shadowing and associated serous retinal detachment. CHIKV-related manifestations are seen lesser in vitreous or anterior parts of the eye. Steroids remain the mainstay of treatment.

In this chapter we presented the commoner virus infections affecting the posterior part of the eye. With lesser available evidence, the COVID-19 pandemic was also associated with retinal vascular occlusions, central serous chorioretinopathy, retinal vascular occlusions, worsened ARN and endophthalmitis. Further manifestations of newer known viruses like EBV, Ebola virus and Marburg virus are also being reported. While the list is likely to expand, aggressive but careful treatment for infective and inflammatory state is warranted, while intrauterine infections need to be prevented and treated to avoid irreparable ocular dysgenesis in a new born.

19.5 Conclusions

A myriad of ocular symptoms from anterior segment disease to posterior segment diseases underpins the majority of the viral infections implicated in ophthalmic diseases. Acute retinal necrosis, cytomegalovirus retinitis and congenital zika virus infections exemplify the more commonly encountered viral afflictions of the eye which are often exacerbated or associated with an underlying immunodeficiency state. Over the years, developments in the imaging modalities used have greatly enhanced our understanding and facilitated the management of these conditions. Antivirals with continuous assessment for complications continue to be among the primary aims of disease management.

Key Points

1. Herpetic keratouveitis and viral scleritis are among the common anterior segment manifestations of viral anterior segment diseases.
2. Retinal necrosis and CMV retinitis are quintessential posterior segment complications, particularly seen in immunocompromised individuals.
3. Rubella, CMV, and Zika virus epitomises transplacental transmission, the need for timely antenatal diagnosis and prevention to avoid lifelong visual impairment.
4. PCR, OCT imaging and fundus photography are vital tools for diagnosis and disease monitoring.
5. Antivirals continue to be the mainstay pharmacological management modalities.

References

1. Acharya M, Dave A, Farooqui JH. Commentary: herpes keratitis: a diagnostic challenge. Indian J Ophthalmol. 2019;67(7):1046–7.
2. Pata R, Datar P. The diagnosis and management of Herpes Simplex Pneumonia in the critical care setting: a comprehensive review. Cureus. 2023;15(8)
3. Babu K, Konana VK, Ganesh SK, Patnaik G, Chan NS, Chee SP, Sobolewska B, Zierhut M. Viral anterior uveitis. Indian J Ophthalmol. 2020;68(9):1764–73.
4. Chan NS, Chee SP. Demystifying viral anterior uveitis: a review. Clin Experiment Ophthalmol. 2019;47(3):320–33.
5. Wensing B, Mochizuki M, De Boer JH. Clinical characteristics of herpes simplex virus associated anterior uveitis. Ocul Immunol Inflamm. 2018;26(3):333–7.
6. Keorochana N, Choontanom R. Efficacy and safety of an extemporaneous preparation of 2% ganciclovir eye drops in CMV anterior uveitis. BMJ Open Ophthalmol. 2017;2(1):e000061.
7. Al Barqi M, Behrens A, Alfawaz AM. Clinical features and visual outcomes of scleritis patients presented to tertiary care eye centers in Saudi Arabia. Int J Ophthalmol. 2015;8(6):1215.
8. Murthy SI, Sabhapandit S, Balamurugan S, Subramaniam P, Sainz-De-La-Maza M, Agarwal M, Parvesio C. Scleritis: differentiating infectious from non-infectious entities. Indian J Ophthalmol. 2020;68(9):1818–28.
9. Ganatra JB, Chandler D, Santos C, Kuppermann B, Margolis TP. Viral causes of the acute retinal necrosis syndrome. Am J Ophthalmol. 2000;129(2):166–72.
10. Lau CH, Missotten T, Salzmann J, Lightman SL. Acute retinal necrosis: features, management, and outcomes. Ophthalmology. 2007;114(4):756–62.
11. Thompson WS, Culbertson WW, Smiddy WE, Robertson JE, Rosenbaum JT. Acute retinal necrosis caused by reactivation of herpes simplex virus type 2. Am J Ophthalmol. 1994;118(2):205–11.
12. Roy R, Pal BP, Mathur G, Rao C, Das D, Biswas J. Acute retinal necrosis: clinical features, management and outcomes – a 10 year consecutive case series. Ocul Immunol Inflamm. 2014;22(3):170–4.
13. Tripathy K, Sharma YR, Gogia V, Venkatesh P, Singh SK, Vohra R. Serial ultra wide field imaging for following up acute retinal necrosis cases. Oman J Ophthalmol. 2015;8(1):71–2.
14. Patel A, Tyagi M. Viral retinitis. Delhi J Ophthalmol. 2021;31(4):19–25.
15. Shantha JG, Weissman HM, Debiec MR, Albini TA, Yeh S. Advances in the management of acute retinal necrosis. Int Ophthalmol Clin. 2015;55(3):1–13.
16. Holland GN. Standard diagnostic criteria for the acute retinal necrosis syndrome. Am J Ophthalmol. 1994;117(5):663–6.
17. Young NJ, Bird AC. Bilateral acute retinal necrosis. Br J Ophthalmol. 1978;62(9):581–90.
18. Palay DA, Sternberg P Jr, Davis J, et al. Decrease in the risk of bilateral acute retinal necrosis by acyclovir therapy. Am J Ophthalmol. 1991;112:250–5.
19. Austin RB. Progressive outer retinal necrosis syndrome: a comprehensive review of its clinical presentation, relationship to immune system status, and management. Clin Eye Vis Care. 2000;12(3-4):119–29.
20. Munro M, Yadavalli T, Fonteh C, Arfeen S, Lobo-Chan AM. Cytomegalovirus retinitis in HIV and non-HIV individuals. Microorganisms. 2019;8(1):55.
21. Rafailidis PI, Mourtzoukou EG, Varbobitis IC, Falagas ME. Severe cytomegalovirus infection in apparently immunocompetent patients: a systematic review. Virol J. 2008;5(1):47.
22. Invernizzi A, Agarwal A, Ravera V, Oldani M, Staurenghi G, Viola F. Optical coherence tomography findings in cytomegalovirus retinitis: a longitudinal study. Retina. 2018;38(1):108–17.
23. Patil AJ, Sharma A, Kenney MC, Kuppermann BD. Valganciclovir in the treatment of cytomegalovirus retinitis in HIV-infected patients. Clin Ophthalmol. 2010;4:111–9.
24. Miller E, Cradock-Watson J, Pollock T. Consequences of confirmed maternal rubella at successive stages of pregnancy. Lancet. 1982;320(8302):781–4.
25. Martínez-Quintana E, Castillo-Solórzano C, Torner N, Rodríguez-González F. Congenital rubella syndrome: a matter of concern. Rev Panam Salud Publica. 2015;37:179–86.
26. Duszak RS. Congenital rubella syndrome – major review. Optometr J Am Optometr Assoc. 2009;80(1):36–43.
27. Rasool I, Azad A, Baradwan S, Salman Bashir M, Al-Jaroudi D. The status of rubella IgG antibody titer between antenatal and postnatal among pregnant non-immune to rubella. Hum Vaccin Immunother. 2021;17(2):377–80.
28. Frank KE, Purnell EW. Subretinal neovascularization following rubella retinopathy. Am J Ophthalmol. 1978;86(4):462–6.
29. Chang TS, Wiener J, Dollard SC, Amin MM, Ellington S, Chasela C, Kayira D, Tegha G, Kamwendo D, Jamieson DJ, Van Der Horst C. Effect of cytomegalovirus infection on breastfeeding transmission of HIV and on the health of infants born to HIV-infected mothers. AIDS. 2015;29(7):831–6.
30. Fernandes ND, Arya K, Syed HA, Ward R. Congenital herpes simplex. InStatPearls [Internet]. StatPearls Publishing; 2024.
31. Buchanan R, Bonthius DJ. Measles virus and associated central nervous system sequelae. In: Seminars in pediatric neurology, vol. 19, No. 3. WB Saunders; 2012. p. 107–14.
32. Garg RK. Subacute sclerosing panencephalitis. J Neurol. 2008;255:1861–71.
33. Garg RK, Mahadevan A, Malhotra HS, Rizvi I, Kumar N, Uniyal R. Subacute sclerosing panencephalitis. Rev Med Virol. 2019;29(5):e2058.

34. Agarwal A, Singh R, Kumar A, Dogra MR, Gupta A. Bilateral subretinal fluid and retinal vasculopathy associated with subacute sclerosing panencephalitis. Retin Cases Brief Rep. 2017;11(2):145–7.
35. Cam F, Dericioğlu V, Celiker H. Spectral domain optical coherence tomography findings of subacute sclerosing panencephalitis presenting with macular necrotizing retinitis: a case report. Ocul Immunol Inflamm. 2023;31(9):1891–6.
36. Besnard M, Lastere S, Teissier A, Cao-Lormeau VM, Musso D. Evidence of perinatal transmission of Zika virus, French Polynesia, December 2013 and February 2014. Eurosurveillance. 2014;19(13)
37. Ventura LO, Ventura CV, Lawrence L, et al. Visual impairment in children with congenital Zika syndrome. J AAPOS. 2017;21:295–9.
38. Singh PK, Guest JM, Kanwar M, Boss J, Gao N, Juzych MS, Abrams GW, Yu FS, Kumar A. Zika virus infects cells lining the blood-retinal barrier and causes chorioretinal atrophy in mouse eyes. JCI Insight. 2017;2(4)
39. Ventura CV, Maia M, Bravo-Filho V, Góis AL, Belfort R. Zika virus in Brazil and macular atrophy in a child with microcephaly. Lancet. 2016;387(10015):228.
40. Chan CY, Au SC. Ocular manifestations of Zika virus: a systematic review. J Ophthalmol Eye Disord Treat. 2021;1(1)
41. Tabbara K. Dengue retinochoroiditis. Ann Saudi Med. 2012;32(5):530–3.
42. Bacsal KE, Chee SP, Cheng CL, Flores JV. Dengue-associated maculopathy. Arch Ophthalmol. 2007;125(4):501–10.
43. Mbu-Nyamsi D, Vincent M, Perez-Fontana M, Best AL, Mesnard C, Villeroy F, Foucher A, Raffray L, Terrier CS, Bertolotti A. Ophthalmic complications during the dengue epidemic in Reunion Island in 2020: a case series and review of the literature. BMC Infect Dis. 2023;23(1):506.
44. Haritoglou C, Dotse SD, Rudolph G, Stephan CM, Thurau SR, Klauβ V. A tourist with dengue fever and visual loss. Lancet. 2002;360(9339):1070.
45. Horwood PF, Buchy P. Chikungunya. Rev Sci Tech. 2015;34(2):479–89.
46. Pfeffer M, Linssen B, Parke MD, Kinney RM. Specific detection of chikungunya virus using a RT-PCR/nested PCR combination. J Vet Med B Infect Dis Vet Public Health. 2002;49:49–54.
47. Martínez-Pulgarín DF, Muñoz-Urbano DM, Zamora-de la Cruz D. The eye and the chikungunya virus. Current Topics in Chikungunya. London: Intech Open; 2016. p. 49–66.
48. Lalitha P, Rathinam S, Banushree K, Maheshkumar S, Vijayakumar R, SatheP. Ocular involvement associated with an epidemic outbreak of chikungunya virus infection. Am J Ophthalmol. 2009;144(4):552–6.
49. Mahendradas P, Ranganna SK, Shetty R, et al. Ocular manifestations associated with chikungunya. Ophthalmology. 2008;115(2):287–91. https://doi.org/10.1016/j.ophtha.2007.03.085.

Neurological Manifestations in Herpes Zoster Ophthalmicus

20

Ritu Arora

Abstract

Herpes zoster Ophthalmicus (HZO) is the second commonest manifestation of Herpes Zoster (HZ). About 50% patients of herpes zoster develop ophthalmic complications. While neurologic complications like cranial nerve palsies are seen in 30% of Herpes zoster patients and optic neuropathy has been reported to occur in less than 1% of HZO patients. Post-herpetic neuralgia (PHN) is the most debilitating sequelae. Other neurological complications, such as cranial nerve palsies, meningitis, contralateral hemiparesis, and acute or chronic encephalitis may also be seen in rare occurrences.

Keywords

Herpes zoster ophthalmicus · Optic neuropathy · Neurotrophic keratitis · Cranial nerve palsies

20.1 Introduction

Herpes zoster ophthalmicus (HZO) is a painful, vesicular skin rash that appears on the dermatome of the first trigeminal branch (V1), and is due to the reactivation of a latent infection by the varicella zoster virus (VZV) in the Gasserian ganglion [1]. It is the second most frequent distribution after the thoracic and accounts for 10–20% of all cases of herpes zoster [1, 2]. Ocular involvement of HZO occurs in 20–70% of cases with various manifestations such as blepharitis, scleritis, keratoconjunctivitis, iridocyclitis, or acute retinal necrosis [2–5]. Neurological complications are less frequent (5–10%) and include oculomotor and facial nerve paresis, optic neuritis, meningoencephalitis, myelitis, and post-herpetic neuralgia [2, 5]. Orbital apex syndrome (OAS) involves the compromise of cranial nerves III, IV and VI and the ophthalmic branch of Vth nerve, as well as optic nerve dysfunction, and is a severe but very rare manifestation of HZO [5]. There are anecdotal reports of OAS available during COVID.

20.2 Pathophysiology of Varicella Zoster Infection

Herpes zoster (HZ) results from reactivation of the varicella zoster virus (VZV) because of decreasing T-cell–mediated immunity in advancing age or immunocompromised conditions. About 10–20% of all HZ involves the ophthalmic division of the trigeminal nerve resulting in herpes zoster ophthalmicus (HZO). About 50% of all HZO have ocular involvement, most commonly of the anterior segment, while posterior segment involvement (vitritis, retinitis, and optic neuritis) is relatively uncommon. Post-herpetic

R. Arora (✉)
Shroff Eye Centre, Delhi, India

B. Sharma et al. (eds.), *Viral Keratitis*, https://doi.org/10.1007/978-981-95-3148-6_20

neuralgia (PHN), a debilitating chronic pain syndrome, is the commonest sequelae of HZ. Other significant neurological complications include meningoencephalitis, myelitis, vasculitis, and cranial neuritis.

VZV is an exclusive human neurotropic alpha herpes virus with an icosahedral nucleocapsid core that contains a double stranded DNA genome. The core is surrounded by an amorphous protein material (tegument) and a lipid-rich envelope embedded with glycoproteins [6]. Viral cycle involves injection of viral DNA into the host nucleus where it replicates forming nucleocapsids, which then bud across the nuclear membrane acquiring the envelope [7].

VZV infects more than 95% of the human population before adolescence, producing the childhood exanthematous illness chicken pox, followed by a lifelong period of latency within neurons of the cranial, dorsal root, autonomic, and enteric ganglia [8]. During latency, the virus exists in the host tissues in with limited gene expression [9, 10]. Whenever host T-cell-mediated immunity diminishes VZV reactivates. The virus replicates in the sensory ganglia and spreads transaxonally to the corresponding mucocutaneous surfaces. This results in an intense inflammatory reaction that produces the painful vesicular dermatomal zoster rash [11]. VZV reactivation along the ophthalmic (V1) division of trigeminal nerve produces HZO. The pathogenesis of HZ-related complications likely involves infectious and inflammatory processes. Intense inflammation with hemorrhagic tissue necrosis and neuritis being evident on histopathology [12]. The pathogenesis of PHN however remains unclear. Proposed mechanisms include altered neuronal excitability and chronic low grade VZV infection of the sensory ganglionic neurons [13]. The neuro-ophthalmic complications result from involvement of the optic and ocular motor nerves, through mechanisms that are not clear. These include direct viral invasion of the nerve through trans-synaptic or vascular routes, extension of inflammation from the meningeal/cerebral tissues, VZV-induced perineuritis, and ischemia secondary to VZV vasculitis [14].

20.3 Herpes Zoster Ophthalmicus

It is a chronic, recurrent disease with a 5-year recurrence rate of 25%. Although frontal branch of the ophthalmic nerve is most commonly affected, involvement of the nasociliary branch produces skin lesions along the side of the nose and increases the risk for corneal denervation and ocular inflammatory disease by 4.02 and 3.35 times, respectively [15, 16]. Common anterior segment manifestations of HZO include conjunctivitis, keratitis, neurotrophic and exposure keratopathy, uveitis, keratouveitis, episcleritis, scleritis, and ocular surface abnormalities [17, 18]. Posterior segment complications such as vitritis, retinitis, and optic neuritis are uncommon. They are commoner in patients with HIV and low CD4 count.

Neurological complications of HZO may be encountered as neurotrophic keratopathy, optic neuritis, ophthalmoplegia, orbital apex syndrome with 3rd nerve and 7th nerve palsy. Another neurologic entity encountered is in the form of post-herpetic neuralgia.

20.4 Management Principles

Although a clinical diagnosis of HZO can be established in cases with classic presentation, diagnostic testing using PCR and serology on paired serum/ocular fluid samples are needed in case of diagnostic uncertainty. Systemic antiviral treatment improves dermatologic healing, decreases pain, viral shedding, adnexal involvement and reduces the rates of severe ocular complications [19]. Antiviral therapy is the mainstay treatment for ongoing HZ affliction. Valacyclovir (1 g 3 times daily for 7–10 days) is preferred in uncomplicated HZO because of simplified dosing, better pharmacokinetics, and better efficacy in decreasing the duration of acute zoster pain and PHN [20]. Other antivirals being acyclovir and famciclovir. A short course of corticosteroids (60 mg/day tapered over 2 weeks) may be used as an adjunct to reduce acute zoster pain. The use of steroids, however, does not decrease frequency of PHN, it can be considered for patients with optic neuropathy and HZ-related ophthalmoplegia especially if there is no significant improvement with antivirals alone within the first 1–2 weeks [20, 21].

20.5 Neurotropic Keratitis

Neurotrophic keratitis is a degenerative disease of corneal epithelium, characterized be absence of corneal sensitivity, which may end in corneal stromal melting and perforation [22].

Pathogenesis
Loss of innervation causes an epithelial defect centrally as the corneal epithelium is persistently regenerated centripetally from the periphery and sheds old cells at its apex as described by **Thoft** (Fig. 20.1).

Clinical Staging According to Mackie's Clinical Staging of Neurotrophic Keratitis, three stages have been defined.

Stage 1: Rose Bengal staining of the palpebral conjunctiva.

Decreased tear break-up time, increased viscosity of tear mucus, Punctate epithelial staining with fluorescein, scattered small facets of dry epithelium (Gaule spots).

Stage 2: Acute loss of epithelium usually under the upper lid, surrounding rim of loose epithelium, stromal edema, aqueous cell and flare and smooth and rolled edges of the defect (Fig. 20.1).

Stage 3: Stromal lysis sometimes resulting in corneal perforation.

Treatment
Selection of the treatment modality depends on the stage of the ulcer which is being treated.

Stage 1
Discontinue epitheliotoxic drugs, copious preservative free lubricants, punctal plugs, Bandage contact lens, and oral tetracycline.

Stage 2
Ocular lubricants, nerve growth factors, topical insulin drops, patching of eye, and tarsorrhaphy.

Stage 3
Collagenase inhibitors in the form of tetracycline, acetylcysteine are helpful. In view of severe corneal thinning tissue adhesives with bandage contact lens, conjunctival flap, amniotic membrane grafting, or tectonic corneal graft may be needed.

Novel Therapy
Certain newer therapies like insulin drops, regenerating agents, substance P, and recombinant neural growth factors have shown promising results [22]. Newer surgical procedures like corneal neurotization restore corneal innervation using nerve transposition or nerve grafting.

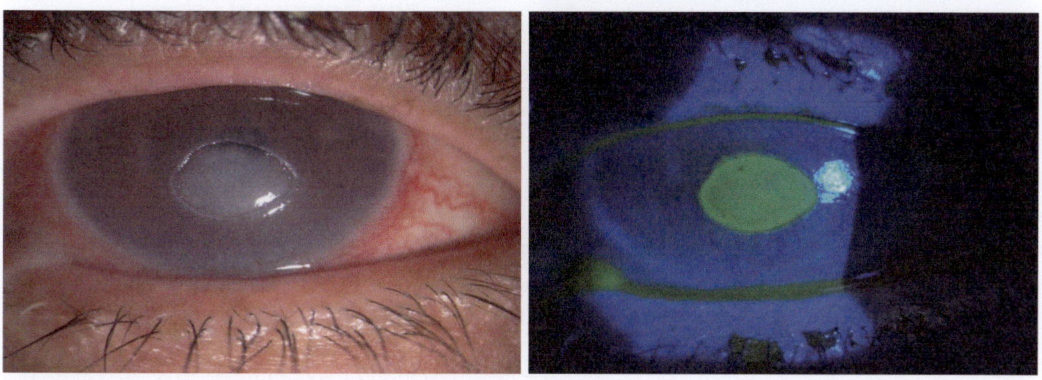

Fig. 20.1 Neuropathic ulcer with rolled-out edges

20.6 Optic Neuropathy

Optic neuropathy is an uncommon sequela of herpes zoster seen in less than 0.5% patients with HZO [23]. Herpes zoster optic neuropathy (HZON) may develop in the acute or late stages of HZO. It may accompany anterior and/or posterior forms of HZO and may present with papillitis, posterior optic neuropathy, or optic atrophy [24]. In B Scan Optic nerve involvement is seen as doubling of optic nerve head shown in Fig. 20.2. The inflammation of optic nerve can cause edema and vascular involvement and hemorrhagic It is rare but serious complication of HZO which can cause vision loss, and is often treated by antiviral medication and steroids.

A clinical diagnosis of HZON is established on the basis of close temporal association of ON with HZO and exclusion of other etiology. Isolated cases of HZON developing before skin rash and in disparate dermatomes as the preceding skin rash (nontrigeminal or contralateral trigeminal) and bilateral HZON also have been reported [25–27].

The pathophysiology of HZON is unclear, and multiple mechanisms have been proposed. These include optic nerve invasion of the VZV through continuous and hematogenous routes and ocular ischemia secondary to vascular inflammation. Other mechanisms for optic neuropathy being indirectly linked like (e.g. inflammatory, demyelination, optic perineuritis, extra orbital infections leading to reactive immune response with subsequent edema of the optic disc) [28–30].

Diagnostic testing using contrast-enhanced MRI and CSF studies have been recommended; however, they were found to be of limited utility in most studies. There are no confirmatory laboratory or imaging tests for HZ-mediated optic neuropathy.

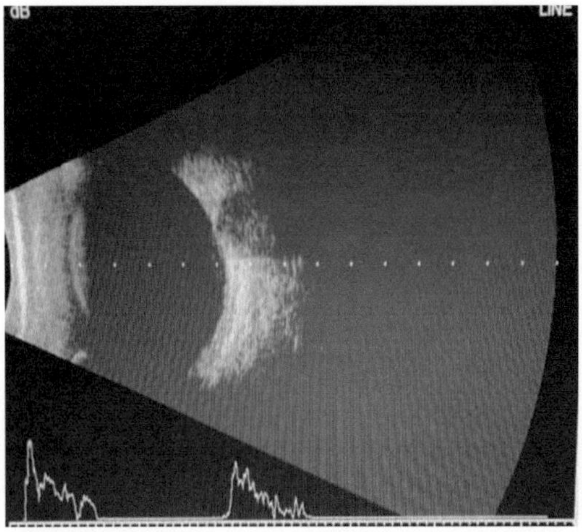

Fig. 20.2 Optic nerve involvement seen in B Scan as doubling of optic nerve head in HZO

Management

All patients with acute optic neuropathy in the setting of HZO should undergo MRI of the brain and orbit with fat suppressed sequences to evaluate optic nerve changes. Confirmatory testing (PCR and serology) should be obtained on paired samples of serum and CSF (in isolated HZON) or intraocular fluid (in patients with uveitis). Patients with evidence of neurological involvement require prompt treatment with intravenous antiviral medications (acyclovir 10–15 mg/kg every 8 hours for 2–3 weeks). Those with isolated optic neuropathy may be managed with oral antiviral medications. Steroid treatment as adjunct is not recommended because of unclear benefits and risk of VZV retinitis. The benefit has not been clearly documented [31]. The use of systemic antiviral treatment may result in modest improvement in visual function in about 50% patients.

20.7 Varicella Orbitopathy and Nonvisual Cranial Neuropathy

VZV can present with ophthalmoplegia from neurological or orbital lesions resulting in internuclear ophthalmoplegia, skew deviation, isolated or combined ocular motor cranial nerve (third, fourth, and sixth) palsy, and orbital myositis [32–35]. Ocular motor cranial neuropathy has been reported to occur in 7%–31% HZO, whereas complete unilateral ophthalmoplegia is a rare manifestation of HZ. Figures 20.3, 20.4 and 20.5 shows a case with VZV-induced third nerve palsy causing ptosis and affecting ocular motility.

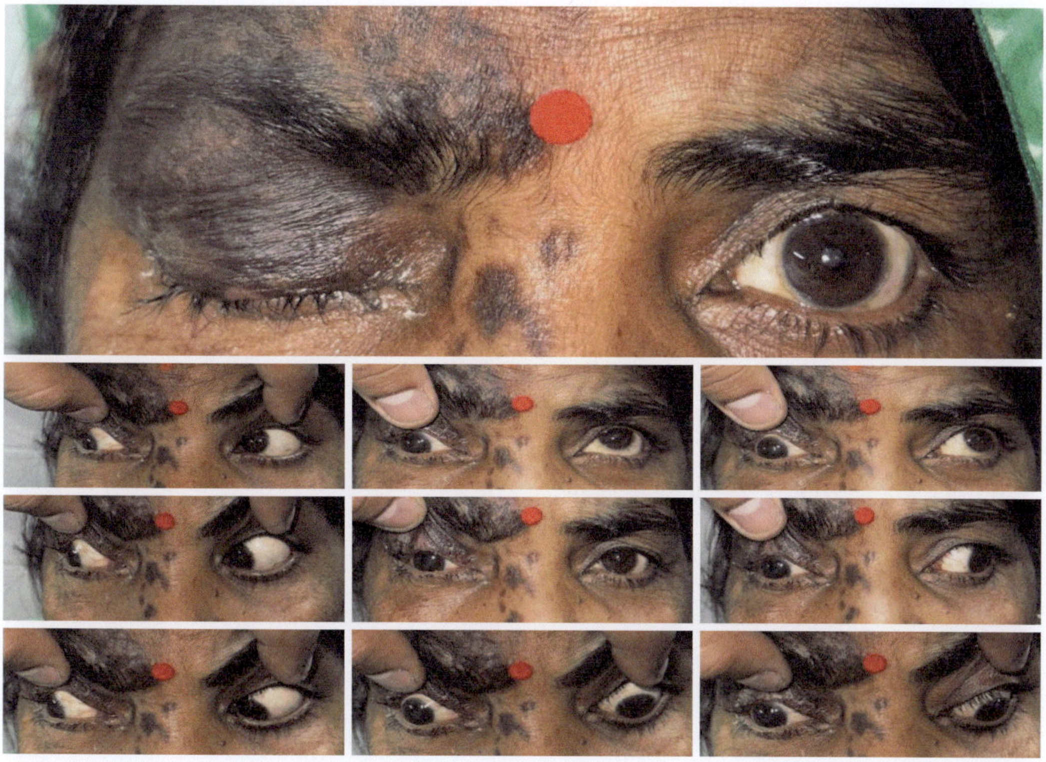

Fig. 20.3 Shows a case with VZV-induced third nerve palsy causing ptosis and affecting ocular motility in nine gazes. (Photo courtesy: Dr Paromita)

Third nerve palsies are most frequent, followed by sixth nerve palsies, and rarely, fourth nerve palsies.

Patients typically complain of binocular diplopia, blurry vision, and partial limitations to ocular motility. HZO can rarely cause orbital signs such as proptosis, ptosis, chemosis, and ophthalmoplegia. Development of cranial neuropathy may be secondary to direct viral invasion, immunologic demyelination, or VZV- associated vasculopathy.

Orbital MRI sequences in these patients may demonstrate enlargement, enhancement of the extraocular muscle and orbital soft tissue. Higher rates of CSF pleocytosis and radiological features of orbital inflammation such as enlarged extraocular muscle and soft-tissue enhancement have also been reported [36]. The prognosis for recovery of ophthalmoplegia is excellent; greater than 90% patients achieve relief from diplopia in primary gaze by 6–12 months [37].

Management

All patients with partial or complete ophthalmoplegia in the setting of HZ should have contrast-enhanced MRI of the brain and orbits to confirm localization of lesion and rule out competing causes. Lumbar puncture with CSF analysis is to be done if imaging depicts intracranial involvement, meningeal enhancement, ischemic stroke, or vasculopathy. Patients with imaging and/or CSF evidence of VZV (VZV DNA or intrathecal antibody production) should be treated with intravenous antiviral medications (acyclovir 10–15 mg/kg every 8 hours for 2–3 weeks). Patients with isolated cranial neuropathy can be managed with oral antiviral medications on an outpatient basis. Adjunctive treatment with a short course (5 days) of corticosteroids may be prescribed. Patients with persistent diplopia and ocular misalignment at 12 months may need optical (prism) or surgical correction.

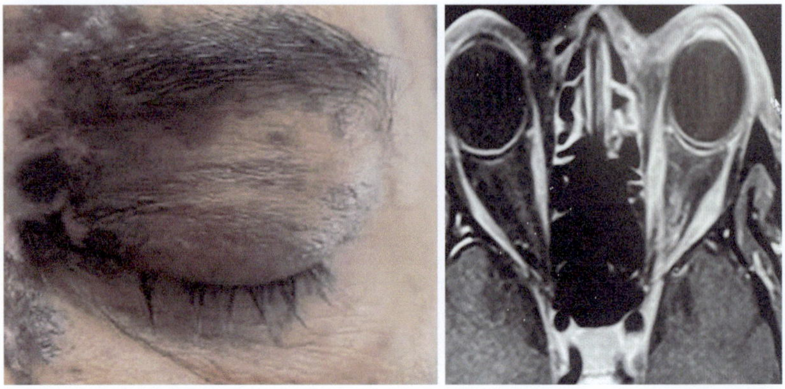

Fig. 20.4 Unilateral total ophthalmoplegia in Herpes Zoster Ophthalmicus due to orbital apex involvement B- MRI image showing edema and infiltration of recti along with optic nerve involvement

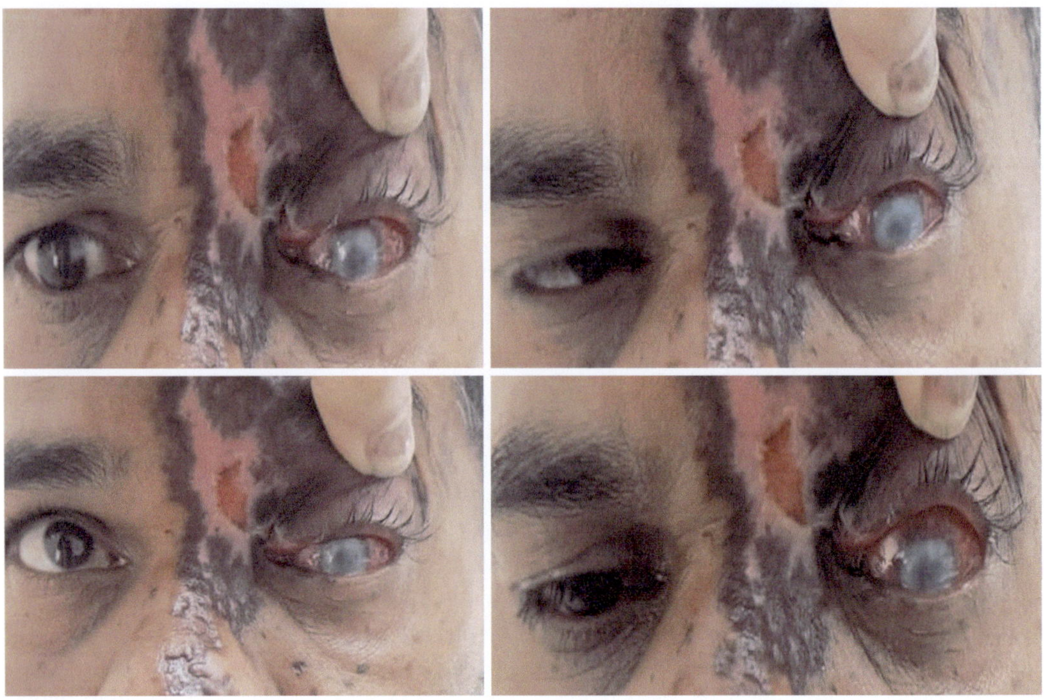

Fig. 20.5 HZO-induced ophthalmoplegia and corneal scar following severe ocular involvement

20.8 Internal Ophthalmoplegia

Rarer neuro-ophthalmic VZV presentations as atypically reduced pupillary reactivity or non-reactive pupils have also been reported. Atypical pupillary involvements are believed to be due to demyelinating, compressive, vasculo-occlusive, direct neuropathic, and/or viral cytotoxic processes. Other reported pupillary abnormalities being light-near dissociation and Horner's syndrome.

20.9 Postherpetic Neuralgia (PHN)

PHN, the most common sequela of HZ, is defined as dermatomal neuropathic pain, which persists at least 3 months after the initial episode of zoster. The prevalence of PHN varies from 5% to 30%. Age is an important risk factor with a three-fold increase in PHN from 50 to 80 years of age [38]. Other risk factors include female sex, increased severity of prodromal or acute zoster pain, premorbid functional status, immunocompromised condition, and involvement of the head and neck regions [39–41].

Pain is typically intermittent or constant burning, aching, or cutting pain accompanied by allodynia and itch in the same dermatomal area as the skin rash. In case of HZO there is moderate to severe pain on the involved half of forehead and head.

PHN results in poor quality of life, psychosocial dysfunction, and loss of independence in the elderly. The pathophysiology of PHN is not well understood and likely multifactorial. The presence of VZV specific protein and DNA in mononuclear cells in patients with chronic recurrent ganglionitis suggests persistent VZV infection after HZ [42, 43]. Peripheral neuronal damage then sets into motion a sequence of events resulting in central neuronal changes, which makes pain management difficult. Peripheral neuronal damage caused by reactivation of varicella zoster virus is suspected to be the common cause. This damage causes nerves in the affected area of the skin to send abnormal electrical signals to the brain which causes pain [44].

Management

Management of PHN is difficult and requires a multidisciplinary approach with a clear plan for escalation depending on responss [45]. Symptom control remains the main goal of treatment. Medications applied to the skin such as capsaicin or topical anaesthetics (e.g., lidocaine) are used for mild pain. Oral anticonvulsants such as gabapentin and pregabalin are also approved for treatment of PHN.

Various treatment options for PHN are shown in graded manner in Table 20.1.

Table 20.1 Showing management options in PHN [45]

Prevention of PHN	1. Vaccination
	2. Oral antiviral (valacyclovir/famciclovir) within 48–72 h of onset
Local application	Lidocaine 5% patch or gel
	Capsaicin 0.075% cream or capsaicin 8% skin patch
	Fentanyl patch
Tricyclic antidepressants	Amitriptyline or nortriptyline (25–150 mg/d)
Antiepileptic drugs	Gabapentin (300–3600 mg/d)
SNRI	Pregabalin (50–600 mg/d) Duloxetine (30–120 mg/d) Venlafaxine 37.5 mg–225 mg/d
Opioids	
Nonpharmacological interventios	1. Nerve block 2. Botulinum injections 3. Intrathecal steroid injection 4. Spinal cord stimulator 5. Pulsated radiofrequency ablation 6. Transcutaneous electrical nerve stimulation

20.10 Varicella Zoster Virus-Related CNS Vasculopathy

VZV vasculopathy results from the transaxonal spread of VZV to the adventitia of cranial arteries. Transmural viral spread is followed by inflammation and intravascular thrombosis. A granulomatous arteritis with transmural inflammation, arterial media necrosis, and giant cell formation is noted on histopathologic examination [46]. Large-vessel VZV vasculopathy is seen as focal and segmental arterial narrowing on angiography. It usually occurs in immunocompetent, older adults who present with stroke like symptoms within few weeks of HZ. Small-vessel vasculitis, on the other hand, typically occurs in immunocompromised individuals. They may have myriad of presentations like, transient ischemic attack (TIA), ischemic or hemorrhagic stroke, seizures, headache, or altered mental status. Multifocal white matter lesions are seen on brain MRI.

Vision loss from anterior ischemic optic neuropathy secondary to VZV vasculopathy also has been reported [29, 30, 47]. A clinical diagnosis of CNS VZV vasculopathy may be evident when neurological signs and symptoms occur in the setting of a classical HZ skin rash. However, 30%–40% patients may have an absence of typical skin rash, a delay between skin rash and neurological symptoms, and normal CSF examination, which makes diagnosis difficult [48].

Diagnostic confirmation should be obtained in all patients with a neurological presentation. This includes an MRI and MR angiography of the brain and CSF examination. Less than a third of patients with VZV vasculopathy have detectable VZV DNA in the CSF. Serologic confirmation is more reliable. Greater than 90% patients have anti-VZV IgG antibody in CSF with a reduced serum/CSF ratio of anti-VZV IgG indicative of intrathecal synthesis of anti-VZV IgG [48].

Management

Patients who develop stroke-like symptoms should be evaluated and managed using standard guidelines for acute stroke management. On confirmation of VZV vasculopathy, patients should be treated aggressively with intravenous antivirals (10–15 mg/kg every 8 h for 2–3 weeks).

Patients with recurrent disease or immunocompromised patients require prolonged oral antivirals for 3–6 months after the induction treatment. A five-day course of oral prednisone at treatment initiation (1 mg/kg/day) (96) may be done.

20.11 Conclusion

Herpes Zoster Ophthalmicus (HZO) is a significant manifestation of varicella zoster virus reactivation, affecting the ophthalmic branch of the trigeminal nerve. It accounts for 10–20% of all herpes zoster cases, with ocular involvement occurring in approximately 50% of HZO patients. The condition can lead to various anterior and posterior segment complications, including conjunctivitis, keratitis, uveitis, and, less commonly, optic neuropathy. Neurological complications such as cranial nerve palsies and postherpetic neuralgia (PHN) further contribute to morbidity. Prompt diagnosis and initiation of antiviral therapy are crucial to mitigate these complications and improve visual outcomes. Vaccination remains a key preventive strategy against HZO and its associated sequelae.

Key Points

1. Approximately half of HZO patients develop ocular complications, commonly affecting the anterior segment (e.g., conjunctivitis, keratitis, uveitis); posterior segment involvement is less frequent.
2. HZO can lead to cranial nerve palsies, optic neuritis, and PHN, with PHN being the most debilitating sequela.
3. Early administration of systemic antiviral agents, such as valacyclovir, acyclovir, or famciclovir, is essential. Adjunctive corticosteroids may be considered to reduce acute pain and inflammation.
4. Vaccination with the recombinant zoster vaccine is recommended for adults over 50 years to prevent HZ and HZO, effectively reducing incidence and severity

References

1. Yawn BP, Gilden D. The global epidemiology of herpes zoster. Neurology. 2013;81:928–30.
2. Yawn BP, Saddier P, Wollan PC, St Sauver JL, Kurland MJ, Sy LS. A population-based study of the incidence and complication rates of herpes zoster before zoster vaccine introduction. Mayo Clin Proc. 2007;82:1341–9.
3. Bricout H, Haugh M, Olatunde O, Prieto RG. Herpes zoster associated mortality in Europe: a systematic review. BMC Public Health. 2015;15:466.
4. Meyers JL, Madhwani S, Rausch D, Candrilli SD, Krishnarajah G, Yan S. Analysis of real-world health care costs among immunocompetent patients aged 50 years or older with herpes zoster in the United States. Hum Vaccin Immunother. 2017;13:1861–72.
5. Yawn BP, Wollan PC, St Sauver JL, Butterfield LC. Herpes zoster eye complications: rates and trends. Mayo Clin Proc. 2013;88:562–70.
6. Zerboni L, Sen N, Oliver SL, Arvin AM. Molecular mechanisms of varicella zoster virus pathogenesis. Nat Rev Microbiol. 2014;12:197–210.
7. Chen JJ, Zhu Z, Gershon AA, Gershon MD. Mannose 6- phosphate receptor dependence of varicella zoster virus infection in vitro and in the epidermis during varicella and zoster. Cell. 2004;119:915–26.
8. Gilden DH, Vafai A, Shtram Y, Becker Y, Devlin M, Wellish M. Varicella-zoster virus DNA in human sensory ganglia. Nature. 1983;306:478–80.
9. Steiner I, Kennedy PG. Herpes simplex virus latent infection in the nervous system. J Neurovirol. 1995;1:19–29.
10. Clarke P, Beer T, Cohrs R, Gilden DH. Configuration of latent varicella-zoster virus DNA. J Virol. 1995;69:8151–4.
11. Steiner I, Kennedy PG, Pachner AR. The neurotropic herpes viruses: herpes simplex and varicella-zoster. Lancet Neurol. 2007;6:1015–28.
12. Mueller NH, Gilden DH, Cohrs RJ, Mahalingam R, Nagel MA. Varicella zoster virus infection: clinical features, molecular pathogenesis of disease, and latency. Neurol Clin. 2008;26:675–97.
13. Mahalingam R, Wellish M, Brucklier J, Gilden DH. Persistence of varicella-zoster virus DNA in elderly patients with postherpetic neuralgia. J Neurovirol. 1995;1:130–3.
14. Kedar S, Lakshman N, Berger JR. Neurological and ophthalmological manifestations of varicella zoster virus. J Neuro-Ophthalmol. 2018;00:1–12.
15. Edgerton AE. Herpes zoster ophthalmicus: report of cases and a review of the literature. Trans Am Ophthalmol Soc. 1942;40:390–439.
16. Zaal MJ, Volker-Dieben HJ, D'Amaro J. Prognostic value of Hutchinson's sign in acute herpes zoster ophthalmicus. Graefes Arch Clin Exp Ophthalmol. 2003;241:187–91.
17. Liesegang TJ. Corneal complications from herpes zoster ophthalmicus. Ophthalmology. 1985;92:316–24.
18. Kaufman SC. Anterior segment complications of herpes zoster ophthalmicus. Ophthalmology. 2008;115(2 suppl):S24–32.
19. Borruat FX, Buechi ER, Piguet B, Fitting P, Zografos L, Herbort CP. Prevention of ocular complications of herpes zoster ophthalmicus by adequate treatment with acyclovir. Klin Monbl Augenheilkd. 1991;198:358–60.
20. McDonald EM, de Kock J, Ram FS. Antivirals for management of herpes zoster including ophthalmicus: a systematic review of high-quality randomized controlled trials. Antivir Ther. 2012;17:255–64.
21. Han Y, Zhang J, Chen N, He L, Zhou M, Zhu C. Corticosteroids for preventing postherpetic neuralgia. Cochrane Database Syst Rev. 2013;3:CD005582.
22. Chang BH, Ewald MD, Groos EB Jr. Neurotrophic keratitis. In: Mannis MJ, Holland EJ, editors. Cornea. 5th ed. Philadelphia: Elsevier; 2022. p. 946.
23. Marsh RJ, Cooper M. Ophthalmic herpes zoster. Eye (Lond). 1993;7(Pt 3):350–70.
24. de Mello VB, Foureaux EC, Porto FB. Herpes zoster optic neuritis. Int Ophthalmol. 2011;31:233–6.
25. Franco-Paredes C, Bellehemeur T, Merchant A, Sanghi P, DiazGranados C, Rimland D. Aseptic meningitis and optic neuritis preceding varicella-zoster progressive outer retinal necrosis in a patient with AIDS. AIDS. 2002;16:1045–9.
26. Mearza AA, Chan JH, Gair E, Jagger J. Herpes zoster ophthalmicus presenting as contralateral disc swelling. Eye (Lond). 2000;2:251–2.
27. Meenken C, van den Horn GJ, de Smet MD, van der Meer JT. Optic neuritis heralding varicella zoster virus retinitis in a patient with acquired immunodeficiency syndrome. Ann Neurol. 1998;43:534–6.
28. Gunduz K, Ozdemir O. Bilateral retrobulbar neuritis following unilateral herpes zoster ophthalmicus. Ophthalmologica. 1994;208:61–4.
29. Mathias M, Nagel MA, Khmeleva N, Boyer PJ, Choe A, Durairaj VD, Bennett JL, Mandava N, Gilden D. VZV multifocal vasculopathy with ischemic optic neuropathy, acute retinal necrosis and temporal artery infection in the absence of zoster rash. J Neurol Sci. 2013;325:180–2.
30. Salazar R, Russman AN, Nagel MA, Cohrs RJ, Mahalingam R, Schmid DS, Kleinschmidt-DeMasters BK, VanEgmond EM, Gilden D. Varicella zoster virus ischemic optic neuropathy and subclinical temporal artery involvement. Arch Neurol. 2011;68:517–20.
31. Nakamoto BK, Dorotheo EU, Biousse V, Tang RA, Schiffman JS, Newman NJ. Progressive outer retinal necrosis presenting with isolated optic neuropathy. Neurology. 2004;63:2423–5.
32. Al-Abdulla NA, Rismondo V, Minkowski JS, Miller NR. Herpes zoster vasculitis presenting as giant cell arteritis with bilateral internuclear ophthalmoplegia. Am J Ophthalmol. 2002;134:912–4.
33. Verhulst E, Van Lammeren M, Dralands L. Diplopia from skew deviation in Ramsey-Hunt syndrome. A case report. Bull Soc Belge Ophtalmol. 2000;278:27–32.

34. Kawasaki A, Borruat FX. An unusual presentation of herpes zoster ophthalmicus: orbital myositis preceding vesicular eruption. Am J Ophthalmol. 2003;136:574–5.
35. Marsh RJ, Dulley B, Kelly V. External ocular motor palsies in ophthalmic zoster: a review. Br J Ophthalmol. 1977;61:677–82.
36. Temnogorod J, Pointdujour-Lim R, Mancini R, Chang SH, Allen RC, Shinder R. Acute orbital syndrome in herpes zoster ophthalmicus: clinical features of 7 cases. Ophthal Plast Reconstr Surg. 2017;33:173–7.
37. Sanjay S, Chan EW, Gopal L, Hegde SR, Chang BC. Complete unilateral ophthalmoplegia in herpes zoster ophthalmicus. J Neuroophthalmol. 2009;29:325–37.
38. Gauthier A, Breuer J, Carrington D, Martin M, Remy V. Epidemiology and cost of herpes zoster and post-herpetic neuralgia in the United Kingdom. Epidemiol Infect. 2009;137:38–47.
39. Gialloreti LE, Merito M, Pezzotti P, Naldi L, Gatti A, Beillat M, Serradell L, di Marzo R, Volpi A. Epidemiology and economic burden of herpes zoster and post-herpetic neuralgia in Italy: a retrospective, population-based study. BMC Infect Dis. 2010;10:230.
40. Drolet M, Brisson M, Schmader K, Levin M, Johnson R, Oxman M, Patrick D, Camden S, Mansi JA. Predictors of postherpetic neuralgia among patients with herpes zoster: a prospective study. J Neuro-Ophthalmol. 2018;00:1–12. 2010;11:1211–21
41. Kawai K, Rampakakis E, Tsai TF, Cheong HJ, Dhitavat J, Covarrubias AO, Yang L, Cashat-Cruz M, Monsanto H, Johnson K, Sampalis JS, Acosta CJ. Predictors of postherpetic neuralgia in patients with herpes zoster: a pooled analysis of prospective cohort studies from North and Latin America and Asia. Int J Infect Dis. 2015;34:126–31.
42. Gilden DH, Cohrs RJ, Hayward AR, Wellish M, Mahalingam R. Chronic varicella-zoster virus ganglionitis – a possible cause of postherpetic neuralgia. J Neurovirol. 2003;9:404–7.
43. Gilden DH, Cohrs RJ, Mahalingam R. VZV vasculopathy and postherpetic neuralgia: progress and perspective on antiviral therapy. Neurology. 2005;64:21–5.
44. Wood M. Understanding pain in herpes zoster: an essential for optimizing treatment. J Infect Dis. 2002;186(suppl 1):S78–82.
45. Oster G, Harding G, Dukes E, Edelsberg J, Cleary PD. Pain, medication use, and health-related quality of life in older persons with postherpetic neuralgia: results from a population-based survey. J Pain. 2005;6:356–63.
46. Linnemann CC Jr, Alvira MM. Pathogenesis of varicella-zoster angiitis in the CNS. Arch Neurol. 1980;37:239–40.
47. Nagel MA, Bennett JL, Khmeleva N, Choe A, Rempel A, Boyer PJ, Gilden D. Multifocal VZV vasculopathy with temporal artery infection mimics giant cell arteritis. Neurology. 2013;80:2017–21.
48. Nagel MA, Cohrs RJ, Mahalingam R, Wellish MC, Forghani B, Schiller A, Safdieh JE, Kamenkovich E, Ostrow LW, Levy M, Greenberg B, Russman AN, Katzan I, Gardner CJ, Hausler M, Nau R, Saraya T, Wada H, Goto H, de Martino M, Ueno M, Brown WD, Terborg C, Gilden DH. The varicella zoster virus vasculopathies: clinical, CSF, imaging, and virologic features. Neurology. 2008;70:853–60.

Prevention

21

Bhavana Sharma, Amit Raj, Parul Mittal, and Arvind Morya

Abstract

Viral diseases of cornea are hallmarked by recurrences and chronicity. The potentially blinding sequelae of viral keratitis due to inflammation vascularization and scarring mainly arise from cycles of frequent relapses. After the primary infection, the implicated virus may lie dormant in neural tissues followed by reactivation due to specific predispositions, which may result into active infection, inflammation or immune response. Hence the most pertinent approach to manage such episodes is to obviate reactivation. Prevention and prophylaxis of viral keratitis is mainly directed against Herpes Simplex-, Varicella Zoster- and Adenovirus-induced chronicity and recurrences. HSV keratitis is hallmarked with recurrences, while HZO with recurrence and chronicity.

This chapter will comprehensively describe the preventive strategies and prophylactic treatment best suited in different disease conditions caused by viral reactivation.

Keywords

Prevention · Prophylaxis · Immunoglobulins

21.1 HSV Keratitis

Repeated reactivation and recurrences are frequent manifestations of HSV keratitis and are mainly seen in epithelial or stromal forms. While epithelial involvement is mainly due to active infection by replicating virus, stromal inflammation is due to replicating virus or recurrent immune-mediated inflammation. Trigeminal ganglion and stromal keratocytes are the most common source of recurrent HSV infection. The viral genome that is retained within the host cell nucleus during latency is responsible for latency-associated transcripts (LATS) and for viral reactivation. Stromal inflammation from HSV keratitis due to altered antigenicity of the stromal cells causes recurrent immune-mediated inflammation [1]. Conditions of impaired host defence, mainly systemic infection, psychological stress, menstruation etc., have been recognized as potential triggers of ocular HSV recurrences. Local factors which act as predisposition are surgical stress, refractive surgeries, collagen cross linking, contact lens overuse or any other minor procedures. Prophylaxis works by preventing virus multiplication, supporting the rhetoric that virus must be actively replicating for acyclovir to be effective.

B. Sharma (✉) · P. Mittal
AIIMS Bhopal, Bhopal, Madhya Pradesh, India

A. Raj
AIIMS Patna, Patna, Bihar, India

A. Morya
AIIMS Bibinagar, Bibinagar, Telangana, India

B. Sharma et al. (eds.), *Viral Keratitis*, https://doi.org/10.1007/978-981-95-3148-6_21

Antiviral prophylaxis reduces the rate of recurrence of epithelial and stromal disease by 50% in HSV keratitis. Acyclovir is the primary drug used for prevention and prophylaxis in addition to Valacyclovir and Famciclovir. Herpetic Eye Disease Study continues to remain the landmark trial, which reported that oral Acyclovir significantly decreased the number of relapses of ocular HSV-1 by 50%–14%. Recurrence rates differ for a first or second episode. It is reported as 36% and 63% at 5 and 20 years respectively after a primary episode [2]. However after second episode, a fairly high recurrence rate of 70–80% within 10 years has been reported [3]. Recurrence rate increases with each episode. HEDS TRIAL has reported an 18% recurrence rate for epithelial and stromal keratitis in patients with ocular HSV over the previous year and 33% within 2 years in patients with two prior episodes [4].

21.1.1 Prophylaxis

Prophylaxis should be considered in patients with frequent recurrences or those with bilateral disease. The prophylactic dose of Acyclovir is 800 mg per day in divided doses, 400 mg twice a day or 200 mg four times daily, for time duration in accordance to the clinical requirement. Oral Valacyclovir, which is the Acyclovir prodrug, increases the bioavailability of Acyclovir three to five times. Additionally, less frequent dosing improves the patient compliance when compared with multiple daily doses. The prophylactic dose of valacyclovir is 500 mg once a day. Several trials have been done to compare the efficacy of low-dose/long-term oral antiviral prophylaxis, high-dose/short-term oral antiviral prophylaxis and comparison of oral Acyclovir and its prodrug, Valacyclovir in the prevention of HSV keratitis. It has been reported that low-dose/long-term oral antiviral prophylaxis in dosing schedule of oral Acyclovir 400 mg BD dose for 1 year is more effective than high-dose/short-term antiviral (400 mg 5 times daily for 3 weeks) in decreasing recurrences [5]. After discontinuation of antiviral the recurrence rate at 6 months was similar in patients without treatment, suggesting absence of prolonged effect of acyclovir [5]. Oral Valaciclovir or Famciclovir are other alternative drugs with standard dose of 500 mg once daily and 250 mg twice daily respectively. For long-term prophylaxis renal and liver functions should be monitored every 6 months to 1 year (Table 21.1).

Table 21.1 Prophylactic management of viral keratitis

Keratitis	Drug
HSV Keratitis	Acyclovir 400 mg BD for 1 year
	Valaciclovir 500 mg OD for 1 year
	Famciclovir 250 mg BD for 1 year
HZO Keratitis	Acyclovir 400 mg BD for 1 year Valaciclovir 500 mg OD for 1 year
Adenoviral keratitis	Hygiene practice

21.1.1.1 Epithelial Disease

HSV dendritic keratitis is reported to have more frequent recurrences, seen in 56.3% of cases, while geographical lesions show recurrences in 9.8% of cases [6]. HEDS trial reported a recurrence rate of 37% for epithelial disease [5]. Prophylaxis is recommended for patients with more than two episodes of epithelial disease per year. Acyclovir 400 mg twice daily over 1–2 years as prophylaxis can reduce the incidence of recurrence.

21.1.1.2 Stromal Disease

Recurrence rate in stromal keratitis has been reported to be 29.5% [7]. While HEDS trial has reported it as 46%. The main pathophysiological event that drives the stromal inflammation is the viral reactivation in the trigeminal ganglion followed by retrograde transmission of virus and subsequent heralding of stromal keratitis. Acyclovir-induced phosphorylation of viral thymidine kinase with subsequent incorporation into viral DNA and its damage is possible only with active viral DNA replication, suggesting that HSV-1 must be multiplying for acyclovir to function. Prophylactic treatment with systemic Acyclovir or Valacyclovir in daily doses of 800–1200 mg and 500 mg, respectively, prevents viral replication within the trigeminal ganglia and, thereby, inhibits the impetus for recurrent stromal inflammation. Long-term suppressive dosing with acyclovir 400 mg twice daily can reduce the recurrence by 45% [6].

21.1.2 Antiviral Prophylaxis in Corneal Transplantation

Surgical stress remains an important predisposition for HSV recurrence in corneal graft leading to potential graft failure. Prophylactic oral antiviral therapy before and after keratoplasty reduces recurrent ocular HSV disease, graft rejection episodes, and, thereby, improves graft survival. Systemic antiviral agents like oral Acyclovir 400 mg BD with adjuvant topical dexamethasone twice daily for 6–12 months after keratoplasty is recommended to mitigate virus reactivation and consequent graft rejection [8].

However, there is no consensus on the regimen of prophylactic antivirals for lamellar corneal transplantation. We recommend 400 mg of oral Acyclovir two times a day, or 500 mg of Valacyclovir once a day, as long as the clinical requirement remains. In long-term administration of systemic antivirals, renal function tests should be done every 6 months to 1 year. Prophylaxis with systemic antiviral over topical is more efficacious in preventing the recurrence, in addition to preventing the toxic keratopathy and conjunctival scarring.

21.1.3 Antiviral Prophylaxis in Surgical Procedures

Recurrence of HSV keratitis after refractive surgery, collagen cross linking and other surgical procedures is a well-known complication. However, some studies have reported good refractive surgery outcomes in patients whose keratitis has been inactive for at least 1 year and in whom perioperative systemic antiviral prophylaxis was used.

We recommend 400 mg of oral Acyclovir two times a day, or 500 mg of Valacyclovir once a day, for 6 months to 1 year to prevent potential recurrences.

21.1.4 Prevention

Preventing recurrence and transmission of HSV keratitis necessitates a multifaceted approach encompassing patient education, lifestyle modifications and targeted interventions. Key preventive strategies include:

- **Avoiding Triggers**: Identifying and avoiding triggers that may precipitate HSV reactivation, such as stress, ultraviolet (UV) exposure and systemic illness.
- **Eye Protection**: Encouraging the use of protective eyewear, such as sunglasses or goggles, to shield the eyes from UV radiation and physical trauma, potentially reducing the risk of HSV reactivation.
- **Hygiene Practices**: Emphasizing good hygiene practices, including regular handwashing and avoiding sharing personal items.

HSV vaccination strategies have been studied to prevent recurrences in predisposed individuals. CD8 T cells-mediated immune mechanism functions against the viral replication in the trigeminal ganglion using non-lytic mechanism [9]. Thus the ongoing research is directed to boost the CD8 T cell response within the dormant ganglia to achieve viral inhibition and subsequent corneal inflammation [10].

Several HSV antigenic products as vaccines have been evaluated with the goal of inhibiting viral reactivation within the trigeminal ganglia and preventing reactivation events. However presently there are no licensed vaccines against either HSV I or II. Two vaccines namely *Heat-inactivated HSV-I & HSV-2 glycoprotein D* have been investigated for efficacy in HSV I & II infections. Heat-inactivated HSV-1 vaccine has been shown to be effective in decreasing both the number and duration of ocular HSV-1 recurrences [10]. While HSV-2 glycoprotein D vaccine was not found to be effective in preventing HSV-2 however was effective in preventing HSV-1 [5]. Further the concerns remain that an increased immune response to HSV after vaccination can exacerbate herpetic stromal keratitis.

21.2 HZO Keratitis

Varicella-zoster virus (VZV) is a double-stranded DNA virus. Primary infection of VZV causes chicken pox in individuals of all age groups. The reactivation of latent virus in the dorsal root ganglion represents a cell-mediated immune response, which manifests as HZO.

Recurrences in HZO are generally seen within 1 year of the initial presentation. Stromal keratitis and uveitis are known to be the most common manifestation among recurred cases [11]. In patients with conjunctivitis, epithelial keratitis, stromal keratitis and raised IOP the incidence of chronic disease and recurrence is reported to be higher.

Several studies indicate that the mean age of HZO onset is decreasing, possibly reflecting a weaker life-long immunity acquired from varicella vaccination in contrast to natural infection [12]. Thus in patients with aforementioned risk factors follow up should be done for at least a year to identify the recurrences of disease [11].

The reported rate of recurrence ranges between 14.6% and 51% in HZO and up to 70% in patients over 80 years of age despite antiviral treatment [11, 13, 14]. Given the high incidence of recurrence and chronicity in HZO, prophylaxis becomes important to mitigate reactivation of virus. Importance of prophylaxis for HZO has been studied in several studies. However the Zoster Eye Disease Study (results are awaited) remains the only RCT undertaken to determine whether prolonged suppressive oral antiviral treatment with valacyclovir reduces the complications of HZO including eye disease and PHN.

Additionally, a study done on patients with autologous transplant using low-dose antiviral prophylaxis with oral Acyclovir 400 mg twice daily or Valacyclovir 500 mg daily for 1 year has been found to be effective in preventing VZV reactivation [15].

21.2.1 Prevention

Preventing VZV keratitis revolves around key strategies like:

1. **Hygiene Practices**: Emphasizing good hygiene practices, including regular handwashing and avoiding contact.
2. **Varicella Vaccination**: Encouraging vaccination against Varicella and Herpes zoster can reduce the risk of VZV infection and subsequent ocular complications, including keratitis.

Two vaccines directed toward VZV have been approved by the US Food and Drug Administration. Zoster vaccine live (ZVL) and recombinant Zoster vaccine (RZV). Attenuated live virus vaccine (Zostavax; Merck & Co, Inc., Whitehouse Station, NJ) was FDA approved in 2006. It decreases the incidence of herpes zoster by 51% and occurrence of postherpetic neuralgia by 66% in immunocompetent people. Being a live virus, it is not recommended in subjects with impaired immunity [16]. All antivirals need to be stopped 1 day before till 2 weeks after the vaccine. Another vaccine i.e. recombinant zoster vaccine (Shingrix, Glaxo-SmithKline, Philadelphia, PA) is recommended for use in adults more than 50 years of age and has an efficacy of approximately 97% in all age group [17]. Being a non-replicating variant it is considered to be safe in immunocompromised persons as well. Effect of vaccination lasts for about 8 years. Current recommendation is to use live attenuated vaccine to prevent chickenpox and recombinant vaccine to prevent herpes zoster [18]. Both vaccines boost cell-mediated immunity against VZV, which then reduces the risk of reactivation [18]. There have been several cases of reactivation of HZ keratitis or uveitis reported within 2 to 5 weeks of Zostavax vaccination [19, 20].

The vaccine has been found to have an efficacy of over 67% in reducing the risk of eye involvement in patients over 60 years [21]. However paradoxically an increase in cell-mediated immunity may also lead to a recurrent stromal keratitis in response to persistent viral antigens in the cornea. Thus, a period of remission of at least 1 year prior to vaccination should be considered in patients with a history of VZV keratitis. Further patients should be closely followed up for any reactivation for at least a year [22]. The efficacy has been shown to wane up to 4% after 8 years.

Recombinant zoster vaccine has been demonstrated to be 97% efficacious for age groups 50 to 69 years and even 91% effective in those aged 70 years and older. The vaccine retains its efficacy at 88% at 4 years, and above baseline at 15 years. CDC recommends adults who received Zostavax to be revaccinated with Shingrix [23, 24].

Zoster Immune Globulin

Zoster immune globulin is a gamma globulin fraction of plasma obtained from a patient recovering from herpes zoster. Zoster immune globulin has provided an effective post-exposure prophylaxis in paediatric age groups in preventing or modifying varicella zoster virus [25].

21.3 Adenoviral Keratitis

Corneal involvement due to Adenovirus occurs in approximately 80% of cases with presentations such as superficial punctate keratitis, focal epithelial punctate keratitis, subepithelial infiltrate and reduced corneal sensitivity [26]. Recurrent infections can present as nummular keratitis [26]. Given the highly infectious nature of adenovirus, hospital setting is often the point of origin for most of the outbreak. Preventive measures should be exercised thoroughly in these locations. Instrument cleaning with hydrogen peroxide, isopropyl alcohol or 1% potassium peroxymonosulfate is effective in eliminating adenovirus [27].

21.4 Conclusion

Viral keratitis is a potential blinding condition of fairly common occurrence. Prophylactic treatment is required to prevent recurrences and chronicity. Oral Acyclovir, Valaciclovir and Famciclovir are effective in preventing HSV recurrences while vaccination has more important role in HZO keratitis than oral drugs.

Key Points

1. Prevention and prophylaxis of viral keratitis is mainly directed against Herpes Simplex-, Varicella Zoster- and Adenovirus-induced chronicity and recurrences.
2. HSV keratitis is hallmarked with recurrences, while HZO with recurrence and chronicity.
3. Preventing recurrence and transmission of HSV keratitis necessitates a multifaceted approach encompassing patient education, lifestyle modifications and targeted interventions.

References

1. Cavanagh HD. The cornea: transactions of the world congress on the cornea III, vol. 3. Raven Press; 1988.
2. Liesegang TJ. Epidemiology of ocular herpes simplex: natural history in Rochester, Minn, 1950 through 1982. Arch Ophthalmol. 1989;107(8):1160–5.
3. Shuster JJ, Kaufman HE, Nesburn AB. Statistical analysis of the rate of recurrence of herpesvirus ocular epithelial disease. Am J Ophthalmol. 1981;91(3):328–31.
4. Predictors of recurrent herpes simplex virus keratitis. Herpetic Eye Disease Study Group. Cornea. 2001;20(2):123–8. https://doi.org/10.1097/00003226-200103000-00001.
5. White ML, Chodosh J. Herpes simplex virus keratitis: a treatment guideline. Hoskins Center for Quality Eye Care and American Academy of Ophthalmology Website; 2014. p. 1–69.
6. Kim TI, Azar DT, Pavan-Langston D. Viral Disease of the Cornea and External Eye. Albert and Jakobiec's Principles and Practice of Ophthalmology; 2022. p. 187–279.
7. Labetoulle M, Auquier P, Conrad H, Crochard A, Daniloski M, Bouée S, El Hasnaoui A, Colin J. Incidence of herpes simplex virus keratitis in France. Ophthalmology. 2005;112(5):888–95.
8. Barney NP, Foster CS. A prospective randomized trial of oral acyclovir after penetrating keratoplasty for herpes simplex keratitis. Cornea. 1994;13(3):232.
9. Knickelbein JE, Khanna KM, Yee MB, Baty CJ, Kinchington PR, Hendricks RL. Noncytotoxic lytic granule–mediated CD8+ T cell inhibition of HSV-1 reactivation from neuronal latency. Science. 2008;322(5899):268–71.
10. Pivetti-Pezzi P, Accorinti M, Colabelli-Gisoldi RA, Pirraglia MP, Sirianni MC. Herpes simplex virus vac-

cine in recurrent herpetic ocular infection. Cornea. 1999;18(1):47–51.
11. Miserocchi E, Fogliato G, Bianchi I, Bandello F, Modorati G. Clinical Features of Ocular Herpetic Infection in an Italian Referral Center. Cornea. 2014;33(6):565.
12. Chan AY, Conrady CD, Ding K, Dvorak JD, Stone DU. Factors associated with age of onset of herpes zoster ophthalmicus. Cornea. 2015;34(5):535.
13. Lee SM, Han J, Yang CM, Choi CY, Khoramnia R, Chung TY, et al. Chronic and recurrent herpes zoster ophthalmicus. Medicina. 2021;57(10):999.
14. Johnson RW, Alvarez-Pasquin MJ, Bijl M, Franco E, Gaillat J, Clara JG, et al. Herpes zoster epidemiology, management, and disease and economic burden in Europe: a multidisciplinary perspective. Ther Adv Vaccines. 2015;3(4):109–20.
15. Fei N, Shah N, Cumpston A, Wen S, Ross KG, Craig M, Kanate AS. Low-dose acyclovir prophylaxis for varicella zoster reactivation in autologous hematopoietic cell transplantation recipients. Clin Hematol Int. 2019;1(2):101–4.
16. Tsui E, Cohen EJ. The importance of vaccination against herpes zoster. Curr Ophthalmol Rep. 2018;6:173–80.
17. Harbecke R, Cohen JI, Oxman MN. Herpes zoster vaccines. J Infect Dis. 2021;224(Supplement_4):S429–42.
18. Tuft S. How to manage herpes zoster ophthalmicus. Commun Eye Health. 2020;33(108):71–2.
19. Khalifa YM, Jacoby RM, Margolis TP. Exacerbation of zoster interstitial keratitis after zoster vaccination in an adult. Arch Ophthalmol. 2010;128(8):1079–80. https://doi.org/10.1001/archophthalmol.2010.142.
20. Jastrzebski A, Brownstein S, Ziai S, Saleh S, Lam K, Jackson WB. Reactivation of herpes zoster keratitis with corneal perforation after zoster vaccination. Cornea. 2017;36(6):740.
21. Tseng HF, Smith N, Harpaz R, Bialek SR, Sy LS, Jacobsen SJ. Herpes zoster vaccine in older adults and the risk of subsequent herpes zoster disease. JAMA. 2011;305(2):160–6.
22. Hassan OM, Farooq AV, Soin K, Djalilian AR, Hou JH. Management of corneal scarring secondary to herpes zoster keratitis. Cornea. 2017;36(8):1018.
23. Hung FT, Harpaz R, Luo Y, Hales CM, Sy LS, Tartof SY, Bialek S, Hechter RC, Jacobsen SJ. Declining effectiveness of herpes zoster vaccine in adults aged ≥60 years. J Infect Dis. 2016;213(12):1872–5.
24. Dooling KL, Guo A, Patel M, Lee GM, Moore K, Belongia EA, et al. Recommendations of the Advisory Committee on Immunization Practices for use of herpes zoster vaccines. Am J Transp. 2018;18(3):756–62.
25. Judelsohn RG, Meyers JD, Ellis RJ, Thomas EK. Efficacy of zoster immune globulin. Pediatrics. 1974;53:476–80.
26. Labib BA, Minhas BK, Chigbu DI. Management of adenoviral keratoconjunctivitis: challenges and solutions. Clin Ophthalmol. 2020;14:837–52.
27. Hashizume M, Aoki K, Ohno S, et al. Disinfectant potential in inactivation of epidemic keratoconjunctivitis-related adenoviruses by potassium peroxymonosulfate. Eur J Ophthalmol. 2021;31(2):379–84.

Section III

Adenoviral Infections

Etiopathogenesis and Clinical Features

22

Abhishek Kumar, Neiwete Lomi, Noopur Gupta, M. Vanathi, and Radhika Tandon

Abstract

Human adenoviruses are the most common cause of conjunctivitis in adults and children. It can cause infection of conjunctiva, gut, lungs and liver. Ocular adenovirus can cause non-specific conjunctivitis, pharyngoconjunctival fever, epidemic keratoconjunctivitis and chronic keratoconjunctivitis. Its genome consists of structural and non-structural proteins that help in the attachment and penetration of the viral genome into host cell and nucleus causing viral replication. Host cells have various defence mechanisms to prevent viral infection and virus has mechanisms to counteract the defence. Mediators such as epithelium of the ocular surface and alpha defensins help build innate immune response, whereas T cells, IL8 and interferon gamma help in adaptive immune response. The virus penetrates and attaches to various cellular receptors, leading to the activation of signalling cascades. Replication of virus occurs in early and late stages. Human adenoviruses have tissue tropism due to which specific species of the viruses interact with specific receptors of the host cells. Characteristic clinical features of adenoviral infection commonly include follicular conjunctivitis, pseudo membrane formation, subepithelial infiltrates and follicular lymphadenitis; however, it depends on the phenotypic type.

Keywords

Adenovirus · Epidemiology · Clinical features · Keratoconjunctivitis

22.1 Introduction

Adenoviruses are among the most common cause of viral conjunctivitis accounting for 75–80% of the cases [1]. Adenoviruses are double-stranded DNA virus, non-enveloped, icosahedral in shape. Human adenoviruses belong to the genus *Mastadenovirus* of the family of *Adenoviridae* and are classified into species A to G. They can cause infections in various human tissues, including the conjunctiva, gastrointestinal tract, myocardium, lungs, and liver [2]. Ocular Adenoviral infection can be in the form of non-specific conjunctivitis, pharyngoconjunctival fever, epidemic keratoconjunctivitis and chronic adenoviral conjunctivitis [3, 4].

A. Kumar · N. Lomi (✉) · N. Gupta · M. Vanathi · R. Tandon
Dr. R P Centre for Ophthalmic Sciences, AIIMS, Delhi, Delhi, India

B. Sharma et al. (eds.), *Viral Keratitis*, https://doi.org/10.1007/978-981-95-3148-6_22

22.2 Epidemiology, Mode of Infection and Preventive Measures

Adenovirus infection can occur throughout the year, most commonly occurring in the early spring or winter. The most common age group affected is from six months to two years of age but is also seen from five to nine years age group. Infection and exposure to infected persons most commonly occur by inhalation of aerosolized droplets, conjunctival inoculation and faecal-oral spread. Adenovirus infection can also occur from exogenous sources (e.g. linens, pillows, lockers, guns) or reactivation of the previous virus (Fig. 22.1) [5]. Incubation period of adenovirus ranges from 2–14 days [6]. Latent Adenovirus may reside in lymphoid tissue, renal parenchyma, or other tissues for years and may get reactivated in severely immunosuppressed patients [7]. Adenovirus is a widespread cause of upper respiratory tract infections and conjunctivitis. Epidemics of the disease may spread rapidly among closed populations such as in hospitals, neonatal nurseries, psychiatric hospitals, boarding schools and public swimming pools. In institutionalized settings, infection control measures and cohorting may help to limit the spread. Adenovirus is resistant to many disinfectants, but 95% ethanol solution is an effective disinfectant [8].

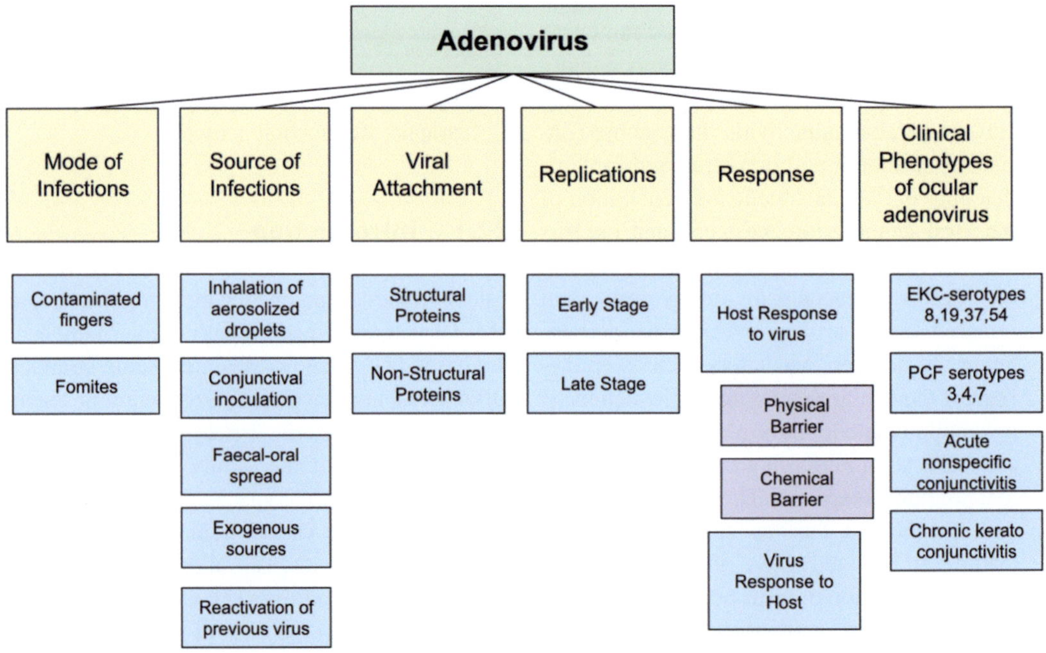

Fig. 22.1 Schematic diagram showing various modes and sources of infection with the pathogenesis and clinical features of adenoviral infections

22.3 Attachment and Penetration of Viral Genome to Host Cells

Adenovirus has 36 Kb genome which encodes structural as well as non-structural proteins [9]. Adenovirus is 90 nm in diameter with an icosahedral capsid that contains 240 trimers of hexon protein and 12 pentamers of penton base proteins. Fibre protein protrudes from the penton base and consists of an N-terminal tail in contact with penton base protein and a C-terminal knob domain that serves as a binding site for host cellular receptors [10].

Major adenoviral structural proteins as shown in Fig. 22.2 include

- Homopentameric penton base that mediates viral internalization into the host [11]
- Homotrimeric fibre protein which plays a role in viral attachment to host cellular receptors [12]
- Hexons that are recognized by neutralizing antibodies [13]

Minor capsid proteins include proteins VI, III, VIII and IX.

Core proteins of human adenovirus include IVa2, V, VII, MU and terminal protein [14].

Primary cellular receptors, such as Coxsackie and Adenovirus receptor (CAR), CD46 (membrane cofactor protein), sialic acid, desmoglein 2, heparin sulfate proteoglycans, CD80, CD86 and GD1a, interact with fibre-knob protein to mediate adenoviral attachment to host cells [11–14].

Adenovirus on the ocular surface leads to activation of IL8 (chemokine) which binds to its receptors CXCR1 and CXCR2 causing subsequent phosphorylation of downstream molecules resulting in translocation of CAR and $\alpha_v\beta_3$ integrin from the basolateral surface of the polarized epithelial cell to the apical surface resulting in adenovirus interaction with epithelial cell of the host [15].

Internalization of adenovirus into an endosome is mediated by the interaction of the homopentameric penton base and vitronectin-binding integrin [16]. Penton base–integrin interaction

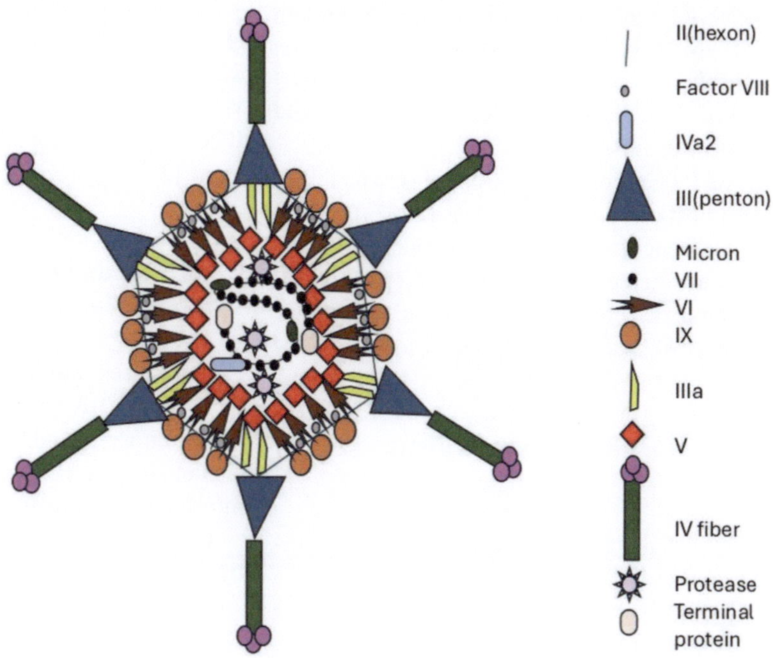

Fig. 22.2 Schematic diagram of human adenovirus 5 virion (HAd5)

activates an intracellular signaling cascade that culminates in the internalization of adenovirus into clathrin-coated vesicles [17]. After internalization of nucleocapsid into endosome, acidification of endosome is required to uncoat adenovirus [18]. This leads to penetration of viral genome into the nucleus following which replication of virus takes place.

22.4 Replication of Human Adenovirus

Replication of virus is divided into Early and Late stages.

- Early stage- It is characterized by E1A protein that activates E1B, E2, E3 and E4 gene [19].
  Adenoviral DNA replication is dependent on viral DNA polymerase, preterminal protein, and DNA-binding protein [11, 20].
  The *E2* gene encodes adenoviral DNA polymerase, precursor terminal protein and DNA-binding protein, which play an important role in viral DNA replication [21].
  The *E3* gene encodes the E3 gp19K protein (E3 Mr 19k glycoprotein), which prevents the display of viral antigen complexed to MHC class 1 molecules on the surface of virally infected cells [22, 23].
  The *E4* gene encodes E4 proteins, which shut off host-cell protein synthesis [22, 23].
- Late stage- It comprises of Adenain (23k cysteine protease), encoded by the *L3* gene which promotes maturation and generation of progeny DNA that is packaged in virions [21].

22.5 Host Response to Virus

- Physical barrier—Epithelium of ocular surface is the primary barrier.
- Chemical barrier—Antimicrobial proteins (defensins) found in tear film. Nguyen et al. demonstrated that human α-defensin blocks the uncoating of viruses [24]. Alpha defensin also inhibits human adenovirus-mediated endosomalysis [25].

Any breach in the above barrier leads to activation of immune response which is innate initially subsequently leading to adaptive immune response.

Mediators are:

- Innate immune response—Natural killer cells (NK), IFN (Interferon) type 1 and Monocytes.
- Adaptive immune response -IL8, TH1 cells, Ig A and IFNγ [26].

Viral proteins bind to pattern recognition receptors on macrophages and dendritic cells leading to their activation and releasing IL1β, IL6, IL8, IL12 and TNFα [27]. Activated dendritic cells traffic to lymphoid tissue activating naïve T cells to CD8 T cells and TH1 cells [28]. NK cells respond to viral infection by promoting and regulating the adaptive immunoresponse via cross talk with dendritic cells and T cells, as well as via production of IFNγ and TNFα [29]. IFNγ secreted by NK cells promotes the upregulation of costimulatory molecules on conventional dendritic cells, priming them for efficient T-cell activation. NK cells are activated by IL12 and type 1 IFN to release IFNγ, TNFα, perforin and granzyme [29].

22.6 Virus Response to Host Defence

Adenoviruses suppress NK cell activity by increasing HLA (Human leukocyte antigen) E, an inhibitory ligand, and decreasing the expression of HLA-A, B, C to modulate MHC class I in infected conjunctival epithelium [30].

Group D human adenovirus evades cytolysis by downregulating expression of ligands (CD112 and CD155) for activating NK cell receptor DNAM1/CD226. This allows virus to remain active on the conjunctival surface and give rise to persistent infection [31].

Virus and Tissue Tropism

Tissue tropism is related to affinity of virus receptors to attachment to host receptors

- Human adenovirus A, C, D, E and F species use CAR [10]
- Human adenovirus B species use CD 46 or membrane glycoprotein desmoglein 2 as cellular receptor for viral attachment.
- Species HAdVD37 utilizes sialic acid and GD1a as cellular receptors
- HAdVD8 and -D19 utilize CAR and sialic acid as cellular receptors to cause ocular infection [10–13].

22.7 Clinical Features of Ocular Adenoviral Infection

Broadly it has four phenotypic types of manifestation.

- Epidemic keratoconjunctivitis
- Pharyngoconjunctival fever
- Acute non-specific follicular conjunctivitis
- Chronic keratoconjunctivitis

22.7.1 Epidemic Keratoconjunctivitis

It is the most serious form of infection.

Serotypes involved [32] are serotypes 8,19,37,54

It occurs in young individuals, usually unilaterally in about two-thirds of cases, without systemic features (c.f PCF) [33]. After 8–10 days of incubation period, patient develops redness of the eyes associated with watering and foreign body sensation.

Signs include Preauricular Lymphadenopathy (50% of the cases) and Tarsal follicular conjunctivitis. Other less common signs include pseudomembranes over the palpebral conjunctiva (Fig. 22.3), chemosis and subconjunctival hemorrhages [34].

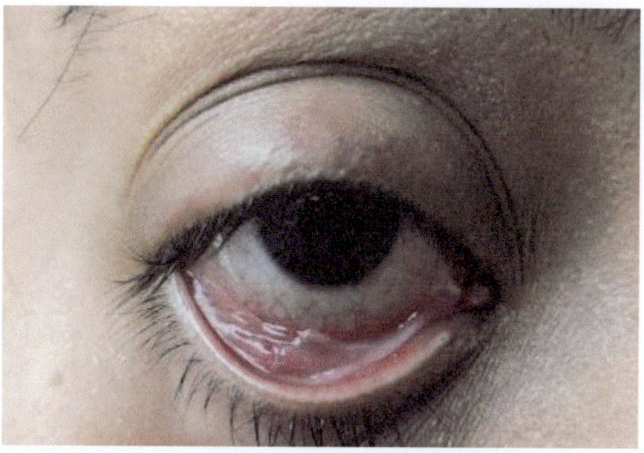

Fig. 22.3 Slit lamp photograph showing pseudomembrane formation in the right inferior palpebral conjunctiva

Stages

Adenoviral keratitis comprises of four stages [34]

Stage 1 Diffuse, fine, superficial epithelial punctate keratitis—worsening symptoms include photophobia, discomfort and lacrimation in this stage

Stage 2 Staining focal punctate white epithelial lesions

Stage 3 Combined epithelial and subepithelial areas

Stage 4 Non-staining subepithelial macular lesions (Fig. 22.4)

Stage 1 is direct infection caused by the live virus; stage 2–4 is caused by the delayed type hypersensitivity reaction [34, 35]. Adenoviral keratitis is usually resolved by 2–3 weeks, however, stage 4 reaches peak at 3–4 weeks. Visual acuity may drop by 1–2 lines, the subepithelial lesions may persist for months to years [36].

Rarely it can present in the form of bilateral disciform keratitis pattern [37].

22.7.2 Pharyngoconjunctival Fever (PCF)

Pharyngoconjunctival fever (PCF) is associated with adenovirus types 3, 4 and 7 [34].

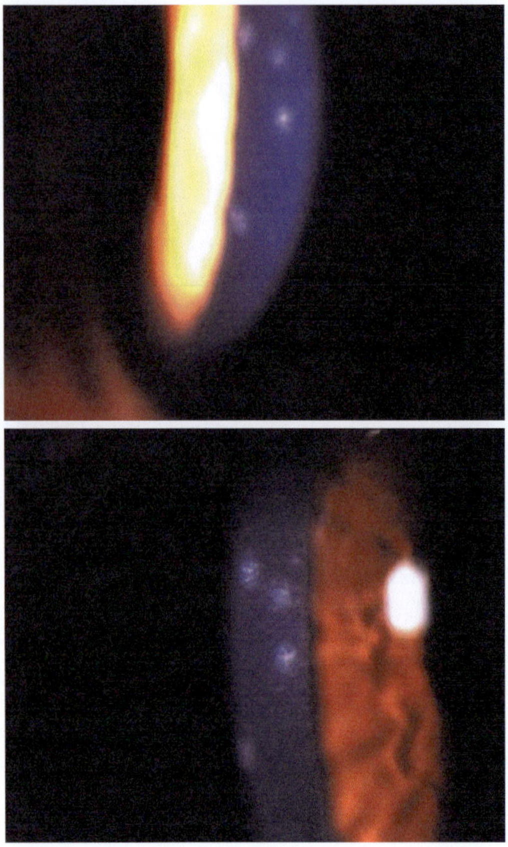

Fig. 22.4 Slit lamp photograph of a 42-year-old patient showing bilateral non staining subepithelial opacities which is persistent even after 2 years post conjunctivitis

It is highly contagious. Systemic symptoms predominate (c.f. EKC), with pharyngitis, tender pre-auricular lymphadenopathy, fever and an acute follicular conjunctivitis [38]. The incubation period is eight days following exposure (range: 5–12 days), when patients develop a high fever with associated muscle pain, malaise and, occasionally, gastrointestinal upset [1, 34]. An acute follicular conjunctivitis develops within few days, initial symptoms are of irritation, burning and lacrimation. The conjunctivitis is usually worse in the lower fornix and can lead to a tender, swollen lower eyelid, occasionally with bruising that can mimic orbital trauma. Both eyes are usually involved; however, there may be a delay of 1–3 days for subsequent eye to get involved. Keratitis is less common in PCF than EKC.

22.7.3 Acute Non-specific Adenoviral Conjunctivitis

It is mild, self-limiting conjunctivitis commonly seen in children and young adults, which resolves within 7–10 days of symptom onset. Conjunctivitis is characterized by soreness and lacrimation, with red conjunctiva and tarsal follicles as shown in Fig. 22.5a–d; the cornea is usually not involved.

22.7.4 Chronic Adenoviral Keratoconjunctivitis

It is rare but reported [37]. It presents as relapsing remitting intermittent redness of eyes with lacrimation and photophobia. History of conjunctivitis is present within 6–9 months previously. Diagnosis is challenging due to presence of papillae instead of follicles of palpebral conjunctiva [38–40].

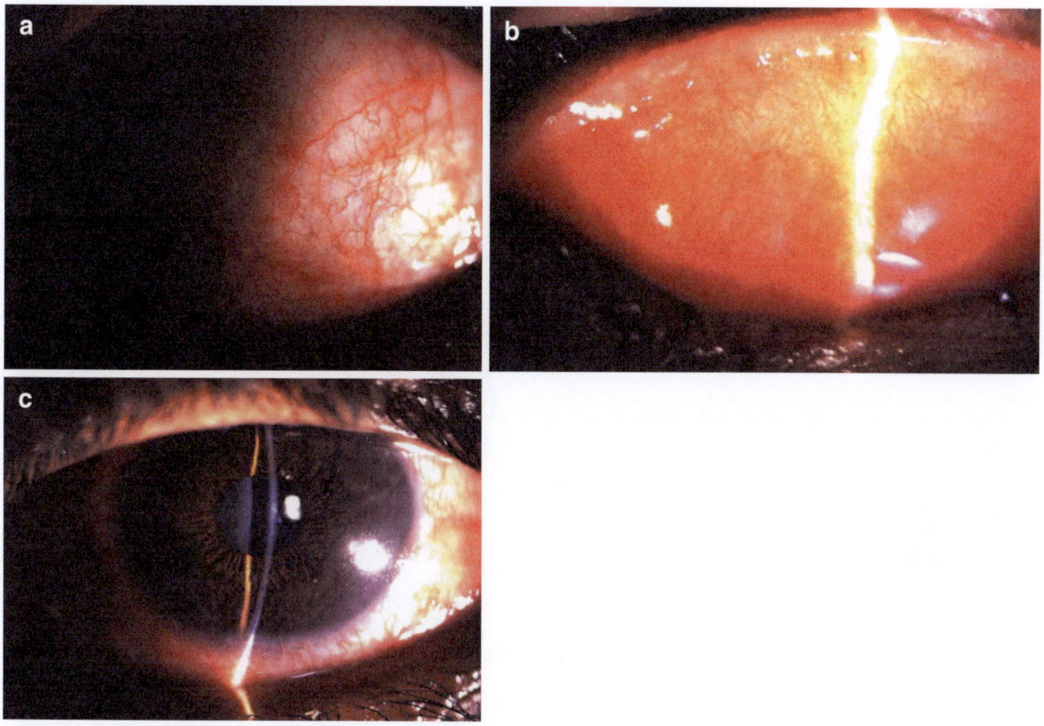

Fig. 22.5 Slit lamp photograph showing (a) an acute non-specific adenoviral conjunctivitis (b) with follicles in the upper palpebral conjunctiva (c) with no cornea involvement

22.8 Conclusion

Adenoviruses are a group of common viruses that can infect airways, lungs, eyes, intestines, urinary tract, and nervous system. They are common causes of fever, coughs, sore throats, diarrhea and pink eye. The infections usually cause only mild symptoms and get better on their own in a few days. But they can be more serious in people with weak immune systems, especially children. Mild adenovirus symptoms clear up within 3–5 days, but a serious infection could last weeks with associated keratitis. Proper hygiene is required to prevent the infection.

Key Points

1. Human Adenovirus are non-enveloped double-stranded DNA viruses which are icosahedral in shape.
2. Its genome has structural and non-structural proteins. Structural proteins consist of 240 trimers of hexon protein and 12 pentamers of penton base proteins.
3. Adenovirus attachment is mediated by interactions between its fiber-knob protein and several cellular receptors, including CAR, CD46, sialic acid, desmoglein 2, heparan sulfate proteoglycans, CD80, CD86, and GD1a.
4. Internalization of adenovirus into an endosome is mediated by the interaction of the homopentameric penton base and vitronectin-binding integrin. Penton base and integrin interaction mediates the signaling cascade and initiate viral replication.
5. Viral replication has early and late stages. Early stage has E1a protein that activates E2,3,4 proteins mediated by DNA polymerase. Late stage helps in maturation of DNA.
6. Host has innate and adaptive immunity to prevent viral infection. Innate immunity comprises of mechanical and chemical barrier and adaptive immunity is by various mediators.
7. Adenovirus has tissue tropism which explains the various serotypes which are responsible for phenotypic variations.

8. Epidemic Keratoconjunctivitis (EKC) is the most serious form and caused by serotype 8,9,37,54 causing acute unilateral conjunctivitis with tender preauricular lymphadenopathy and pseudomembrane formation. Risk of keratitis is high in EKC.
9. Pharyngoconjunctival fever is caused by serotype 3,4,7 causing acute bilateral follicular conjunctivitis with systemic features such as pharyngitis, preauricular lymphadenopathy and fever.

References

1. Muto T, Imaizumi S, Kamoi K. Viral conjunctivitis. Viruses. 2023;15(3):676.
2. Logan JS, Shenk TH. Transcriptional and translational control of adenovirus gene expression. Microbiol Rev. 1982;46(4):377–83.
3. Jhanji V, Chan TC, Li EY, Agarwal K, Vajpayee RB. Adenoviral keratoconjunctivitis. Surv Ophthalmol. 2015;60(5):435–43.
4. Kuo IC. Adenoviral keratoconjunctivitis: diagnosis, management, and prevention. Curr Ophthalmol Rep. 2019;7:118–27.
5. Guadalupe-Fernández V, Martínez-Solanas E, Sabrià-Sunyé A, et al. Investigating epidemiological distribution (temporality and intensity) of respiratory pathogens following COVID-19 de-escalation process in Catalonia, September 2016-June 2021: Analysis of regional surveillance data. PLoS One. 2024;19(2):e0285892.
6. Ison MG. Adenovirus infections in transplant recipients. Clin Infect Dis. 2006;43(3):331–9.
7. Garnett CT, Erdman D, Xu W, Gooding LR. Prevalence and quantitation of species C adenovirus DNA in human mucosal lymphocytes. J Virol. 2002;76(21):10608–16.
8. Guner A, Sarınoglu RC, Aydın FO, Turhan SA, Kuskucu MA, Toker AE, Yagcı AK. Molecular analysis of human adenoviral keratoconjunctivitis cases: results of a 2-year survey. Marmara Med J. 2023;36(1):1–6.
9. Schaar K, Röger C, Pozzuto T, Kurreck J, Pinkert S, Fechner H. Biological antivirals for treatment of adenovirus infections. Antivir Ther. 2016;21(7):559–66.
10. Gonçalves MA, de Vries AA. Adenovirus: from foe to friend. Rev Med Virol. 2006;16(3):167–86.
11. Wickham TJ, Mathias P, Cheresh DA, Nemerow GR. Integrins αvβ3 and αvβ5 promote adenovirus internalization but not virus attachment. Cell. 1993;73(2):309–19.
12. Walters RW, Freimuth P, Moninger TO, Ganske I, Zabner J, Welsh MJ. Adenovirus fiber disrupts CAR mediated intercellular adhesion allowing virus escape. Cell. 2002;110(6):789–99.
13. Nagarajan T, Rupprecht CE. History of rabies and rabies vaccines. Rabies Rabies Vaccines. 2020:11–43.
14. Nemerow GR, Pache L, Reddy V, Stewart PL. Insights into adenovirus host cell interactions from structural studies. Virology. 2009;384(2):380–8.
15. Bergelson JM, Cunningham JA, Droguett G, Kurt-Jones EA, Krithivas A, Hong JS, Horwitz MS, Crowell RL, Finberg RW. Isolation of a common receptor for Coxsackie B viruses and adenoviruses 2 and 5. Science. 1997;275(5304):1320–3.
16. Wu E, Trauger SA, Pache L, Mullen TM, Von Seggern DJ, Siuzdak G, Nemerow GR. Membrane cofactor protein is a receptor for adenoviruses associated with epidemic keratoconjunctivitis. J Virol. 2004;78(8):3897–905.
17. Wang H, Li ZY, Liu Y, Persson J, Beyer I, Möller T, Koyuncu D, Drescher MR, Strauss R, Zhang XB, Wahl JK III. Desmoglein 2 is a receptor for adenovirus serotypes 3, 7, 11 and 14. Nat Med. 2011;17(1):96–104.
18. Nilsson EC, Storm RJ, Bauer J, Johansson SM, Lookene A, Ångström J, Hedenström M, Eriksson TL, Frängsmyr L, Rinaldi S, Willison HJ. The GD1a glycan is a cellular receptor for adenoviruses causing epidemic keratoconjunctivitis. Nat Med. 2011;17(1):105.
19. Wolfrum N, Greber UF. Adenovirus signalling in entry. Cell Microbiol. 2013;15(1):53–62.
20. Yousuf MA, Zhou X, Mukherjee S, Chintakuntlawar AV, Lee JY, Ramke M, Chodosh J, Rajaiya J. Caveolin-1 associated adenovirus entry into human corneal cells. PLoS One. 2013;8(10):e77462.
21. Rodriguez E, Everitt E. Adenovirus uncoating and nuclear establishment are not affected by weak base amines. J Virol. 1996;70(6):3470–7.
22. Chung YS, Kim MK, Lee WJ, Kang C. Silencing E1A mRNA by RNA interference inhibits adenovirus replication. Arch Virol. 2007;152:1305–14.
23. Kneidinger D, Ibrišimović M, Lion T, Klein R. Inhibition of adenovirus multiplication by short interfering RNAs directly or indirectly targeting the viral DNA replication machinery. Antivir Res. 2012;94(3):195–207.
24. Bos JL, ten Wolde-Kraamwinkel HC. The E1b promoter of Ad12 in mouse L tk-cells is activated by adenovirus region E1a. EMBO J. 1983;2(1):73–6.
25. Hoeben RC, Uil TG. Adenovirus DNA replication. Cold Spring Harb Perspect Biol. 2013;5(3):a013003.
26. Ginsberg HS, Lundholm-Beauchamp U, Horswood RL, Pernis B, Wold WS, Chanock RM, Prince GA. Role of early region 3 (E3) in pathogenesis of adenovirus disease. Proc Natl Acad Sci. 1989;86(10):3823–7.
27. Evans JD, Hearing P. Distinct roles of the Adenovirus E4 ORF3 protein in viral DNA replication and inhibition of genome concatenation. J Virol. 2003;77(9):5295–304.
28. Nguyen EK, Nemerow GR, Smith JG. Direct evidence from single-cell analysis that human α-defensins block adenovirus uncoating to neutralize infection. J Virol. 2010;84(8):4041–9.

29. Smith JG, Nemerow GR. Mechanism of adenovirus neutralization by human α-defensins. Cell Host Microbe. 2008;3(1):11–9.
30. Calcedo R, Vandenberghe LH, Roy S, Somanathan S, Wang L, Wilson JM. Host immune responses to chronic adenovirus infections in human and nonhuman primates. J Virol. 2009;83(6):2623–31.
31. Lütschg V, Boucke K, Hemmi S, Greber UF. Chemotactic antiviral cytokines promote infectious apical entry of human adenovirus into polarized epithelial cells. Nat Commun. 2011;2(1):391.
32. McSharry BP, Burgert HG, Owen DP, Stanton RJ, Prod'homme V, Sester M, Koebernick K, Groh V, Spies T, Cox S, Little AM. Adenovirus E3/19K promotes evasion of NK cell recognition by intracellular sequestration of the NKG2D ligands major histocompatibility complex class I chain-related proteins A and B. J Virol. 2008;82(9):4585–94.
33. Yawata N, Selva KJ, Liu YC, Tan KP, Lee AW, Siak J, Lan W, Vania M, Arundhati A, Tong L, Li J. Dynamic change in natural killer cell type in the human ocular mucosa in situ as means of immune evasion by adenovirus infection. Mucosal Immunol. 2016;9(1):159–70.
34. Rajaiya J, Saha A, Ismail AM, Zhou X, Su T, Chodosh J. Adenovirus and the cornea: more than meets the eye. Viruses. 2021;13(2):293.
35. Russell WC. Adenoviruses: update on structure and function. J Gen Virol. 2009;90(1):1–20.
36. Chigbu DI, Labib BA. Pathogenesis and management of adenoviral keratoconjunctivitis. Infect Drug Resist. 2018:981–93.
37. Laibson PR, Dhiri S, Oconer J, Ortolan G. Corneal infiltrates in epidemic keratoconjunctivitis: response to double-blind corticosteroid therapy. Arch Ophthalmol. 1970;84(1):36–40.
38. Hoffman J. Adenovirus: ocular manifestations. Commun Eye Health. 2020;33(108):73.
39. Boniuk M, Phillips CA, Friedman JB. Chronic adenovirus type 2 keratitis in man. N Engl J Med. 1965;273(17):924–5.
40. Altan-Yaycioglu R, Poyraz S. Bilateral disciform keratitis of presumed adenoviral etiology. Indian J Ophthalmol. 2018;66(1):132–4.

Management of Adenoviral Keratoconjunctivitis

23

Navneet Sidhu, Yogita Gupta, Neiwete Lomi, and Radhika Tandon

Abstract

Adenoviral infections are the commonest cause of acute keratoconjunctivitis globally, manifesting as red eye. Adenoviral keratoconjunctivitis presents with redness, lacrimation, ocular discomfort and photophobia. In later stages, it can present with epithelial and subepithelial corneal lesions. Nummular corneal opacities are the most common sequelae seen in most cases. Epidemic keratoconjunctivitis (EKC) is the commonest clinical manifestation of adenoviral keratitis that is highly contagious and known to spread rapidly in the community. Management of adenoviral infections is mostly supportive. Most adenoviral infections are self-limiting in nature. Though most cases resolve spontaneously and require no intervention, few cases developing vision-threatening complications which need to be managed aggressively.

N. Sidhu
Centre for Sight, New Delhi, India

Y. Gupta (✉)
Dept of Ophthalmology, Deen Dayal Upadhyay Hospital, Delhi, India

N. Lomi · R. Tandon
Dr R P Centre for Ophthalmic Sciences, All India Institute of Medical Sciences (AIIMS) Delhi, Delhi, India

Keywords

Adenoviral keratitis, Adenoviruses, keratoconjunctivitis, conjunctivitis, · Viral keratitis · Nummular keratitis

23.1 Introduction

Adenoviruses are the commonest cause of acute viral conjunctivitis and lead to nearly three-fourths of conjunctivitis cases worldwide. Adenoviruses can lead to: *epidemic keratoconjunctivitis (EKC)*, *pharyngoconjunctival fever (PCF)*, *isolated follicular conjunctivitis* and *chronic keratoconjunctivitis*. EKC is the most frequently seen manifestation of ocular adenoviral infections [1, 2]. It is commonly caused by adenovirus serotypes 8, 19 and 37, although associations with other serotypes have been reported.

Adenoviruses, spread by fomite transfer through agents like contaminated hands, linen, cosmetics and other shared objects; inadequately chlorinated swimming pools, contaminated eye examination instruments and eye solutions. The incubation period is 3–7 days.

Adenoviral keratitis can be categorized into four stages: **first stage** of discomfort, photophobia and lacrimation; **second stage** of larger, fluorescein-staining white punctate epithelial corneal lesions; **third stage** with areas of combined epithelial and subepithelial lesions; and the

B. Sharma et al. (eds.), *Viral Keratitis*, https://doi.org/10.1007/978-981-95-3148-6_23

fourth stage is the resolving stage with non-staining subepithelial lesions.

23.2 Clinical Features

Adenovirus commonly manifests as **follicular conjunctivitis**. This is seen clinically as palpebral conjunctival oedema, conjunctival injection with folliculitis, particularly on the inferior palpepral conjunctiva and chemosis. Occasionally, few pinpoint subconjunctival haemorrhages may develop. In severe cases corneal involvement in the form of epithelial, subepithelial infiltrates, corneal erosions, superficial keratopathy and nummular corneal opacities are seen in addition to formation of pseudomembrane and preauricular lymphadenopathy (Figs. 23.1a–c and 23.2).

Symptoms usually begin in one eye, and later spread to the contralateral eye. A history of antecedent upper respiratory tract infection or close contact with patient of conjunctivitis is common. Symptoms may range in severity with complaints of redness, watering, burning or gritty foreign body sensation, watery, mucoid discharge and crusting of eye lashes (occuring due to mucus and pus-mixed discharge which dries and forms a crust along the lash line). The lids may become red and edematous. When adenoviral eye infections further involve the cornea, patients present with photophobia, blurring or diminution of vision.

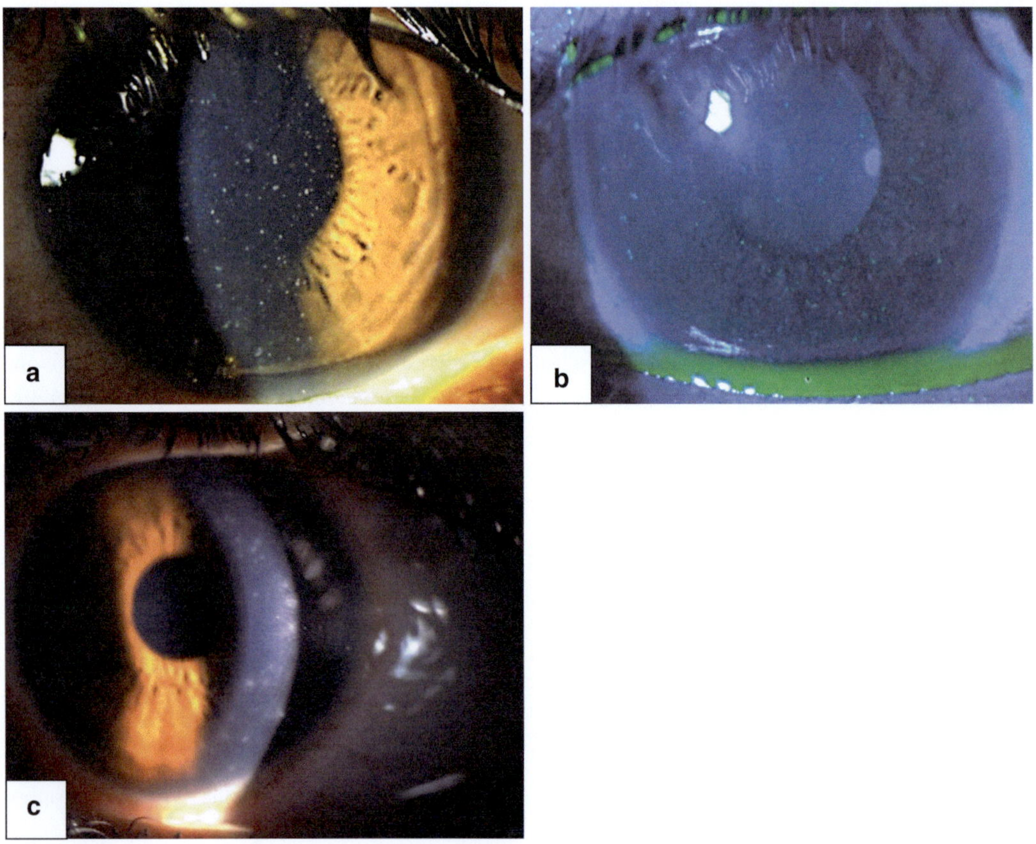

Fig. 23.1 (**a** and **b**) Slit and fluorescein-stained images showing **early** epithelial infiltrate seen in Adenoviral keratoconjunctivitis. (**c**) Slit lamp image showing epithelial infiltrates with surrounding haze in early phase of adenoviral keratoconjunctivitis

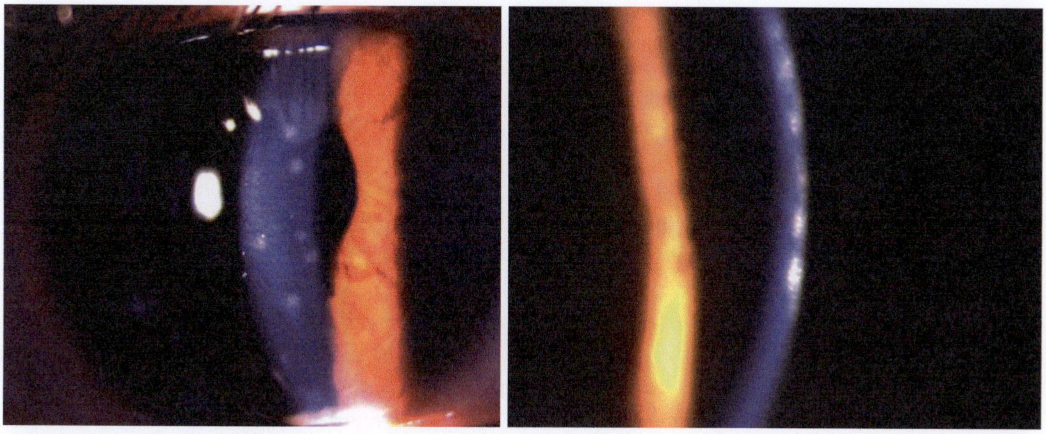

Fig. 23.2 Slit lamp image showing circular white epithelial and subepithelial infiltrates consolidated in **late** phase of adenoviral keratoconjunctivitis

23.3 Diagnosis

Adenoviral infections are usually diagnosed based on clinical features. For management and follow-up, investigative modalities which are employed are anterior segment optical coherence tomography (AS-OCT) and in vivo confocal microscopy (IVCM). Anterior segment imaging techniques like AS-OCT and IVCM are helpful for detecting sub-epithelial lesions with good sensitivity and can guide treatment in cases of adenoviral keratitis threatening central vision. Visual acuity assessment and slit-lamp examination must be performed at first and follow-up visits. The intraocular pressure assessment (non-contact tonometry) is usually avoided in viral conjunctivitis, especially during the pandemic times so as to avoid viral transmission with aerosols generated during air pulse release.

Laboratory tests mainly Polymerase Chain Reaction (PCR) may be required to confirm the diagnosis in patients with prolonged illness and those not responding to standard treatment. These laboratory tests also save health care costs by timely diagnosis and help clinicians decide suitability of starting antimicrobial therapy.

Adenoviruses are double-stranded deoxyribose nucleic acid (dsDNA) viruses. Adenoviruses are classified into seven species and different serotypes based on their structural and functional properties. While EKC is caused by adenovirus serotypes 8, 19 and 37, PCF has association with serotypes 3, 5, 7 and 11 and serotypes 1–11 cause isolated follicular conjunctivitis [3–6].

The laboratory tests include:

1. **Polymerase chain reaction (PCR)**: Deoxyribose nucleic acid (DNA) amplification using PCR of tear film sample helps in confirming adenoviral infection of the eye. This test has very high sensitivity.
2. **Rapid antigen detection tests**: These are immunoassays which quickly detect adenoviruses within few minutes in the test sample (e.g. tear film sample). These rapid diagnostic tests are now being increasingly used to decrease unnecessary use of antibiotics [2].
3. **Cell culture**: Sample taken from the eye with high-yield conjunctival swabs can be processed using cell cultures to look for adenoviruses serotypes which grow in particular human cell lines. This cell culture method can be coupled with tests like direct and indirect immunofluorescence staining tests.

Differential diagnoses include allergic conjunctivitis, viral conjunctivitis caused by non-adenoviral species, infections by herpes simplex virus, varicella/zoster virus, bacterial conjunctivitis, *Acanthamoeba* keratitis, bacterial and fungal keratitis.

23.4 Management

Adenoviral infections are usually self-limited with complete resolution in most of the cases without any treatment. Frequent hand washing, avoidance of contaminant objects and supportive treatment is the standard of care. Complications associated with adenoviral infections such as subepithelial corneal infiltrates, visual axis involvement, pre-existing ocular surface disease may present with deterioration of vision and require aggressive management.

23.4.1 Management Principles

Treatment for ocular adenoviral infections is mainly conservative. Symptomatic management is done for ocular pain, photophobia and ocular discomfort using cold compresses, topical lubricants, cycloplegics and other anti-inflammatory agents in most cases. Complications like subepithelial infiltrates, ocular surface inflammation, pseudomembrane and/or symblepharon formation should be detected and managed promptly and aggressively. Subepithelial infiltrations are treated using topical soft corticosteroids after resolution of acute phase, which hasten clearing of subepithelial haze. However topical steroids should be avoided in acute disease due to potential progression of disease [7].

23.4.2 Management of Specific Types

(a) Management of epidemic keratoconjunctivitis (EKC): Transmission of adenoviruses during epidemics as EKC is through contact with infected fomites and respiratory droplets. It can also spread from contact with medical personnel and medical instruments shared between different patients. EKC usually resolves on its own. Symptomatic and supportive treatment is given for pain and photophobia. An important aspect of management is to control the spread of infection in cases of EKC outbreaks. Careful history of any affected family member or occupational exposure must be taken to identify pockets of population infected with adenovirus in community, followed by complete examination of any affected person with whom patient has come in close contact. In EKC, most cases complain of a viral prodrome presenting with fever, malaise, myalgia, nausea and vomiting prior to the ocular infection. Adenoviruses are highly contagious pathogens and thus family members living in close contact with infected cases may also be affected [2].

(b) Management of Pharyngoconjunctival Fever: PCF is characterized by acute follicular conjunctivitis and preauricular lymphadenopathy. Besides topical medications to manage follicular or papillary reaction, conjunctival chemosis, subconjunctival haemorrhage and ocular surface inflammation, local ointments may be required to take care of the crusting and swelling of eyelids, which may be a common presentation in PCF cases [2]. Steroids and cyclosporine may be required to treat pseudomembrane and/or symblepharon formation in complicated cases to reduce disease progression and arrest subepithelial infiltration and prevent further fibrosis.

23.5 Medical Management

23.5.1 Topical Therapy

Medical management includes symptomatic relief with artificial tears like 0.5% CMC or 0.3% HPMC. Povidone Iodine 2–5% has been shown to reduce adenoviral load if individuals present $\leq$4 days of symptom onset and hasten resolution of signs and symptoms [8]. Topical Ciprofloxacin 0.3% in BD-QID dosage is used in patients with secondary infection. Cycloplegic agents such as homatropine 2% may be added in cases with significant photophobia. Topical antihistaminic and vasoconstrictor agents may help reduce discomfort and redness.

In patients with sub-epithelial involvement particularly involving the visual axis, topical steroids like Loteprednol 0.5% or Fluorometholone

0.1% are started in BD-QID dosage. Cyclosporine 0.1% eye drops can also be used as a steroid-sparing agent for the treatment in cases of adenoviral conjunctivitis with subepithelial infiltrates [9]. They can reduce the formation of subepithelial infiltrates and reduces symptoms [10, 11].

Subepithelial infiltrates in adenoviral keratitis are hypothesized to arise from a delayed hypersensitivity immune reaction to the viral antigens in the corneal stroma. The use of steroids and cyclosporine is found to reduce the immune reaction and hence clear the infiltrates [9–12].

In cases with ocular surface inflammation, pseudomembrane and/or symblepharon formation, anti-inflammatory agents have a beneficial role. Topical interferon β (IFN β) 1 MIU /ml has been shown to be useful in cases of acute conjunctivitis as it reduces the length of disease and prevents corneal complications [2, 13]. Povidone-iodine is an antiseptic agent with broad spectrum antimicrobial activity, which can be used to reduce viral load, thereby reducing spread of infection and disease progression of cases [14]. However, it is effective also in the disinfection of free adenoviruses, but not the intracellular viral particles [15, 16]. Topical povidone-iodine 2–5% BD is usually coupled with steroids to reduce ocular surface inflammation [14].

23.5.2 Oral Therapy

The use of oral anti-viral therapy has been widely studied in the treatment of adenoviral conjunctivitis. Since the virus also infects other mucosal surfaces involving upper and lower respiratory tract, gastrointestinal system and the urinary bladder, anti-viral therapy against the same is already being used [1]. The use of ganciclovir, ribavirin and cidofovir has been widely reported in severe adenoviral infections [17].

Oral ganciclovir (50% effective concentration (EC_{50}) of ganciclovir, which ranged from 2.64 to 5.10 μg/mL (10.3 to 19.9 μM), indicating a dose-dependent, inhibits the replication of the adenoviruses [18]. Significant dose-dependent reduction in the viral load in the ocular tissues has been seen with the use of oral ganciclovir, with limited local and systemic side effects. Ribavirin and cidofovir (5 mg/kg administered once weekly for two consecutive weeks (induction phase), followed by 5 mg/kg every other week (maintenance phase) have also shown efficacy in the resolution of adenoviral keratitis [17]. Cidofovir may cause allergic skin reactions, while Ribavirin may cause systemic side effects like anaemia, bone marrow suppression or extravascular hemolysis [18]. In patients with adenoviral pneumonia with keratitis, early systemic administration of cidofovir has shown efficacious results [19].

Cidofovir causes significant systemic toxicity and many virus strains may also be resistant to it. Hence, a new lipid-linked derivative of the same, brincidofovir, (100 mg twice weekly for adults or 2 mg/kg twice weekly in pediatric patients) has been investigated [20]. It is more readily absorbed orally, thereby increasing bioavailability of the drug and has shown to reduce the nephrotoxicity of the drug.

23.5.3 Adjunctive Therapy

Anti-adenovirus immunoglobulin G (IgG (0.5–1 g/kg/day for 2 consecutive days) has been shown to target the adenoviral capsid proteins, thus limiting the viral infection [21]. When given topically, Ig offers the same effect on ocular tissues, thus preventing the transmission and replication of the virus [1]. Ig also has anti-inflammatory properties, hence helps in early resolution of the symptoms [22]. Ig was comparable to cidofovir in its antiviral activity in one of the studies [22]. Cidofovir acts intracellularly to block viral DNA replication, Ig neutralizes the virus on the ocular surface, so a combination therapy may be effective in severe cases of keratitis caused by the virus.

23.6 Surgical Management and Management of Complications

Surgery is rarely required in cases of adenoviral keratitis. However, consequences like corneal scarring and severe fibrosis may need surgical management. The pseudomembranes should be removed with a blunt forceps or a cotton swab. Removal of membranes may lead to tiny bleeding points to be seen. Prolonged presence of pseudomembrane causes subepithelial fibrosis of conjunctiva, symblepharon formation and occlusion of lacrimal puncta with scarring of the ocular surface [23]. This would require surgical intervention to release the symblepharon, conjunctival excision with amniotic membrane graft (AMG) placement and even fornix formation surgeries. Severe cases with ocular surface fibrosis may require extensive resection of fibrotic tissue with AMG transplantation to repair the ocular surface.

Patients with subepithelial corneal scars affecting their visual acuity after resolution of the infection may require removal of the superficial layers of the cornea. This can be done using phototherapeutic keratectomy (PTK) in which the epithelium, Bowman's layer and superficial stroma is removed precisely using femtosecond laser. Transepithelial PTK with low dose mitomycin C has also shown promising results in cases of healed adenoviral keratitis presenting with nummular corneal opacities post EKC [12]. There is a significant improvement in the best corrected visual acuity, photophobia, glare and contrast sensitivity, along with significant reduction in higher order aberrations [24–26]. Phototherapeutic keratectomy is done for anterior 10–20% corneal scars, as deeper scars need deeper ablations and may result in hyperopic shift.

A transepithelial approach allows to remove the epithelial thickness variability and hence refractive outcomes are more consistent with a defined refractive target, which is usually emmetropia [24, 25].

23.7 Follow-Up and Monitoring of Treatment

Treatment protocol majorly involves symptomatic treatment since the infection is usually self-resolving. The use of topical steroids has been advocated to reduce inflammation and scarring. Serial follow-ups are essential to monitor the progress. The patient should be followed up at 3 days, 1 week and then weekly or monthly as per the clinical picture to look for disease resolution and presence of any complications that may require early interventions. Steroids should be tapered weekly depending on the response. Close monitoring must be done for cases on topical steroids to detect any steroid-related complications like glaucoma and cataract in time.

23.8 Patient Education and Preventing Spread in Community

Adenoviral infections are usually self-limiting; however, being highly contagious, with potential long-term visual complications a management protocol is essential to prevent spread in the community. Individuals at high risk due to viral dissemination include children, elderly and the immunocompromised. Health education in the community with regards to effective disinfection, hand hygiene and prevention protocols need to be advocated. Patients with respiratory and urinary tract infection should be timely and appropriately tested for adenovirus and treated accordingly.

23.9 Recent Advances

Adenovirus keratitis also has a high propensity for reactivation later in life. This nature of the virus to reactivate and the easy transmissibility has led to additional research for an effective and prophylactic therapy.

New therapies under consideration include sialic acid analogues, cold atmospheric plasma

(CAP), N- chlorotaurine and benzalkonium chloride (BAK) [27, 28]. Sialic acid analogues block sialic acid containing glycans which act as cellular receptors and hence decrease the replication of the virus. CAP also has demonstrated antiviral effects in various skin diseases and might be effective in ocular tissues as well. BAK, which is a common preservative in many ophthalmic formulations, in concentrations of more than 0.1% has been found to be effective against adenovirus [29]. However, it is associated with ocular side effects. Newer adjunctive agents are being explored and these may be promising in future to reduce viral load in infected cases especially in the immunocompromised individuals, in whom persistence of the virus and a usually high load of the infection is noted.

23.10 Conclusion

Adenoviral keratitis is usually a self-limited disease, but the high rate of transmission, risk of reactivation and potential long-term side effects necessitate compliance to established treatment protocol. Children, elderly and immunocompromised individuals are majorly at risk and so timely treatment is essential. Use of lubricants like 0.5% CMC or 0.3% HPMC and 2% povidone Iodine are efficacious in early phase of disease. Topical steroids have been effective in managing the corneal complications after the acute infection is resolved. The use of topical anti-virals is also under consideration in alleviating the symptoms and to prevent recurrence.

Key Points

1. Adenovirus has a high risk of transmission, causing a high epidemic burden in communities.
2. It is persistently secreted in the tears, causing rapid spread of viral particles.
3. Viruses may reactivate later in life.
4. Symptopmatic treatment is given as soon as diagnosis is made. Early treatment has proven to be useful in preventing complications and visual impairment and thus reduces ocular morbidity.

References

1. Labib BA, Minhas BK, Chigbu DI. Management of Adenoviral Keratoconjunctivitis: challenges and Solutions. Clin Ophthalmol. 2020;14:837–52.
2. Jhanji V, Chan TCY, Li EYM, Agarwal K, Vajpayee RB. Adenoviral keratoconjunctivitis. Surv Ophthalmol. 2015;60(5):435–43.
3. Ariga T, Shimada Y, Shiratori K, et al. Five new genome types of adenovirus type 37 caused epidemic keratoconjunctivitis in Sapporo, Japan, for more than 10 years. J Clin Microbiol. 2005;43(2):726–32.
4. Erdman DD, Xu W, Gerber SI, et al. Molecular epidemiology of adenovirus type 7 in the United States, 1966–2000. Emerg Infect Dis. 2002;8(3):269–77.
5. Schrauder A, Altmann D, Laude G, et al. Epidemic conjunctivitis in Germany, 2004. Euro Surveill. 2006;11(7):185–7.
6. Adlhoch C, Schöneberg I, Fell G, Brandau D, Benzler J. Increasing case numbers of adenovirus conjunctivitis in Germany, 2010. Euro Surveill. 2010;15(45):19707.
7. Laibson PR, Dhiri S, Oconer J, Ortolan G. Corneal infiltrates in epidemic keratoconjunctivitis. Response to double-blind corticosteroid therapy. Arch Ophthalmol. 1970;84(1):36–40.
8. Than T, et al. Efficacy of a single administration of 5% povidone-iodine in the treatment of adenoviral conjunctivitis. Am J Ophthalmol. 2021;231:28–3.
9. Hillenkamp J, Reinhard T, Ross RS, et al. Topical treatment of acute adenoviral keratoconjunctivitis with 0.2% cidofovir and 1% cyclosporine: a controlled clinical pilot study. Arch Ophthalmol. 2001;119(10):1487–91.
10. Jeng BH, Holsclaw DS. Cyclosporine A 1% eye drops for the treatment of subepithelial infiltrates after adenoviral keratoconjunctivitis. Cornea. 2011;30(9):958–61.
11. Levinger E, Slomovic A, Sansanayudh W, Bahar I, Slomovic AR. Topical treatment with 1% cyclosporine for subepithelial infiltrates secondary to adenoviral keratoconjunctivitis. Cornea. 2010;29(6):638–40.
12. Yamazaki ES, Ferraz CA, Hazarbassanov RM, Allemann N, Campos M. Phototherapeutic keratectomy for the treatment of corneal opacities after epidemic keratoconjunctivitis. Am J Ophthalmol. 2011;151(1):35–43.e1.
13. Wilhelmus KR, Dunkel EC, Herson J. Topical human fibroblast interferon for acute adenoviral conjunctivitis. Graefes Arch Clin Exp Ophthalmol. 1987;225(6):461–4.
14. Clement C, Capriotti JA, Kumar M, et al. Clinical and antiviral efficacy of an ophthalmic formulation of dexamethasone povidone-iodine in a rabbit model of adenoviral keratoconjunctivitis. Invest Ophthalmol Vis Sci. 2011;52(1):339–44.
15. Kawana R, Kitamura T, Nakagomi O, et al. Inactivation of human viruses by povidone-iodine

in comparison with other antiseptics. Dermatology. 1997;195(Suppl 2):29–35.
16. Monnerat N, Bossart W, Thiel MA. Povidone-iodine for treatment of adenoviral conjunctivitis: an in vitro study. Klin Monbl Augenheilkd. 2006;223(5):349–52.
17. Wold WSM, Toth K. New drug on the horizon for treating adenovirus. Expert Opin Pharmacother. 2015;16(14):2095–9.
18. Huang J, Kadonosono K, Uchio E. Antiadenoviral effects of ganciclovir in types inducing keratoconjunctivitis by quantitative polymerase chain reaction methods. Clin Ophthalmol. 2014;8:315–20.
19. Kim SJ, Kim K, Park SB, Hong DJ, Jhun BW. Outcomes of early administration of cidofovir in non-immunocompromised patients with severe adenovirus pneumonia. PLoS One. 2015;10(4):e0122642.
20. Grimley MS, Chemaly RF, Englund JA, et al. Brincidofovir for asymptomatic adenovirus viremia in pediatric and adult allogeneic hematopoietic cell transplant recipients: a Randomized Placebo-Controlled Phase II Trial. Biol Blood Marrow Transplant. 2017;23(3):512–21.
21. Goossens PH, Vogels R, Pieterman E, et al. The influence of synovial fluid on adenovirus-mediated gene transfer to the synovial tissue. Arthritis Rheum. 2001;44(1):48–52.
22. Nwanegbo EC, Romanowski EG, Gordon YJ, Gambotto A. Efficacy of topical immunoglobulins against experimental adenoviral ocular infection. Invest Ophthalmol Vis Sci. 2007;48(9):4171–6.
23. Chintakuntlawar AV, Chodosh J. Cellular and tissue architecture of conjunctival membranes in epidemic keratoconjunctivitis. Ocul Immunol Inflamm. 2010;18(5):341–5.
24. Kepez Yildiz B, Urvasizoglu S, Yildirim Y, et al. Changes in higher-order aberrations after phototherapeutic keratectomy for subepithelial corneal infiltrates after epidemic keratoconjunctivitis. Cornea. 2017;36(10):1233–6.
25. Spadea L, Visioli G, Mastromarino D, Alexander S, Pistella S. Topography-guided trans-epithelial no-touch photorefractive keratectomy for high irregular astigmatism after penetrating keratoplasty: a prospective 12-months follow-up. Ther Clin Risk Manag. 2021;17:1027–35.
26. Dausch D, Schröder E, Dausch S. Topography-controlled excimer laser photorefractive keratectomy. J Refract Surg. 2000;16(1):13–22. https://doi.org/10.3928/1081-597X-20000101-03.
27. Gonzalez G, Yawata N, Aoki K, Kitaichi N. Challenges in management of epidemic keratoconjunctivitis with emerging recombinant human adenoviruses. J Clin Virol. 2019;112:1–9.
28. Nilsson EC, Storm RJ, Bauer J, et al. The GD1a glycan is a cellular receptor for adenoviruses causing epidemic keratoconjunctivitis. Nat Med. 2011;17(1):105–9.
29. Romanowski EG, Yates KA, Shanks RMQ, Kowalski RP. Benzalkonium chloride demonstrates concentration-dependent antiviral activity against adenovirus in vitro. J Ocul Pharmacol Ther. 2019;35(5):311–4.

Section IV

Other Viral Infections

Keratitis Associated with Other Viral Infections

24

Bhavana Sharma, Nikhil Agrawal, Priyanka, and A. P. Mohammed Sabir

Abstract

Corneal infections are significant threats to ocular health, often leading to severe complications if not promptly identified and treated. While bacterial pathogens and common viruses like herpes simplex virus type 1 (HSV-1) are well-known causes, numerous other less common viral agents can also induce serious corneal disease. This chapter aims to describe the diverse array of such viruses, offering comprehensive details of their clinical presentations, diagnostic challenges, and treatment options. Emphasis is placed on the unique characteristics of these viruses and the critical need for healthcare professionals to recognize and manage their often atypical presentations. Covered are DNA viruses from the families Poxviridae, Herpesviridae (beyond HSV and zoster viruses), and Papovaviridae, along with RNA viruses from the families Picornaviridae, Togaviridae, Paramyxoviridae, and Orthomyxoviridae. Additionally, it provides detailed insights into the ocular complications associated with each virus, ranging from severe conditions like smallpox-induced corneal perforation to less common manifestations such as Zika virus-associated conjunctivitis. Given the varied and sometimes severe ocular complications, treating clinicians should ensure early detection and tailored therapeutic approaches to prevent vision loss and other serious outcomes.

Keywords

Uncommon · EBV · Rubella · Rare

24.1 Introduction

Corneal infections pose significant risks to eye health and can lead to severe complications if not properly identified and treated promptly. While bacterial infections and prevalent viruses like herpes simplex virus type 1 (HSV-1) are well-recognized causes, a variety of less common viral pathogens also exist that can induce serious corneal disease. This chapter addresses the diverse group of such viruses, providing in-depth knowledge on clinical features, diagnostic challenges, and treatment options. Special emphasis is placed on the unique characteristics of these viruses and the critical need for healthcare professionals to recognize and manage their often unusual presentations. The chapter will cover DNA viruses from the families Poxviridae, Herpesviridae (beyond the common herpes simplex and zoster viruses), and Papovaviridae. Additionally, it will discuss RNA viruses from the families Picornaviridae, Togaviridae, Paramyxoviridae,

B. Sharma (✉) · Priyanka · A. P. Mohammed Sabir
AIIMS Bhopal, Bhopal, Madhya Pradesh, India

N. Agrawal
AIIMS Jodhpur, Jodhpur, Rajasthan, India

B. Sharma et al. (eds.), *Viral Keratitis*, https://doi.org/10.1007/978-981-95-3148-6_24

and Orthomyxoviridae that are known to affect ocular health.

24.2 DNA Viruses

Various DNA viruses with their ocular and systemic manifestations have been described in Flow Diagram 24.1.

24.2.1 Poxviridae

24.2.1.1 Variola Virus (Smallpox)

Variola virus, responsible for smallpox, was a major cause of morbidity and mortality until its eradication was declared by the World Health Organization in May 1980, following extensive global vaccination campaigns [1]. Despite its eradication, there have been some reports of isolated resurgences [2, 3]. The disease is heralded by a viremic phase lasting 2–3 days with constitutional symptoms due to multiplication of the virus in lymphoid tissues, followed by potential spread to other body tissues. The disease is characterized by a maculopapular rash that evolves into vesicles and pustules, eventually healing with depigmented scars and pits.

Ocular Involvement

Ocular involvement can be severe owing to active viral replication and reactionary severe inflammation, with vesicles on the eyelids, severe periorbital edema, preseptal cellulitis, and complete closure of the lids. Secondary infection leading to orbital cellulitis can be seen in complicated cases. Scarring at the ciliary border can result in cicatricial entropion, madarosis, trichiasis, and punctal stenosis. There may be catarrhal, follicular, pustular, purulent, or membranous conjunctivitis in addition to corneal complications such as ulceration, interstitial or disciform keratitis, and necrosis and perforation of the globe in severe cases.

Treatment

Treatment of smallpox generally involves supportive care with anti-inflammatory and nutritional supplements in addition to isolation and adherence to infection control. Antiviral drugs

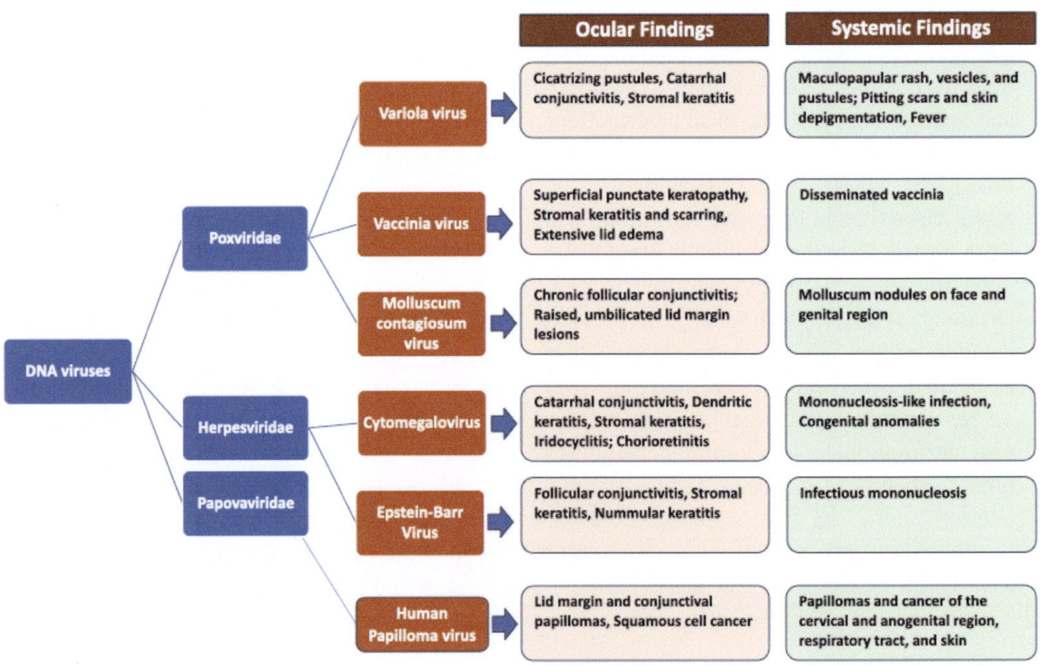

Flow Diagram 24.1 Showing classification of DNA viruses with their ocular and systemic manifestations

approved by the FDA for treatment include Tecovirimat and Brincidofovir. Although long-term efficacy data in humans is limited, the FDA Antimicrobial Drugs Advisory Committee has reported that the benefits of Tecovirimat treatment for smallpox outweigh its risks. Further, cidofovir has been found to be efficacious in treating patients with orthopoxvirus infection based on individual risk-benefit assessment [4]. Ocular involvement should be treated as per the anatomical structure involved. Ocular surface lubricants are to be prescribed in uncomplicated cases with conjunctival inflammation. They can be supplemented with broad-spectrum antibiotics in 4–6 times dosing to prevent potential secondary infections. In cases of severe involvement with tissue necrosis, appropriate medical or surgical intervention should be initiated to minimize complications.

24.2.1.2 Vaccinia Virus

The vaccinia virus, primarily known for its role in the smallpox vaccine, generally causes mild infections and confers immunity against smallpox, monkeypox, and cowpox. However, certain subjects, including pregnant women, immunocompromised individuals, and persons with eczema or chronic dermatitis, are at risk of developing disseminated vaccinia [5]. Cutaneous lesions from vaccinia typically appear 3–5 days after inoculation. Hence, all patients with a history of exposure should be kept under observation for prompt intervention and prevention of further infection [6].

Ocular Involvement

Ocular involvement with the vaccinia virus typically occurs through autoinoculation when the virus is transferred from the vaccination site to the eye by hand-to-eye contact. Patients present with varying symptoms ranging from itching, tearing, conjunctival injection, severe pain in the periorbital and orbital region, and visual deprivation due to corneal and deeper tissue involvement. Once autoinoculation occurs, there is an eruption of vaccinial vesicles on the eyelids. These vesicles may coalesce to form larger lesions with severe inflammation, accompanied by edema and erythema of the eyelids and periorbita, in addition to blepharitis, madarosis, secondary scarring, entropion, and ectropion. Other ocular manifestations may include chemosis of varying severity, membranous conjunctivitis, and consequent symblepharon. Secondary infection may result in orbital cellulitis and potential complications. Corneal infiltration can lead to stromal keratitis, melting, and consequent scarring if not treated promptly.

Treatment

Treatment options include intramuscular hyperimmune vaccinia immunoglobulin to control systemic disease. Ocular involvement is treated with topical antiviral agents such as Vidarabine, Trifluorothymidine, and Idoxuridine to decrease the viral load [5, 6]. Adjuvant treatment with systemic doxycycline, vitamin C, topical lubricants, cycloplegics, and IOP-lowering drugs should be initiated according to clinical involvement.

24.2.1.3 Molluscum Contagiosum

Molluscum contagiosum is a viral infection caused by the Molluscum contagiosum virus, a DNA virus from the poxvirus group. The virus is transmitted by skin contact or sexual intercourse. It generally occurs in children and is characterized by distinctive small, raised, flesh-colored or clear papules with a pitted center, seen on the face, abdomen, and genital regions. Severe involvement over multiple sites or disseminated form may be seen in individuals with immune deficiencies [7].

Ocular Involvement

Patients generally present with complaints of multiple swellings over the eyelids along with redness, gritty sensation, watering, photophobia, and visual impairment of varying severity. Ocular involvement typically manifests as multiple warty nodules with pitted centers seen on the eyelids. Figure 24.1 Viral proteins shed from the lid lesions into the tear film can lead to a hypersensitivity reaction with secondary chronic follicular conjunctivitis, punctate keratopathy, subepithelial infiltrates, and corneal pannus. Rarely primary lesions may be seen on the

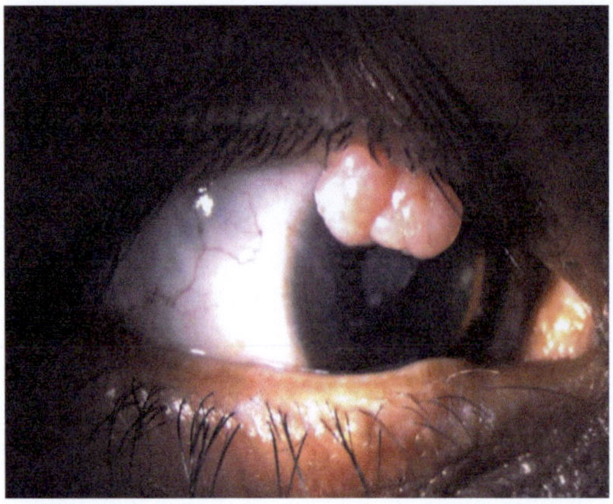

Fig. 24.1 Molluscum contagiosum viral wart showing clustered white-colored, dome-shaped, pearly papules

conjunctiva and cornea. The condition needs to be differentiated from other ocular surface disorders like trachoma, DED, rosacea keratitis, and allergic keratoconjunctivitis owing to similar presentation. Careful ocular examination to identify viral warts over eyelids remains the most important diagnostic differentiator. Diagnosis is usually based on clinical findings, while histopathological examination and laboratory tests are often not necessary. However, diagnosis can be confirmed by expressing the core of a molluscum lesion onto a slide for microscopic examination which reveals eosinophilic intracytoplasmic viral inclusion bodies.

Treatment

Although molluscum contagiosum is usually self-limiting with resolution over 2–3 months, treatment is initiated to prevent further infection, accelerate recovery, and minimize complications. Surgical options include excision, curettage followed by cryotherapy to the base of the lesion, while smaller lesions can be directly cauterized at the base. For reactionary keratoconjunctivitis, adjuvant treatment comprising lubricants, cycloplegics, and anti-inflammatory drops can be initiated, and the lesions resolve within weeks of surgical removal of primary eyelid lesions. Newer therapies such as immunomodulatory medications like Imiquimod, photodynamic therapy, electron beam radiation, carbon dioxide laser, and topical Cidofovir offer effective alternatives, especially in cases involving extensive or persistent lesions [7, 8].

24.2.2 Herpesviridae

The Herpesviridae is a large family of double-stranded DNA viruses with nine herpesvirus types known to primarily infect humans [9]. It can cause a wide spectrum of ocular infections ranging from anterior segment involvement to more severe posterior segment affections. While herpes simplex and herpes zoster are the commonly recognized pathogens affecting the eye, other members of this virus family, such as cytomegalovirus (CMV) and Epstein-Barr virus (EBV), also pose significant risks, albeit less frequently involving the anterior segment of the eye [10].

24.2.2.1 Cytomegalovirus

Cytomegalovirus (CMV) is a ubiquitous herpesvirus that infects over 90% of humans by their lifetime, and thus the seropositivity in humans exceeds 50% of the population. Infection is spread through saliva, sexual contact, transplacental spread, or breast milk. CMV causes subclinical infection in children and a nonspecific febrile illness in adults. The viremia transmits the virus to the bone marrow, where it becomes latent until its activation, expression, and shedding of the virus. CMV causes a wide range of ocular involvement, from subclinical to fulminant infection. Ocular disease can manifest as keratitis, chorioretinitis, optic atrophy, cataract, Peters anomaly, microphthalmia, and anophthalmia. In immunocompromised subjects, there can be extensive ocular involvement with devastating sequelae. Interestingly, CMV retinitis is present among the immunocompromised, while CMV endotheliitis is observed in the immunocompetent [11, 12].

Ocular Involvement

Anterior segment affection of CMV includes acute catarrhal conjunctivitis, stromal keratitis, endothelitis, and iritis. CMV keratitis is charac-

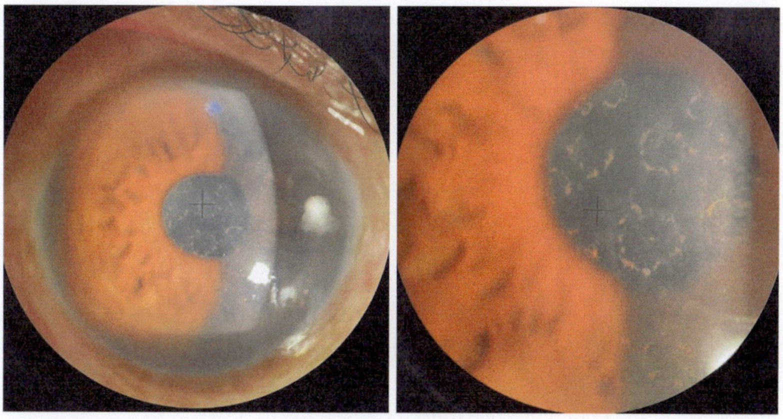

Fig. 24.2 CMV keratitis with characteristic coin-shaped lesions on endothelium. (Figure courtesy: Dr. Praveen Dhanapal DNB, Director Cornea and refractive surgery services, Ratan Jyoti Netralaya Institute of Ophthalmology and Research Centre Gwalior)

terized by an intact epithelium as opposed to HSV keratitis where an epithelial defect is commonly seen. CMV endothelitis is characterized by coin-shaped keratic precipitates and corneal edema, while some patients may present with linear keratic precipitates (Fig. 24.2). Other ocular manifestations include acute anterior uveitis with elevated IOP, anterior chamber cells, flare, and KPs. Such presentations may be misdiagnosed as Posner-Schlossman syndrome. Chronic uveitis with iris atrophy resembling Fuch's heterochromic iridocyclitis (FHI) may also be seen. The Japanese Corneal Endothelitis Study Group has proposed a diagnostic criteria and classified the disease into typical and atypical CMV endotheliitis, combining both clinical features and laboratory tests [12].

Diagnosis

Diagnosis is confirmed by careful slit lamp examination showing typical coin-shaped lesions with confirmatory PCR of aqueous tap reporting CMV DNA. Concurrent serum testing should also be performed to rule out systemic viremia. In addition, concomitant testing for other herpesviruses can be performed. Nonresponsive cases may require histologic examination of corneal biopsy or other surgical specimens. In vivo confocal microscopy shows pathognomonic large cells with a prominent nucleus and high reflection, surrounded by a halo of low reflection, typically described as owl's eye morphology at the level of the corneal endothelium.

CMV Keratitis and Keratoplasty

CMV endotheliitis, being increasingly common now, is often misdiagnosed as herpetic eye disease. In addition, CMV reactivation following corneal transplant presents with diffuse corneal edema and keratic precipitates can mimic endothelial graft rejection or graft failure [13]. Differentiating corneal graft rejection from CMV reactivation in post-keratoplasty eyes remains a diagnostic and therapeutic challenge. Postoperative steroid administration can predispose reactivation of latent CMV and increased risk of graft failure. Raised IOP, sudden drop in cell count, localized corneal edema, linear pigmented KPs, and nummular or coin-shaped endothelial lesion involving both donor and recipient cornea are the differentiating features from allograft rejections.

Treatment

Ganciclovir, Valganciclovir, Foscarnet, and Cidofovir are FDA-approved antiviral agents for CMV infections. However, there is a paucity of standardized treatment regimens for CMV endotheliitis. Current treatment regimens in CMV endotheliitis aim at targeting both the infectious and inflammatory components. Treatment recommendations include oral Valganciclovir 900 mg twice daily for 2–4 weeks. Valganciclovir is a prodrug of ganciclovir which transforms into ganciclovir after hydrolyzation. It has a better oral bioavailability of 60% compared to 6% of ganciclovir. For resistant CMV cases, second-line antiviral agents like Foscarnet and Cidofovir could be considered. In post-keratoplasty reactivation, oral Valganciclovir 900 mg twice daily for 6 weeks, followed by 900 mg daily for another 6 weeks, has shown to be efficacious [13]. Topical Ganciclovir 0.15–2% 3–5 times is effective when used as an adjunct to systemic therapy and in maintenance regimens along with topical NaCl 5%, cycloplegics, and lubricants as adjuvants.

Antiviral prophylaxis is prudent in cases with a prior history of CMV-associated anterior uveitis or endotheliitis who are planned for keratoplasty. Systemic Ganciclovir 5 mg/kg twice daily, topical Ganciclovir 0.15% 4–8 times daily, and Fluorometholone 0.1% 2–4 times daily for 2 weeks has been reported to be effective in preventing recurrences [14]. However, up to 35–40% of cases may show recurrences, requiring reinstated antiviral regimens, thus long-term surveillance for recurrences is needed. Anterior uveitis can be treated with systemic ganciclovir along with topical corticosteroids, cycloplegics, and anti-glaucoma medications as per the therapeutic requirement [14, 15].

24.2.2.2 Epstein-Barr Virus

Epstein-Barr Virus (EBV), best known for causing infectious mononucleosis, is also implicated in a range of other diseases including nasopharyngeal carcinoma, Sjogren's syndrome, Perinaud's oculoglandular syndrome, oral hairy leukoplakia, and Burkitt's lymphoma [16].

Ocular Involvement

EBV commonly leads to monocular follicular conjunctivitis, presenting as an inflamed, gritty sensation along with watering and redness. Additionally, some patients may develop conjunctival nodules, episcleritis, and uveitis. Corneal involvement is mainly stromal and occurs in two distinct forms: first as multifocal pleomorphic sharply demarcated ring-shaped granular opacities in the anterior stroma, and second as ill-defined, blotchy, pleomorphic, and multifocal infiltrates predominantly involving the peripheral cornea [16]. Furthermore, subepithelial infiltrates, stellate microdendrites, and nummular keratitis have also been reported [17–19]. Diagnosis of EBV infection is confirmed by the detection of serum antibodies to virus-specific antigens.

Treatment

EBV infection is generally a self-limited condition, hence treatment is typically supportive. The role of antivirals has not been fully established. Topical corticosteroids are reserved for patients with stromal keratitis causing visual impairment [20].

24.2.3 Papovaviridae

Human Papillomavirus

Papillomaviruses (HPV) belong to the family of Papovaviridae and are known for their affinity for epithelial tissues, leading to both benign and malignant neoplasms in various body sites such as the cervix, anogenital region, respiratory tract, and skin. Ocular involvement in HPV manifests in the form of conjunctival papillomas, recurrent pterygiums, dysplasia, and ocular surface squamous neoplasia, reflecting its potential for serious ocular complications. The histological hallmark for diagnosis is the identification of koilocytosis, which is an intermediate mature squamous cell characterized by perinuclear vaculation, densely staining peripheral cytoplasm, and a nucleus with an undulating nuclear membrane and a rope-like chromatin pattern [21].

Treatment

Treatment includes surgical resection to remove papillomas or malignant growths. This can be supplemented with other techniques such as carbon dioxide laser cauterization or cryotherapy to ensure complete removal and prevent recurrence. In addition to surgical methods, immunotherapy plays a crucial role, particularly systemic interferon alpha, which is often administered postsurgery to enhance the immune response and reduce the likelihood of recurrence [22, 23].

24.3 RNA Viruses

24.3.1 Picornaviridae

Acute Hemorrhagic Conjunctivitis (AHC)

AHC is primarily caused by certain picornavirus subtypes, most commonly enterovirus 70 and coxsackievirus A24 [24–26]. The infection typically begins with the sudden onset of severe conjunctivitis in one eye, followed by involvement of the other eye. The most distinctive feature of AHC is subconjunctival hemorrhages on the bulbar conjunctiva, which are visible as variably sized bright red blotches ranging from pinpoint petechiae to larger, flat hemorrhages (Fig. 24.3a, b). Additionally, superficial punctate keratopathy or subepithelial infiltrates may be seen in the inferior half of the cornea [27]. Ocular symptoms are often accompanied by systemic symptoms such as lymphadenopathy, fever, malaise, and signs of an upper respiratory infection, reflecting the virus's impact beyond the eyes. The course of the disease is generally short, with most cases resolving within 1–2 weeks without any long-term effects. However, rare but serious systemic complications can occur, including radiculomyelitis, muscle dysfunction, and Bells palsy [28, 29].

24.3.2 Togaviridae

Rubella (German Measles) Virus

Acquired rubella primarily affects children and young adults, typically presenting as mild catarrhal or follicular conjunctivitis. Rarely, it may also manifest as bilateral, fine, punctate, central epithelial keratopathy. Both keratitis and conjunctivitis associated with acquired rubella generally resolve within 7 days without long-term effects [30]. Congenital rubella is acquired through maternal fetal transmission of the rubella virus. The presence of constitutional symptoms such as fever, malaise, and lymphadenopathy in the mother during the viremic phase remains a differentiating feature; however, it may not be accompanied by a morbilliform rash [31]. Congenital rubella poses more serious risks and can lead to a variety of ocular and systemic abnormalities. Ocular manifestations of congenital rubella include salt-and-pepper retinopathy, which is a distinctive pattern of pigmentation seen on the retina. Other possible complications include microphthalmos, strabismus, congenital cataracts, transient corneal leukoma, iris atrophy, iris hypoplasia, and glaucoma, all of which can significantly impact vision and overall eye health [32].

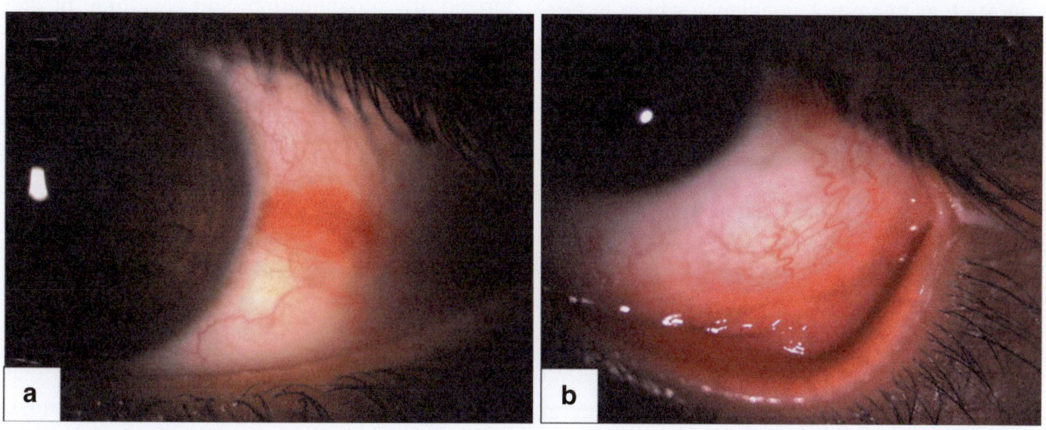

Fig. 24.3 (**a**, **b**) Subconjunctival hemorrhage seen over bulbar conjunctiva with follicles in inferior tarsal conjunctiva in Acute Hemorrhagic Conjunctivitis

24.3.3 Paramyxoviridae

24.3.3.1 Rubeola (Measles)

Rubeola, commonly known as measles, is a highly contagious virus transmitted through inhalation of aerosolized respiratory secretions from an infected individual. Classic symptoms of measles include cough, coryza, Kopliks spots, fever, and a characteristic morbilliform rash. Ocular involvement in measles typically manifests as mild conjunctivitis, subconjunctival hemorrhage, and ocular surface involvement including fine, superficial punctate epithelial erosions and subepithelial infiltrates [32]. Additionally, Koplik's spots may be seen on the caruncle. Patients usually complain of tearing, photophobia, decreased vision, and a recent onset of foreign body sensation. Treatment of conjunctival involvement is symptomatic with complete resolution in 1–2 weeks. However, the keratitis may take a longer time to heal. Culture-guided antimicrobial treatment along with adjuvants should be started at the earliest along with the management of the systemic condition [33, 34].

While there is no specific treatment or cure for measles, immunization remains the most effective prophylaxis against the virus. In developing countries, such as India, measles infections can lead to complications exacerbated by malnutrition, such as vitamin A deficiency which in turn is a significant risk factor for ocular complications, including Keratomalacia with potential secondary infections. Thus, addressing nutritional deficiencies and ensuring vaccination are crucial in preventing the severe outcomes of measles, particularly in vulnerable populations [35, 36].

24.3.3.2 Mumps

Mumps is a contagious viral infection transmitted primarily through the inhalation of airborne secretions. It is well-known for causing bilateral swelling and tenderness of the parotid and other salivary glands [37].

Ocular Involvement

Ocular involvement in mumps is varied but generally mild. The most common ocular manifestation is dacryoadenitis, an inflammation of the lacrimal gland. Patients may also experience mild follicular conjunctivitis, characterized by mild hyperemia (redness) and edema (swelling) of the conjunctiva and eyelids. Corneal involvement is rare in mumps [38]. In addition to these, mumps can lead to more serious ocular conditions such as extraocular muscle palsies, tenonitis, iritis, and scleritis. Secondary infections can also complicate the ocular presentation of mumps, necessitating vigilant monitoring and management to prevent long-term visual impairment [39, 40].

24.3.3.3 Newcastle Disease

Newcastle disease is a highly contagious viral disease primarily affecting birds, but it can occasionally infect humans, particularly those in close contact with infected birds, such as poultry workers. In humans, the disease manifests with a range of symptoms including diarrhea, intestinal hemorrhage, respiratory distress, and nasal and ocular discharge. Complications can include encephalitis and gastroenteritis, indicating a systemic viral impact [41, 42].

Ocular Involvement

Ocular involvement in Newcastle disease typically presents as follicular conjunctivitis, characterized by inflammation and swelling of the conjunctival follicles. Additionally, affected individuals may experience superficial punctate keratitis. Subepithelial infiltrates may also occur, appearing as cloudy areas under the cornea's surface, which can affect vision [43].

24.3.4 Orthomyxoviridae

Influenza

Influenza is an acute respiratory infection that typically causes symptoms like fever, chills, myalgia, and headache, and can lead to complications such as viral or bacterial pneumonia. Ocular manifestations are generally mild, most often presenting as catarrhal conjunctivitis. However, more severe ocular conditions such as keratitis, uveitis, retinal hemorrhages, and optic neuritis can occur, though these are rare. Monitoring for eye symptoms in flu patients is important, especially in severe cases [44, 45].

24.4 Other Rare Viruses Causing Corneal Infections

24.4.1 SARS-CoV-2

COVID-19 and Corneal Infection: COVID-19, caused by the SARS-CoV-2 virus, primarily impacts the respiratory system but can also affect other organs, including the eyes [46]. Ocular manifestations, though less common, can range from mild conjunctivitis (Fig. 24.4) to more severe conditions like keratitis, which involves inflammation of the cornea. Symptoms of corneal involvement may include eye pain, blurred vision, light sensitivity, and a gritty sensation. The virus's entry into ocular tissues is facilitated by ACE2 receptors, leading to potential infection and inflammation. Diagnosis involves PCR testing of ocular swabs and thorough eye examinations, while treatment is supportive, focusing on symptom management and preventing secondary infections with measures like artificial tears, topical antibiotics, and, in severe cases, antiviral medications and corticosteroids [47, 48].

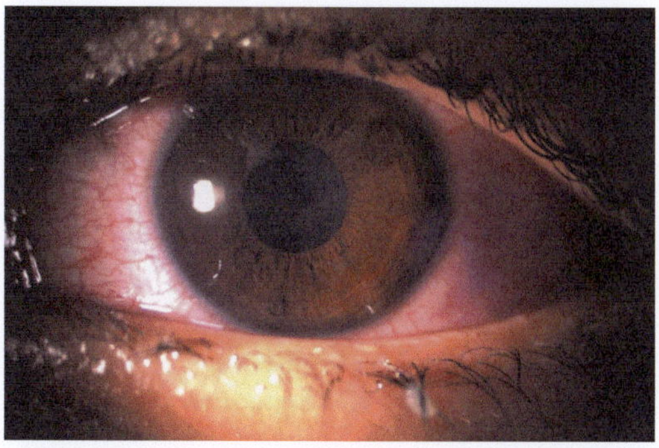

Fig. 24.4 Reactionary conjunctivitis in a patient with COVID-19 infection

24.4.2 Zika Virus and Corneal Infection

The Zika virus, transmitted by Aedes mosquitoes, is known for causing congenital abnormalities, but it can also affect the eyes, including the cornea [49]. Ocular complications such as conjunctivitis, uveitis, and, rarely, corneal infections have been reported. Conjunctivitis is more common, presenting as redness and discomfort, while uveitis can cause pain, redness, and blurred vision. Although direct corneal infections are rare, the virus's presence in ocular tissues can lead to inflammation. Diagnosis involves detecting viral RNA through PCR testing of ocular samples and thorough eye examinations. Treatment is primarily supportive, with anti-inflammatory medications used to manage symptoms, as there is no specific antiviral treatment for Zika virus infections [50].

24.5 Conclusion

Uncommon viral pathogens pose significant challenges in diagnosing and managing corneal infections and can lead to severe ocular complications if not promptly identified and treated. Therefore, healthcare professionals must be vigilant and carefully evaluate the patient's history, systemic features, and pattern of ocular involvement. Continuous research and heightened awareness are essential to enhance understanding and improve the management of these rare yet impactful viral infections affecting the cornea.

Key Points

- Atypical viral infections pose a diagnostic challenge due to their varied clinical presentations, necessitating the use of diverse diagnostic techniques and treatments, including antiviral agents, immunoglobulins, corticosteroids, and supportive care.

- Immunocompromised individuals, including those with AIDS or undergoing immunosuppressive treatments, are at a higher risk for severe and atypical presentations of these viral infections, requiring vigilant monitoring and tailored therapeutic approaches.
- Early detection and appropriate management of these viral infections are essential to prevent severe complications, highlighting the need for healthcare professionals to be aware of uncommon pathogens affecting the cornea.

References

1. Strassburg MA. The global eradication of smallpox. Am J Infect Control. 1982;10(2):53–9. https://doi.org/10.1016/0196-6553(82)90003-7. PMID: 7044193.
2. Drazen JM. Smallpox and bioterrorism. N Engl J Med. 2002;346(17):1262–3.
3. Shchelkunov SN, Shchelkunova GA. We should be prepared to smallpox re-emergence. Vopr Virusol. 2019;64(5):206–14.
4. Centers for Disease Control and Prevention. Smallpox vaccination and adverse reactions: guidance for clinicians. MMWR Recomm Rep. 2003;52(RR-4):1–28.
5. Cono J, Casey CG, Bell DM. Smallpox vaccination and adverse reactions. Morb Mortal Wkly Rep. 2003;52(RR-4):1–28.
6. Rotz LD, Dotson DA, Damon IK, Becher JA; Advisory Committee on Immunization Practices. Vaccinia (smallpox) vaccine: recommendations of the Advisory Committee on Immunization Practices (ACIP), 2001. MMWR Recomm Rep. 2001; 50(RR-10):1–25; quiz CE1-7. PMID: 15580803.
7. Hanna D, Hatami A, Powell J. Surgical treatment of molluscum contagiosum. J Am Acad Dermatol. 2006;55(2):321–7.
8. Zabawski EJ Jr, Cockerell CJ. Topical and intralesional cidofovir: a review of pharmacology and therapeutic effects. J Am Acad Dermatol. 1998;39:741–5.
9. Ding SC. Virology: principles and applications. Yale J Biol Med. 2008;81(3):155–6.
10. Roizman B, Pellett PE. The family Herpesviridae: a brief introduction. In: Knipe DM, Howley PM, editors. Fields virology. 4th ed. Lippincott Williams & Wilkins; 2001. p. 2381–97.
11. Jabs DA. Cytomegalovirus retinitis and the acquired immune deficiency syndrome bench to bedside: LXVII Edward Jackson Memorial Lecture. Am J Ophthalmol. 2011;151(2):198–216.e1.
12. Koizumi N, Inatomi T, Suzuki T, et al. Japan Corneal Endotheliitis Study Group. Clinical features and management of cytomegalovirus corneal endotheliitis: analysis of 106 cases from the Japan corneal endotheliitis study. Br J Ophthalmol. 2015;99(1):54–8.
13. Anshu A, Chee SP, Mehta JS, Tan DT. Cytomegalovirus endotheliitis in Descemet's stripping endothelial keratoplasty. Ophthalmology. 2009;116(4):624–30.
14. Kitazawa K, Jongkhajornpong P, Inatomi T, et al. Topical ganciclovir treatment post-Descemet's stripping automated endothelial keratoplasty for patients with bullous keratopathy induced by cytomegalovirus. Br J Ophthalmol. 2018;102(9):1293–7.
15. Landolfo S, Gariglio M, Gribaudo G, Lembo D. The human cytomegalovirus. Pharmacol Ther. 2003;98(3):269–97.
16. Alfieri C, Tanner J, Carpentier L, Perpate C, Powers A, Ghibu F. Epstein-Barr virus. N Engl J Med. 2015;372:1236–45.
17. Matoba AY, Jones DB. Corneal subepithelial infiltrates associated with systemic Epstein-Barr viral infection. Ophthalmology. 1987;94(12):1669–71.
18. Wilhelmus KR. Ocular involvement in infectious mononucleosis. Am J Ophthalmol. 1981;91(1):117–8.
19. Pinnolis M, McCulley JP, Urman JD. Nummular keratitis associated with infectious mononucleosis. Am J Ophthalmol. 1980;89(6):791–4.
20. Niederer RL, Lightman S. The Epstein-Barr virus and ocular disease. Int Ophthalmol Clin. 2007;47(2):47–63.
21. Rosai J. Ackerman's surgical pathology. 9th ed. St. Louis: Mosby; 1996. p. 1358.
22. Lass JH, Foster CS, Grove AS, et al. Interferon-alpha therapy of recurrent conjunctival papillomas. Am J Ophthalmol. 1987;103(3 Pt 1):294–301.
23. Muralidhar R, Sudan R, Bajaj MS, Sharma V. Topical interferon alpha-2b as an adjunctive therapy in recurrent conjunctival papilloma. Int Ophthalmol. 2009;29(1):61–2.
24. Wolken SH. Acute hemorrhagic conjunctivitis. Surv Ophthalmol. 1974;19:71–84.
25. Yin-Murphy M. Acute hemorrhagic conjunctivitis. Prog Med Virol. 1984;29:23–44. PMID: 6199813.
26. Lin KH, et al. Molecular epidemiology of a variant of coxsackievirus A24 in Taiwan: two epidemics caused by phylogenetically distinct viruses from 1985 to 1989. J Clin Microbiol. 1993;31:1160–6.
27. Christopher S, et al. An epidemic of acute hemorrhagic conjunctivitis due to coxsackievirus A24. J Infect Dis. 1982;146:16–28.
28. Kono R, et al. Neurologic complications associated with acute hemorrhagic conjunctivitis virus infection and its serologic confirmation. J Infect Dis. 1974;129:590–3.
29. Chopra JS, et al. Neurological complications of acute hemorrhagic conjunctivitis. J Neurol Sci. 1986;73:177–91.
30. Smolin G. Report of a case of rubella keratitis. Am J Ophthalmol. 1972;74:436–647.
31. Centers for Disease Control and Prevention (CDC). Rubella and congenital rubella syndrome–United

States, January 1, 1991–May 7, 1994. MMWR: Morb Mortal Wkly Rep. 1994;43(21):391–401.
32. Lambert N, Strebel P, Orenstein W, Icenogle J, Poland GA. Rubella. Lancet. 2015;385(9984):2297–307.
33. Végh M, Hári Kovács A, Roth HW, Facskó A. A kanyaró szemészeti tünetei és kezelése (Ophthalmological symptoms of measles and their treatment). Orv Hetil. 2017;158(39):1523–7.
34. Eddine I, Sana S, Achraf F, Chiraz A, Walid Z. Ocular manifestations of measles in adults: about three cases. J Fr Ophtalmol. 2020;43(5):392–6.
35. Bester JC. Measles and measles vaccination: a review. JAMA Pediatr. 2016;170(12):1209–15.
36. Sommer A, West KP Jr. Vitamin A deficiency: health, survival, and vision. Oxford University Press; 1996.
37. Hviid A, Rubin S, Mühlemann K. Mumps. Lancet. 2008;371(9616):932–44.
38. Pomeroy C, Jordan MC. Mumps. In: Hoeprich PD, Jordan MC, Ronald AR, editors. Infectious diseases: a treatise of infectious processes. 5th ed. Philadelphia: JB Lippincott; 1994.
39. Riffenburgh RS. Ocular manifestations of mumps. Arch Ophthalmol. 1961;66(5):739–43.
40. Sutphin JE. Mumps keratitis. Ophthalmol Clin N Am. 1994;7:557–66.
41. Alexander DJ. Newcastle disease and other avian paramyxoviruses. Rev Sci Tech l'OIE. 2000;19(2):443–62.
42. Beard CW, Hanson RP. Newcastle disease. In: Hofstad MS, editor. Diseases of poultry. 8th ed. Iowa State University Press; 1984. p. 452–70.
43. Hales RH, Ostler HB. Newcastle disease conjunctivitis with subepithelial infiltrates. Br J Ophthalmol. 1973;57:694–7.
44. Fiore AE, Uyeki TM, Broder K, Finelli L, Euler GL, Singleton JA, Iskander JK, Wortley PM, Shay DK, Bresee JS, Cox NJ. Prevention and control of influenza with vaccines: recommendations of the Advisory Committee on Immunization Practices (ACIP), 2010. MMWR Recomm Rep. 2010;59(RR-8):1–62.
45. Fiore AE, et al. Prevention and control of influenza with vaccines: recommendations of the Advisory Committee on Immunization Practices (ACIP). Morb Mortal Wkly Rep. 2010;59(RR-8):1–62.
46. Wu P, Duan F, Luo C, Liu Q, Qu X, Liang L, Wu K. Characteristics of ocular findings of patients with coronavirus disease 2019 (COVID-19) in Hubei Province, China. JAMA Ophthalmol. 2020;138(5):575–8.
47. Cheema M, Aghazadeh H, Nazarali S, Ting A, Hodges J, McFarlane A, Kanji JN, Zelyas N, Damji KF, Solarte C. Keratoconjunctivitis as the initial medical presentation of the novel coronavirus disease 2019 (COVID-19). Can J Ophthalmol. 2020;55(4):e125.
48. Sen M, Honavar SG, Sharma N, Sachdev MS. COVID-19 and eye: a review of ophthalmic manifestations of COVID-19. Indian J Ophthalmol. 2021;69(3):488–509.
49. Marquezan MC, Ventura CV, Sheffield JS, Golden WC, Omiadze R, Belfort R Jr, May W. Ocular effects of Zika virus-a review. Surv Ophthalmol. 2018;63(2):166–73.
50. Ventura CV, Maia M, Bravo-Filho V, Gois AL, Belfort R Jr. Zika virus in Brazil and macular atrophy in a child with microcephaly. Lancet. 2016;387(10015):228.

Corneal Non-infectious Manifestations of Systemic Viral Disorders

25

Saloni Gupta and Sahil Agrawal

Abstract

The cornea, susceptible to various systemic diseases including viral infections, can suffer from direct and immune-mediated effects, often impacting vision significantly if not promptly diagnosed and managed. This chapter describes the various non-infectious manifestations of systemic viral disorders on the cornea, highlighting their clinical presentations, underlying mechanisms and management strategies. Corneal vulnerability to systemic diseases including herpes simplex, varicella-zoster, Epstein-Barr virus (EBV), cytomegalovirus (CMV), human immunodeficiency virus (HIV), Hepatitis C, Hepatitis B, Sars-Covid, adenoviral pharyngoconjunctival fever and measles is elaborated.

Keywords

Viral keratitis · Noninfectious keratitis · Immune keratitis · Corneal opacity · Systemic viral disorder

S. Gupta (✉)
Indian Railway Post Graduate Institute of Medical Sciences and Research, New Delhi, India

S. Agrawal
RP Centre, AIIMS Delhi, New Delhi, India

25.1 Introduction

Cornea is vulnerable to several systemic diseases, including viral infections. They can cause both direct and immune-mediated effects. Non-infectious corneal manifestations have a significant impact on vision if not diagnosed and managed timely. They can also be the first indicator of an and undiagnosed systemic condition [1, 2]. Although, many of them may not be exclusive to a specific disease, they can be diagnosed along with other symptoms. This chapter will discuss clinical presentation, underlying mechanism and management of various non-infectious corneal manifestations associated with systemic viral infection.

25.2 Herpes Simplex

Herpes Simplex is a ubiquitous human pathogen that has strong affinity for neural tissue, often leading to recurrence. Non-infectious, corneal sequelae can largely result from immunologic response and neural damage associated with its episodes. Both cellular and humoral host response may occur and be responsible for pathological sequelae in cornea like immune stromal keratitis, endothelitis.

B. Sharma et al. (eds.), *Viral Keratitis*, https://doi.org/10.1007/978-981-95-3148-6_25

25.2.1 Immune Stromal Keratitis

Immune stromal keratitis is a fairly common chronic recurrent manifestation of HSV. The inflammation is thought to be due to retained viral antigen within the stroma and an antigen-antibody-complement (AAC) cascade. The overlying epithelium is almost always intact while the stromal tissue is damaged with infiltration of immune cells and release of inflammatory cytokines. Immune stromal keratitis may present several days to months after an incident of infectious epithelial keratitis [3, 4].

Clinical Features Patients typically present with symptoms such as blurred vision, photophobia and pain. The deposition of antigen antibody complex may manifest as punctate stromal opacities or as a circular deposition known as the immune ring of Wessely. The ring may be incomplete or complete and is usually seen in mid-stroma of central and paracentral area. Stromal haze due to cellular infiltration and neovascularization may accompany (Fig. 25.1). Persistent and recurrent inflammation may lead to lipid keratopathy, further scarring and vision loss [3, 4].

Management Topical corticosteroids are the mainstay of treatment along with anti-viral cover in the usual dose 4–6 times of Prednisolone 1%; Dexamethasone 0.1%; Loteprednol 0.5% eye drops. The dose of corticosteroid should be adjusted according to the level of inflammation. Also, abrupt discontinuation or rapid tapering should be avoided to prevent rebound inflammation. Oral corticosteroids may be useful in severe cases in the dose of 1 mg/kg body weight [4].

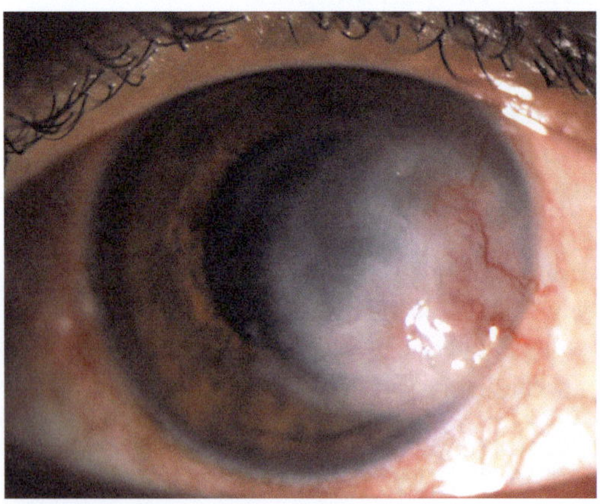

Fig. 25.1 A case of HSV Stromal keratitis, figure showing stromal scarring and neovascularization

25.2.2 Endothelitis

Immune-mediated inflammation at the level of the endothelium remains the main pathologic entity of HSV endothelitis; however, the role of live virus-mediated inflammation has also been speculated as contributing to this clinical entity [5–7].

Clinical Features Patient presents with watering, photophobia, discomfort and blurred vision. Clinically, there is epithelial and stromal oedema along with underlying keratic precipitates and iritis (Fig. 25.2a, b). It can be classified into three forms disciform, diffuse and linear endothelitis based on the shape of overlying oedema and distribution of keratic precipitates. Disciform endothelitis is the most common presentation amongst them. Stromal infiltration and neovascularization are typically absent [5].

Management Topical corticosteroids along with adjunctive treatment of 5% hypertonic saline, cycloplegics and ocular surface lubricants usually result in complete resolution of oedema and inflammation [6, 7].

25.2.3 Neurotropic Keratitis

Neurotropic keratitis can develop in patients with previous HSV epithelial disease. It arises from impaired corneal innervation secondary to HSV induced damage to the corneal nerves. HSV has a predilection for neural tissues, its reactivation can cause direct damage to trigeminal ganglion that disrupts corneal innervation leading to decreased sensation and impaired healing. It may be further exacerbated by chronic use of topical anti-viral treatment [8].

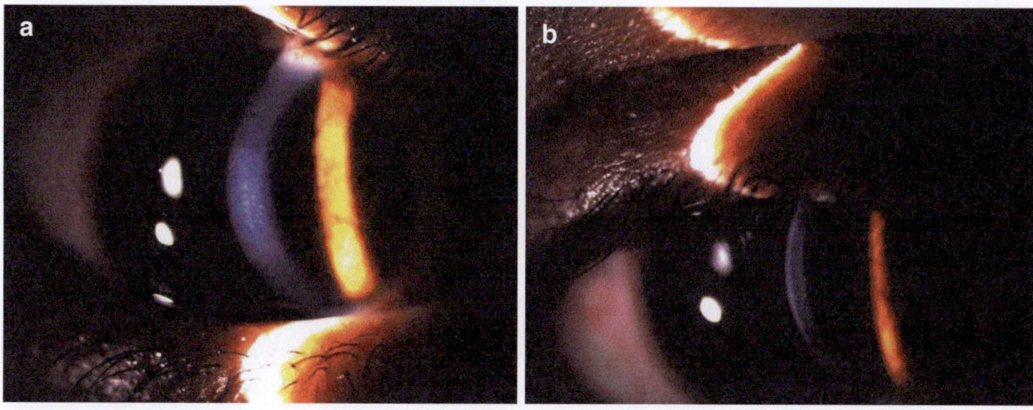

Fig. 25.2 HSV endothelitis showing (**a**) stromal oedema with (**b**) underlying keratic precipitates

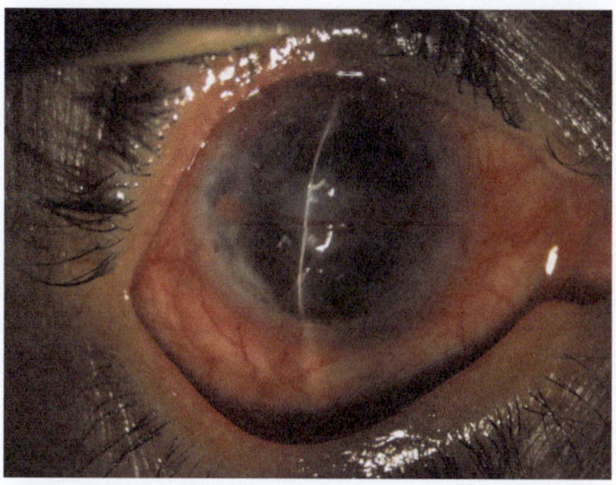

Fig. 25.3 Clinical picture showing HSV neurotrophic keratopathy

Clinical Features Neuropathic keratopathy is initially, characterized by punctate epithelial erosions along with decreased tear secretion. They may then progress to persistent epithelial defect and eventually lead to non-healing, sterile ulceration known as neurotropic ulcer. Clinically neurotropic ulcer is round or oval in shape with smooth borders usually located in central, inferior or inferonasal cornea (Fig. 25.3). The edges appear to be thickened and rolled up due to heaped up epithelium and ulcer bed typically has grey-white appearance. They can be distinguished from geographical ulcers which have scalloped borders with irregular shape and stain with Rose Bengal dye [8].

Management Treatment focuses on promoting epithelial healing and preventing secondary infections. Medical management include frequent use of non-preserved lubricants in the form of drops, gels and ointments. Discontinuation of all unnecessary topical medications should be done. Additional treatment options in severe cases to prevent progression include bandage contact lens, amniotic membrane application or surgical tarsorrhaphy. When left untreated or mistreated it may lead to progressive stromal scarring, perforation and necrosis [8].

25.3 Varicella Zoster

Varicella zoster virus can cause disease either through a primary infection or by reactivation of a dormant virus residing in a sensory nerve ganglion. Among patients diagnosed with herpes Zoster, about 8–20% are complicated by Herpes Zoster Ophthalmicus. Patients with HZO present with prodromal unilateral pain along V1 dermatomal distribution [9]. Besides direct viral invasion, corneal involvement can also occur due to immune response virus.

Clinical Features In acute phase of involvement, disease may present as nummular lesions in anterior stroma. Later in disease course, deep stromal keratitis may occur in the form of disciform keratitis. Similar to HSV, clinically it presents with stromal oedema with overlying intact epithelium. It may also be associated with immune ring in central or paracentral cornea [9] (Fig. 25.4).

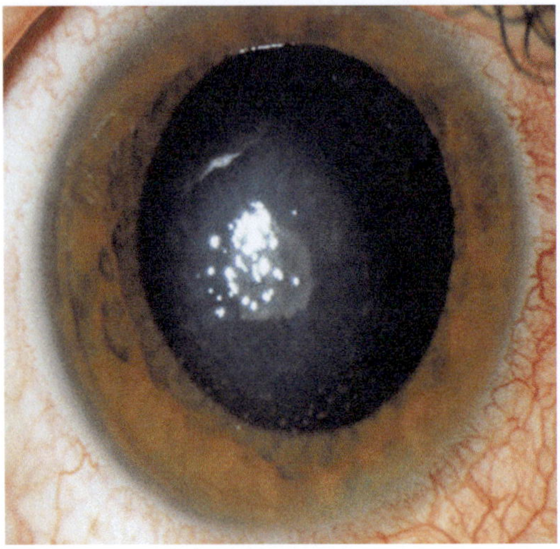

Fig. 25.4 Showing sectoral corneal oedema with enothelial keratic precipitates and mild anterior chamber inflammation in HZO endothelitis

Decreased corneal sensitivity due to persistent inflammation can cause neurotropic keratopathy. It starts with mild punctate epithelial erosions and may finally develop into horizontal oval defects which stromal ulcers. Chronic stromal inflammation can cause corneal scarring, vascularization and lipid deposition [10].

Management Systemic Acyclovir 800 mg 5 times, Valacyclovir 1000 mg twice and Famciclovir 500 mg twice daily are the available treatment options. Topical corticosteroids in tapering doses are beneficial in decreasing the inflammation and immune reaction in stromal keratitis. However, they should be used once the active viral disease is controlled [9, 10].

25.4 Epstein Bar Virus

Epstein-Barr virus, a member of herpes family, is a ubiquitous virus. Primary EBV infection may affect during childhood and is mainly asymptomatic. If acquired later in life, it can cause the classical symptoms of Infectious Mononucleosis syndrome [11].

Pathophysiology Epstein-Barr virus antigens may generate immune response in the host and lead to the formation of immune complexes which get deposited in cornea. These may cause inflammation and sub epithelial infiltrates [12].

Clinical Features Acute phase is associated with stromal oedema and neovascularization followed by corneal scarring and thinning in chronic phase. Besides, these typical patterns, they may present in other distinct forms [11, 12].

1. Sharply, demarcated, multifocal or ring-shaped, granular, anterior stromal opacities within normal intervening stroma.
2. Peripheral cornea is mainly involved with soft pleomorphic infiltrates.

Management Treatment of choice in EBV-related stromal keratitis is topical steroids either Prednisolone 1% or Dexamethasone 0.1% to reduce stromal inflammation and thus reduce scarring [12].

25.5 Cytomegalovirus

Cytomegalovirus, another member of herpes family, is an important cause of corneal endothelitis especially in immunocompromised patients [13]. CMV endothelitis is an inflammation specific to corneal endothelium triggered by CMV [13].

Clinical Features Patients usually complain of photophobia and visual disturbances. Presentation may vary from focal endothelitis to diffuse bullous keratopathy. It is characterized by presence of endothelial cell loss, keratic precipitates with overlying corneal oedema, mild anterior chamber inflammation and increase in intraocular pressure (Fig. 25.5). Coin-shaped or disc-shaped keratic precipitates are frequently observed. Based on the pattern of keratic pre-

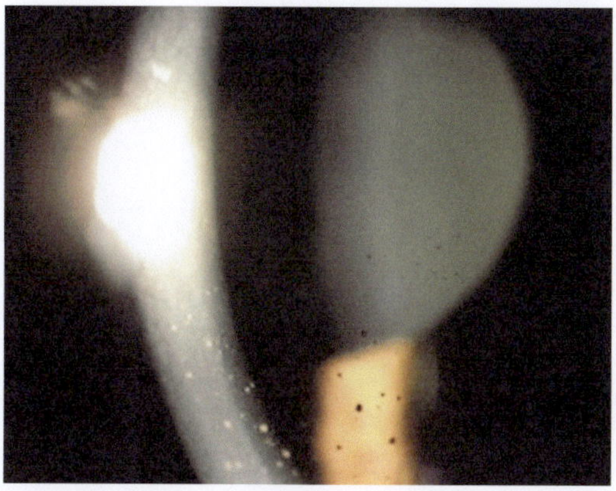

Fig. 25.5 Demonstrating keratic precipitates with overlying oedema in a case of CMV endothelitis

cipitates and overlying stromal oedema, it can be divided into four types, namely, linear, sectoral, disciform and diffuse [14].

Management Besides, clinical suspicion, laboratory confirmation is usually established by PCR testing in aqueous fluid. PCR testing for CMV, HSV and VZV can be useful in guiding for further treatment. Non-invasive imaging tests like confocal microscopy and Anterior segment OCT can also assist in diagnosis and monitoring of disease progression. Different patterns can be demonstrated in ASOCT depending on the causative organism. Kobayasi et al. demonstrated a sawtooth appearance of protruding structures and high reflectivity of posterior cornea in CMV endothelitis [15].

Japan Endotheliitis study group reported that combined systemic and topical therapy appeared to be more effective in reducing KPs and corneal oedema [16]. After treatment, a considerable portion of patients (36%) experienced a recurrence and needed to be placed back on therapy. The study also reported that 5.8% of patients did not respond to any treatment, signifying that severe corneal endothelial damage in CMV endotheliitis may be irreversible even with antiviral treatment.

Treatment is mainly aimed at controlling both the infectious and inflammatory components with topical/systemic antivirals; topical corticosteroids and anti-glaucoma medication if required. Apply topical 0.15% ganciclovir gel five times daily, gradually tapering to a prophylactic dose of three times daily. Administer oral valganciclovir 900 mg twice daily, reducing to a prophylactic dose of 900 mg once daily for at least three months after clinical resolution. In cases with inadequate response or high viral CMV load, Foscarnet 60 mg/kg TID or Cidofovir can be considered with timely evaluation of liver and kidney functions.

Topical steroids are used to reduce the inflammation usually combined with anti-CMV regimen. Prednisolone 1% or Dexamethasone 0.3% in dosing schedule of 4–6 times daily remains the usual dosing schedule [13, 14].

25.6 HIV

Human immune deficiency virus is a retro virus manifesting as a multisystem disease, AIDS.

In HIV patients, the majority of ocular complications result from opportunistic infections, most commonly caused by HSV, VZV, and CMV [17].

Though majority of the corneal manifestations of HIV are in infectious category, non-infective inflammatory involvement should also be kept in mind. They include keratoconjunctivitis sicca (KCS), peripheral ulcerative keratitis (Fig. 25.6) and squamous cell carcinoma of the conjunctiva that may involve cornea [17].

KCS Approximately 20% of HIV patients develop KCS or severe dry eye disease. It occurs due to HIV-mediated inflammatory destruction of accessory and main lacrimal glands. Management of keratoconjunctivitis sicca include frequent use of non-preserved lubricating drops and anti-inflammatory drugs. Carboxymethylcellulose, dextran, glycerin, hypomellose, polyethylene glycol 400 (PEG 400), polysorbate, polyvinyl alcohol, povidone or propylene glycol are the common preparations,

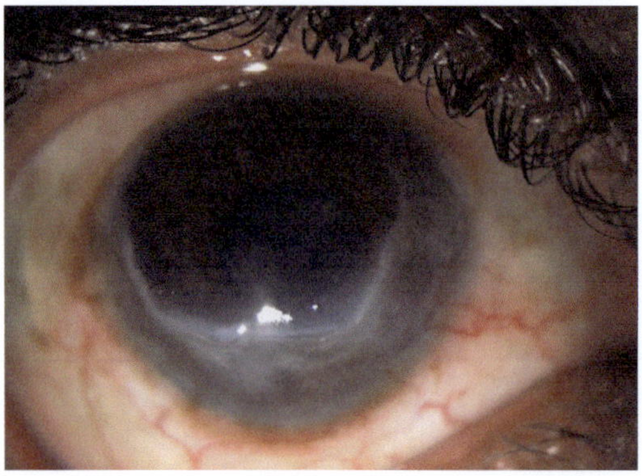

Fig. 25.6 Slit-lamp photograph displaying peripheral corneal thinning, surrounding neovascularization, and inflammatory infiltrates in HIV-related peripheral ulcerative keratitis

among others, that can be used in frequent dosing schedule.

Keratitis It is rare and may present as punctate epithelial keratitis, neurotropic keratopathy or PUK. Neurotropic keratitis can cause epithelial defects and corneal ulceration due to impaired corneal healing. Though rare, PUK may be the initial manifestation in a patient with asymptomatic human immunodeficiency virus (HIV) infection, due to increased predisposition to other infective conditions, which themselves may be associated with PUK or chronic HIV infection-induced high levels of circulating immune complexes which can precipitate in the peripheral cornea, initiate an inflammatory cascade and consequent keratolysis. Treatment of keratitis is done depending upon the involved microbial infection, sensitivity pattern and structural involvement [17]. Moreover, some medications used in ART, especially protease inhibitors, have been associated with keratopathy that can manifest as corneal epithelial microcysts, stromal deposits or endothelial changes affecting vision [17].

25.7 Hepatitis C

Hepatitis C Virus is an important cause of both hepatic and extrahepatic Sequalae.

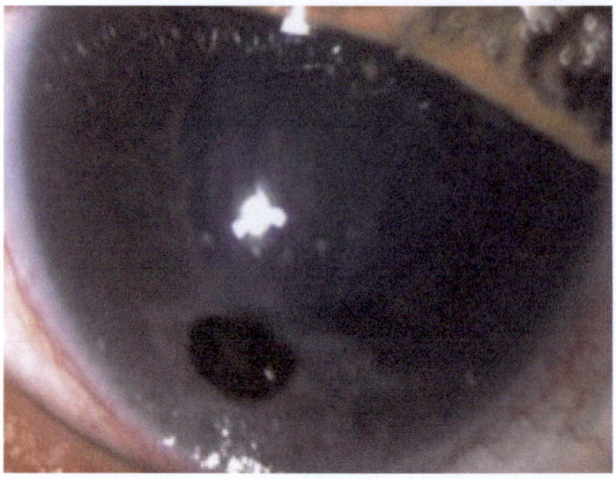

Fig. 25.7 Slit-lamp photograph illustrating HCV-associated severe keratoconjunctival sicca

Pathophysiology It has been associated with many ocular pathologies which may be due to direct invasion of virus or immunological reaction to certain viral antigens and even immune complex deposition causing inflammation [18].

Clinical Features Keratoconjunctivitis Sicca is the most common ocular finding of Chronic Hep C Virus infection (Fig. 25.7). It can result from HCV-induced inflammation of lacrimal gland. It usually improves with topical lubricants [18].

Infection with HCV has also been associated with Moorens ulcer. It is a chronic relentlessly progressive peripheral ulcerative keratitis (PUK) (Fig. 25.8). The main pathophysiology of the disease is autoimmune causing chronic systemic inflammation and Mixed Cryoglobulinemia, characterized by deposition of insoluble immune complexes in small and medium blood vessels causing vasculitis. More than half of the patients with PUK and Hepatitis C have associated Mixed Cryoglobulinemia. Thus, in all patients presenting with inflammatory peripheral keratitis without systemic rheumatological disease it is important to screen for HCV [18, 19]. Patients present with pain, photophobia and peripheral corneal ulceration [18, 19].

Management The treatment for Moorens ulcer involves topical or oral corticosteroids or topical cyclosporine 1–2%. Stronger immunosuppressive agents can be used in severe disease or in

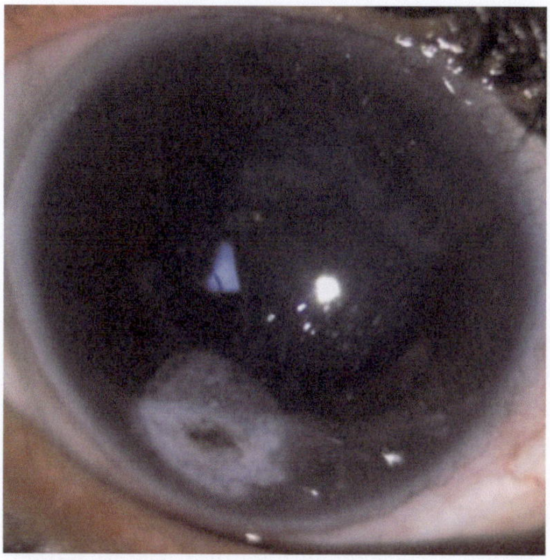

Fig. 25.8 Clinical photograph showing crescent-shaped peripheral corneal thinning, adjacent stromal infiltration, and neovascularization in HCV peripheral ulcerative keratitis

progression. Immunosuppressive agent interferon alpha b2b given subcutaneously is effective as it helps to reduce systemic inflammation. In severe cases, surgical procedures like conjunctival resection, Amniotic membrane transplant may help to promote healing and prevent complications [18, 19]. Other surgical options include keratoplasty, keratoepithelioplasty, delimiting keratotomy, and conjunctival flap and patch grafts.

25.8 Hepatitis B

Hepatitis B can cause potentially life-threatening hepatitis and is a major cause of morbidity and mortality throughout the world.

Pathophysiology One of the most common extrahepatic manifestations is Sjogren like syndrome which mainly causes aqueous tear deficient dry eye. It is postulated to be an autoimmune-mediated local lymphocytic infiltration that affects function of lacrimal glands [20, 21].

Similar to Hepatitis C, Hepatitis B has also been associated with PUK due to direct vessel inflammation or hepatitis-associated cryoglobulinemia. However, it is more commonly observed with Hepatitis C [22, 23].

Management Management mainly involves treating the underlying Hepatitis B infection along with specific intervention for ocular manifestations like lubricants, topical and systemic anti-inflammatory drugs and immunosuppressive therapy [21–23].

25.9 Adenoviral Pharyngoconjunctival Fever

Adenoviral PCF is most commonly found in children and is usually caused by adenovirus serotype 3, but has also been associated with types 1, 4, 5, 6, 7 and 14. Patient usually presents with fever lasting for about 10 days along with pharyngitis and tender pre-auricular lymphadenopathy [24].

Clinical Features On corneal examination, superficial punctate keratitis (SPK) and subepithelial infiltrates may be commonly present and are caused by immune-mediated responses to the viral antigens. Subepithelial infiltrates usually appear as grey-white lesions beneath the corneal surface (Fig. 25.9). These lesions are accumulation of lymphocytes, macrophages/monocytes, and activated fibroblasts in reaction to adenoviral-infected corneal keratocytes and is a key characteristic. These corneal opacities can last from a few weeks to a few years and can lead to reduced vision, glare, sensitivity to light and irregular astigmatism. Inflammatory response triggered by adenoviral infection can also lead to corneal oedema and corneal opacities in case of intense inflammation [24].

Management Treatment typically involves supportive care, such as lubricating eye drops, cold

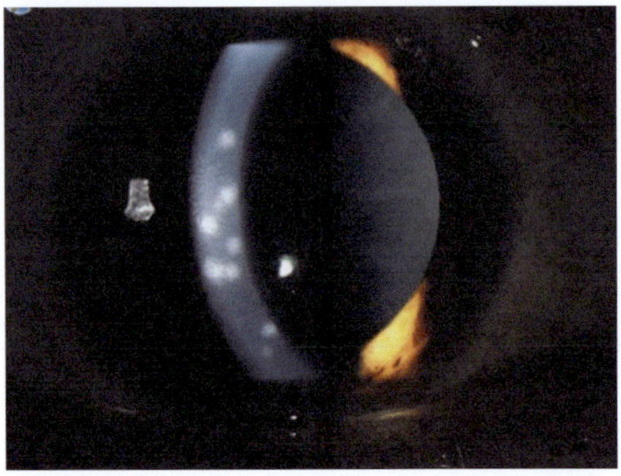

Fig. 25.9 A case of adenoviral keratitis demonstrating discrete sub-epithelial and stromal opacities

compresses and sometimes topical steroids to reduce inflammation and manage symptoms [24].

25.10 SARS COVID

December 2019 saw the start of COVID-19 developing into a global pandemic caused by the highly transmissible SARS-CoV-2. Conjunctivitis and keratoconjunctivitis were the most prevalent ocular symptoms in adults. They may be the presenting finding or develop several weeks after recovery [25, 26].

Pathophysiology They can result from direct effect of virus, immune-mediated tissue damage, and activation of the coagulation cascade. The infection or its comorbidities and medications used in its treatment can induce prothrombotic state and cause ocular manifestations [25].

Interstitial Keratitis Besides direct invasion, immune-mediated tissue damage and inflammation can also affect cornea. Though rare, interstitial keratitis and acute corneal graft rejection have also been reported after both COVID-19 infection and its vaccination, as its pathophysiology involves systemic immune responses, with massive production of inflammatory mediators. Interstitial keratitis involves chronic and non-ulcerative inflammation of the corneal stroma usually without epithelial or endothelial involvement. It may be associated with neovascularization and also lead to corneal scarring and decreased vision. Corticosteroids are the treatment of choice [27, 28].

25.11 Measles

Ocular manifestations of Rubeola are predominantly limited to conjunctive and cornea. It may cause disturbances of vitamin A metabolism and absorption [29].

Clinical Features This reduced availability of vitamin A and malnutrition may lead to xerophthalmia, corneal ulceration and vitamin A-dependent keratomalacia. Chronic and severe deficiency of vitamin A may cause punctate keratitis, oedema and vascularization. Keratomalacia may cause acute liquefactive necrosis of the cornea [30, 31].

Management Treatment requires supplementation with systematic vitamin to halt the progression of corneal melting [30, 31].

25.12 Conclusion

The cornea can be affected by a myriad of systemic viral afflictions with bearings on visual acuity. Amongst the various viral etiologies implicated with non-infectious afflictions of the cornea, Herpes simplex virus, Cytomegalovirus, and Epstein-Barr virus continue to be the most prominent ones with the occasional afflictions of hepatitis C, HIV and adenovirus amongst other rarer causes. The recent pandemic of COVID-19 has also reported the involvement of corneal tissue.

Key Points

1. Ocular manifestations of systemic viral infections can range from non-specific involvement to corneal manifestations of disciform keratitis; neurotrophic keratitis; stromal keratitis or PUK.

2. Awareness of the possible associations of ocular diseases with systemic viral diseases is important to ask relevant history, look for specific clinical signs, advice appropriate investigations to diagnose and initiate early treatment for life and vision-threatening complications.
3. Besides clinical diagnosis, diagnostic testing for viral infections may include blood testing or nose and throat sample for serologic studies and viral detection.
4. HIV or other immunocompromising conditions may simultaneously have more than one active secondary infection and thus have signs that are atypical.
5. Timely diagnosis and management with corticosteroids are usually required in non-infectious corneal manifestations of systemic viral diseases to decrease inflammation and prevent long-term ocular morbidity.

References

1. Darougar S, Hunter PA, Viswalingam M, et al. Acute follicular conjunctivitis and keratoconjunctivitis due to herpes simplex virus in London. Br J Ophthalmol. 1978;62:843–9. https://doi.org/10.1136/bjo.62.12.843.
2. Darougar S, Wishart MS, Viswalingam ND. Epidemiological and clinical features of primary herpes simplex virus ocular infection. Br J Ophthalmol. 1985;69:2–6. https://doi.org/10.1136/bjo.69.1.2.
3. Wishart MS, Darougar S, Viswalingam ND. Recurrent herpes simplex virus ocular infection: epidemiological and clinical features. Br J Ophthalmol. 1987;71:669–72. https://doi.org/10.1136/bjo.71.9.669.
4. Wilhelmus KR. Diagnosis and management of herpes simplex stromal keratitis. Cornea. 1987;6:286–91. https://doi.org/10.1097/00003226-198706040-00011.
5. Vannas A, Ahonen R, Mäkitie J. Corneal endothelium in herpetic keratouveitis. Arch Ophthalmol. 1983;101:913–5. https://doi.org/10.1001/archopht.1983.01040010913011.
6. Kaufman HE, Kanai A, Ellison ED. Herpetic iritis: demonstration of virus in the anterior chamber by fluorescent antibody techniques and electron microscopy. Am J Ophthalmol. 1971;71:465–9. https://doi.org/10.1016/0002-9394(71)90119-x.
7. Olsen TW, Hardten DR, Meiusi RS, et al. Linear endotheliitis. Am J Ophthalmol. 1994;117:468–74. https://doi.org/10.1016/s0002-9394(14)70006-6.
8. Liesegang TJ. Corneal complications from herpes zoster ophthalmicus. Ophthalmology. 1985;92:316–24. https://doi.org/10.1016/s0161-6420(85)34034-4.
9. Mackie IA. Role of the corneal nerves in destructive disease of the cornea. Trans Ophthalmol Soc UK. 1962;1978(98):343–7.
10. Yu DD, Lemp MA, Mathers WD, et al. Detection of varicella-zoster virus DNA in disciform keratitis using polymerase chain reaction. Arch Ophthalmol. 1993;111:167–8. https://doi.org/10.1001/archopht.1993.01090020021010.
11. Matoba AY, Jones DB. Corneal subepithelial infiltrates associated with systemic Epstein-Barr viral infection. Ophthalmology. 1987;94:1669–71. https://doi.org/10.1016/s0161-6420(87)33260-9.
12. Wilhelmus KR. Ocular involvement in infectious mononucleosis. Am J Ophthalmol. 1981;91:117–8. https://doi.org/10.1016/0002-9394(81)90358-5.
13. Garau J, Kabins S, DeNosaquo S, et al. Spontaneous cytomegalovirus mononucleosis with conjunctivitis. Arch Intern Med. 1977;137:1631–2.
14. Wilhelmus KR, Font RL, Lehmann RP, et al. Cytomegalovirus keratitis in acquired immunodeficiency syndrome. Arch Ophthalmol. 1996;114:869–72. https://doi.org/10.1001/archopht.1996.01100140083016.
15. Kobayashi R, Hashida N, Soma T, et al. Clinical findings of anterior segment spectral domain optical coherence tomography images in cytomegalovirus corneal endotheliitis. Cornea. 2017;36:411–4. https://doi.org/10.1097/ICO.0000000000001103.
16. Koizumi N, Inatomi T, Suzuki T, et al. Clinical features and management of cytomegalovirus corneal endotheliitis: analysis of 106 cases from the Japan corneal endotheliitis study. Br J Ophthalmol. 2015;99:54–8. https://doi.org/10.1136/bjophthalmol-2013-304625.
17. Shah R, Amador C, Tormanen K, et al. Systemic diseases and the cornea. Exp Eye Res. 2021;204:108455. https://doi.org/10.1016/j.exer.2021.108455.
18. Jain AK, Sukhija J, Saini JS, et al. Hepatitis C virus-associated keratitis. Eye (Lond). 2004;18:131–4. https://doi.org/10.1038/sj.eye.6700604.
19. Li S, Li A, Ruan F, et al. Evaluation of the clinical characteristics of dry eye secondary to different types of liver diseases. Ophthalmol Ther. 2023;12:2493–503. https://doi.org/10.1007/s40123-023-00747-4.
20. Cuşnir V, Slepova O, Dumbravă V, et al. Ocular manifestations of hepatitis B. Oftalmologia. 1997;41:25–7.
21. Guvenir M, Arikan A. Hepatitis B virus: from diagnosis to treatment. Pol J Microbiol. 2020;69:391–9. https://doi.org/10.33073/pjm-2020-044.
22. Hassanpour K, H ElSheikh R, Arabi A, et al. Peripheral ulcerative keratitis: a review. J Ophthalmic Vis Res. 2022;17:252–75. https://doi.org/10.18502/jovr.v17i2.10797.
23. Höllhumer R. Peripheral ulcerative keratitis: a review of aetiology and management. Afr Vision Eye Health. 2022;81:697. https://doi.org/10.4102/aveh.v81i1.697.

24. Chigbu DI, Labib BA. Pathogenesis and management of adenoviral keratoconjunctivitis. Infect Drug Resist. 2018;11:981–93. https://doi.org/10.2147/IDR.S162669.
25. Oren B, Kocabas DO. Assessment of corneal endothelial cell morphology and anterior segment parameters in COVID-19. Ther Adv Ophthalmol. 2022;14:25158414221096057. https://doi.org/10.1177/25158414221096057.
26. Sarkar D, Soni D, Nagpal A, et al. Ocular manifestations of RT-PCR-confirmed COVID-19 cases in a large database cross-sectional study. BMJ Open Ophthalmol. 2021;6:e000775. https://doi.org/10.1136/bmjophth-2021-000775.
27. Khan TA, Sidhu N, Khan L, et al. Bilateral immune-mediated keratolysis after immunization with SARS-CoV-2 recombinant viral vector vaccine. Cornea. 2021;40:1629–32. https://doi.org/10.1097/ICO.0000000000002844.
28. Douglas KAA, Douglas VP, Moschos MM. Ocular manifestations of COVID-19 (SARS-CoV-2): a critical review of current literature. In Vivo. 2020;34:1619–28. https://doi.org/10.21873/invivo.11952.
29. Bonamour G. Role of the cornea in cutaneous eruptions of the face in infectious eruptive diseases in childhood; measles and scarlet fever. Bull Soc Ophtalmol Fr. 1953;3:258–61.
30. Guad F. Ocular complications of eruptive infectious diseases of children. Arch Ophtalmol Rev Gen Ophtalmol. 1958;18:25–56.
31. Kayikçioglu O, Kir E, Söyler M, et al. Ocular findings in a measles epidemic among young adults. Ocul Immunol Inflamm. 2000;8:59–62. https://doi.org/10.1076/0927-3948(200003)811-sft059.

Section V

Surgical Interventions

Decision-Making in Corneal Transplantation

26

Radhika Natarajan and Madhuvanthi Mohan

Abstract

Keratoplasty following healed Herpes simplex viral (HSV) keratitis presents sizeable challenges at various stages, namely diagnosis, decision between medical and surgical treatment, preoperative assessment, intraoperative management, and postoperative care. This chapter details an overview of the key considerations in such cases, detailing both common and atypical features of HSV keratitis and their impact on surgical decision-making. It discusses the clinical examination, relevant investigations, indications for keratoplasty, and the intraoperative challenges that may arise, along with strategies to manage them effectively. Additionally, it outlines a structured approach to preoperative and postoperative care for high-risk grafts, emphasizing the importance of careful planning and execution to improve outcomes. By addressing these aspects, it aims to provide a comprehensive guide for corneal transplantation in patients with healed HSV keratitis.

Keywords

Herpes keratitis · HSV · Keratoplasty

26.1 Introduction

Keratoplasty after healed Herpes simplex viral (HSV) keratitis poses a challenge to corneal surgeons due to difficulties arising preoperatively, intraoperatively and postoperatively. HSV keratitis predisposes the corneal graft to a higher likelihood of rejection and failure [1]. Corneal surgeons are faced with a distinct set of challenges ranging from accurately diagnosing HSV infection and its sequelae to deciding the optimal timing for keratoplasty and managing the postoperative complications.

This chapter will examine the typical and atypical features of HSV keratitis in relation to preoperative diagnosis, the criteria for deciding when keratoplasty is indicated, intraoperative problems and their management and approach of these high-risk grafts postoperatively. By following structured approaches, decision-making before corneal transplantation in HSV grafts can become more systematic, thereby improving surgical and postoperative outcomes.

R. Natarajan (✉)
Department of Cornea and Refractive Surgery, Sankara Nethralaya, Medical Research Foundation, Chennai, Tamil Nadu, India

M. Mohan
Cornea & Refractive Services, Rajan Eye Care Hospital, Chennai, Tamil Nadu, India

B. Sharma et al. (eds.), *Viral Keratitis*, https://doi.org/10.1007/978-981-95-3148-6_26

26.2 Clinical Diagnosis

26.2.1 Diagnostic Confirmation

When making pre-surgical decisions for a patient with HSV keratitis, accurate diagnosis is essential due to the high recurrence rate and potential for severe complications.

The diagnosis of HSV keratitis is largely clinical in the early stage. Accurate diagnosis is critical due to its high recurrence rate, may require antiviral cover and grafts for HSV keratitis are considered high-risk making their diagnosis even more crucial. HSV keratitis can present as epithelial keratitis (Fig. 26.1), stromal immune keratitis (Fig. 26.2) and endothelitis (Fig. 26.3). Healing results in vascularisation or presence of ghost vessels,degeneration of corneal nerves, decreased corneal sensations and scarring [2].

As grafts for HSV keratitis are considered high-risk [3], the surgeon must be prepared to address both the infectious aspects of the condition and the risk of graft rejection or failure. The different forms of HSV keratitis, such as epithelial, stromal, and endotheliitis, each pose unique challenges to corneal healing. Stromal inflammation, immune responses, and the potential for corneal thinning or neovascularisation can complicate graft outcomes. Therefore, understanding the specific type of keratitis and its impact on the cornea is vital for determining the appropriate treatment strategy and anticipating possible complications during and after surgery.

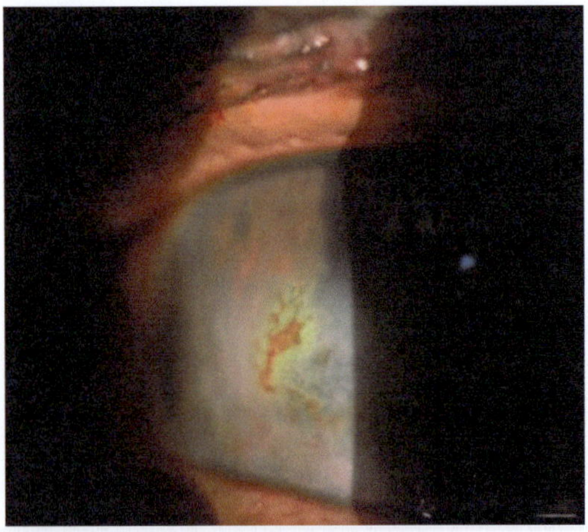

Fig. 26.1 Slit-lamp photo of viral dendritic keratitis

26.2.2 Need for Further Investigation

Though diagnosis of primary and recurrent ocular HSV infection primarily relies on a thorough clinical evaluation, viral culture can provide a definitive diagnosis when done early and in suspicious cases. Traditional viral culture may take up to a week for the results, but rapid assays like enzyme-linked or shell vial cultures offer similar sensitivity in just 24 hours. Polymerase chain reaction (PCR), while more sensitive and specific, requires specialised equipment and is therefore less accessible as it requires special equipment and a skilled technician. Cytologic methods using Giemsa or Wright stains can pro-

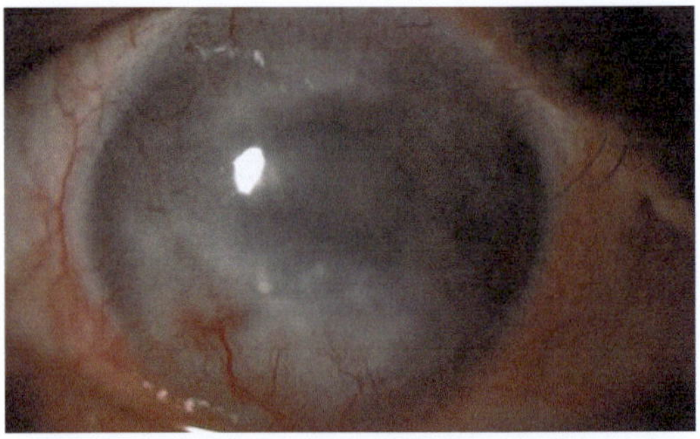

Fig. 26.2 Diffuse slit-lamp photo of stromal immune keratitis with vascularisation

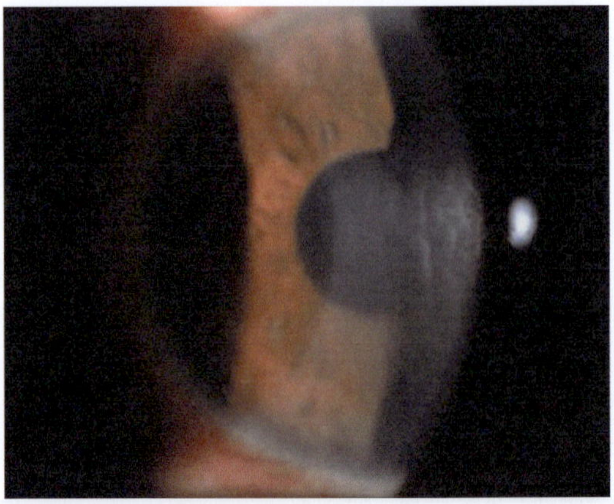

Fig. 26.3 Slit image of viral endothelitis

vide clues by identifying multinucleated giant cells and intranuclear inclusions, though these findings are not specific to HSV. Immunologic tests like Herpchek can offer quicker results, but studies have mentioned that clinical examination is equally effective [4]. Other diagnostic tools include electron microscopy to directly view herpes virions, DNA hybridisation techniques using HSV nucleic acid probes and testing of serum antibody titres.

26.2.3 Evaluating and Diagnosing Quiescence

The eye must remain quiet at least for 6 months before surgery in patients with healed HSV keratitis. What may seem like a straightforward scar with vascularisation could conceal deeper issues or even a dendrite, which can be detected through fluorescein staining (Fig. 26.4). Any signs of inflammation in the eye indicate that it is not yet quiet.

26.2.4 Atypical Presentations

In some cases, healed HSV keratitis presents with atypical features, for example, steel wool keratopathy [5] (Fig. 26.5). These refer to greyish-white metallic deposits in individual or multifocal areas with a feathery pattern and a polychromatic sheen.

If scarred lesions are peripheral, they are more suggestive of healed autoimmune disease, whereas central involvement (Fig. 26.6) indicates a higher likelihood of healed HSV keratitis which has to be recognised preoperatively. The presence of nummular corneal scars in the fellow eye can point towards adenoviral keratitis [6] (Fig. 26.7).

One of the most common differentials of active HSV marginal keratitis is Staphylococcal marginal keratitis. Staphylococcal marginal keratitis usually has an associated dry blepharitis with mild perilimbal immune infiltrate, whereas HSV marginal ulcer is a primary infectious disease characterised by active viral replication [7, 8].

Presence of lid inflammation and discharge is usually indicative of HSV rather than staphylococcal immune disease [9, 10]. HSV blepharitis can be diagnosed based on its characteristic clinical presentation, including a recurrent focal vesicular lesion, and confirmed through viral culture.

It is important to distinguish between these two as the treatment differs significantly. If left untreated, HSV marginal ulcers tend to progress

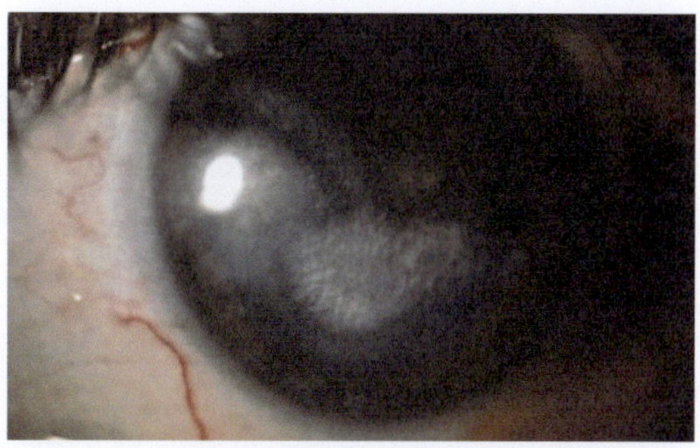

Fig. 26.5 Appearance of 'steel wool keratopathy' on the cornea

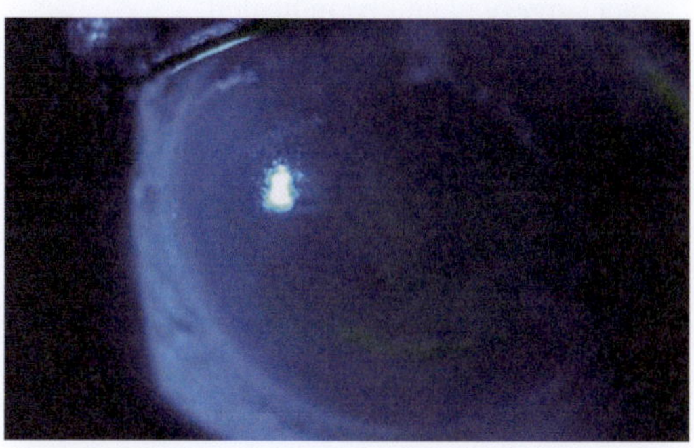

Fig. 26.4 Slit-lamp image of a quiet eye showing a dendrite on fluorescein staining

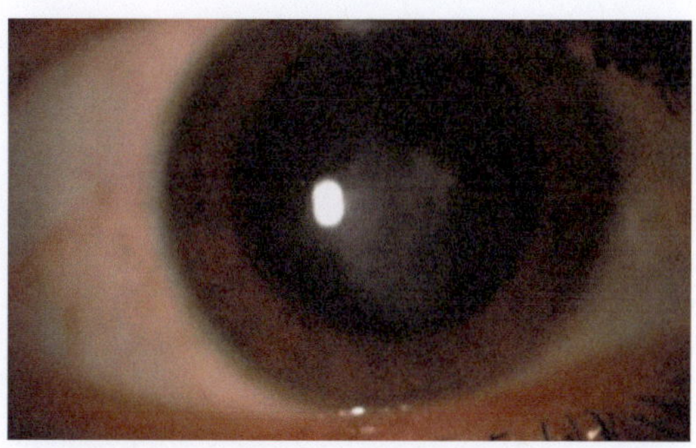

Fig. 26.6 Diffuse slit-lamp image of central healed HSV keratitis

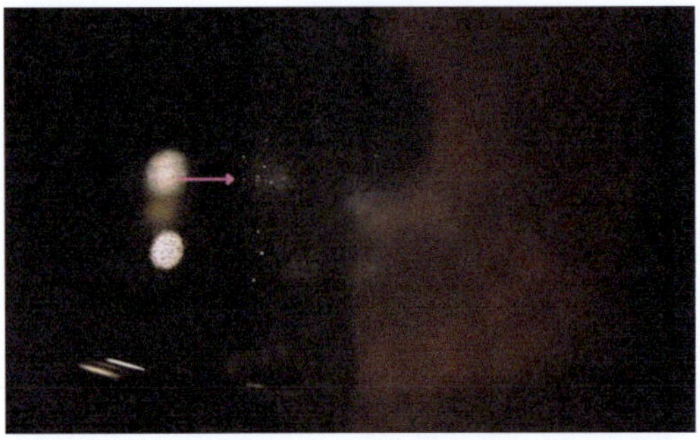

Fig. 26.7 Nummular scars (marked by pink arrow) suggestive of post-adenoviral keratitis

centrally, whereas staphylococcal marginal infiltrates typically spread circumferentially without central involvement. If treated improperly with topical antibiotics, and particularly with topical corticosteroids in the absence of antivirals, the lesion may progress centrally, leading to ulceration and subepithelial infiltration. This central progression often manifests with a dendritic pattern, which is a hallmark feature aiding in accurate diagnosis. Steroids are usually the first line management for staphylococcal immune disease which suppresses the immune reaction whereas use of steroids can exacerbate HSV blepharoconjunctivitis where the mainstay of treatment is antiviral agents [11].

Herpetic scars can cause irregularity and dry eye and in cases where there is sub-tarsal fibrosis in dry eyes, it appears to mimic cicatrizing diseases and presence of the quite rare herpetic sclerokeratitis can also be seen in patients.

26.3 Surgical Considerations: When Is Keratoplasty Required?

Scarring sequelae in HSV keratitis is a potentially sight-threatening complication. These scars can vary from faint, grey-white subepithelial opacities to dense stromal scars associated with corneal thinning and significant vision loss [12]. They are best observed during slit-lamp examination using diffuse or broad, oblique illumination.

Table 26.1 Summary of preoperative considerations of herpetic scars

Type of scarring	Identification feature	Management
Faint post-herpetic scars	Superficial dendritic scars that do not impair vision	No keratoplasty needed; cataract surgery indicated if cataract is present
Moderate scarring	Diffuse nebulomacular scarring with visible iris and pupil, causing glare and distortion but reasonable vision.	PROSE lenses recommended to improve vision and reduce discomfort; surgery avoided
Severe scarring with vascularisation	Severe stromal necrosis or scarring with vascularisation	Keratoplasty required; Fine Needle Diathermy (FND) may be performed before surgery to regress vasculature

One of the major decisions in managing post-herpetic eye disease is determining whether keratoplasty is necessary. This decision depends on several factors (Table 26.1):

1. *Faint Post-Herpetic Scars*: In cases where the post-herpetic scar is faint (Fig. 26.8) such as a scarred superficial dendrite and does not impair vision, keratoplasty is usually not necessary. However, if the patient presents with a cataract in conjunction with a faint scar, cataract surgery would be indicated.
2. *Moderate Scarring*: Diffuse nebulomacular scarring with the iris and pupil architecture still clearly seen (Fig. 26.9a, b) constitutes moderate scarring. When this causes significant glare and distortion but reasonable vision remains, contact lenses such as PROSE lenses may be an effective solution, avoiding the need for invasive surgery. Prosthetic Replacement of the Ocular Surface Ecosystem (PROSE)

lenses are custom-designed therapeutic scleral lenses used to manage a range of ocular surface diseases, including corneal scars and play a significant role in improving visual acuity and reducing surface discomfort. PROSE lenses create a smooth refractive surface by vaulting over the irregular cornea, thereby creating a more uniform refractive surface and improving vision. The fluid reservoir created by PROSE lenses helps in maintaining a stable tear film and protects the cornea by preventing direct contact with the eyelids, reducing friction and promoting healing. They are also highly oxygen permeable, thereby reducing risk of long-term hypoxia-related complications and ensuring comfort to the patient.

3. *Severe Scarring with Vascularisation*: In cases of severe stromal necrosis or scarring with vascularisation (Fig. 26.10), keratoplasty becomes necessary [13]. Fine needle diathermy (FND) may be performed before keratoplasty to regress the vasculature, leaving only the scar [14].

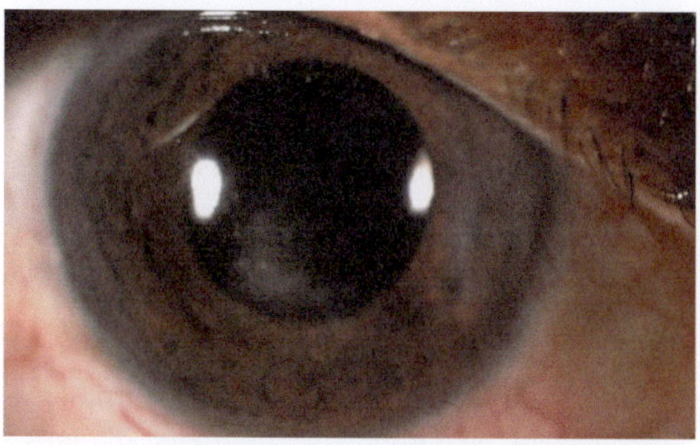

Fig. 26.8 Faint herpetic scar away from the visual axis

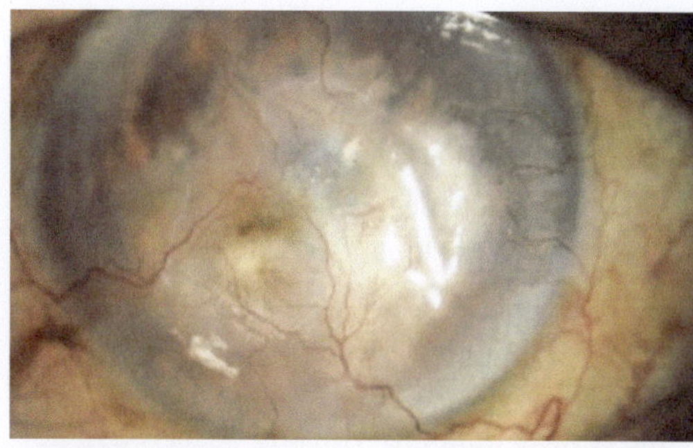

Fig. 26.10 Diffuse dense scarring of the cornea with vascularisation hindering anterior chamber details

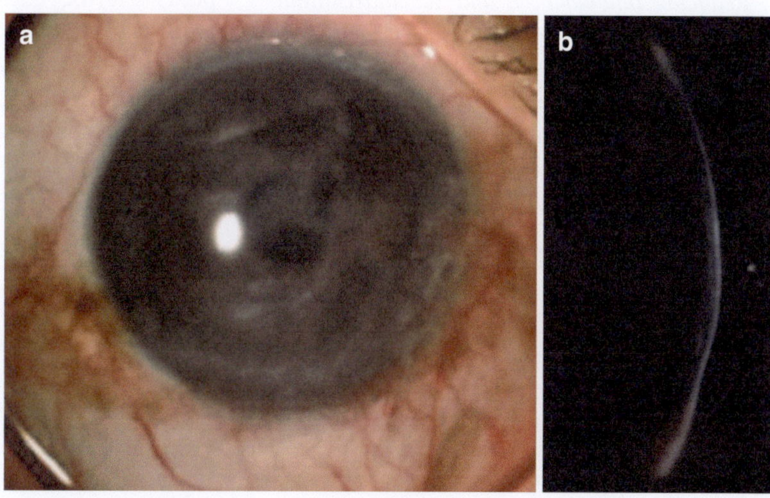

Fig. 26.9 (**a**) Diffuse nebulomacular stromal scarring with clear view of anterior chamber details suggestive of moderate scarring. (**b**) Slit view of the same image showing a nebulomacular scarring

26.4 Preoperative Considerations

Before undergoing keratoplasty for healed HSV keratitis, several preoperative factors need to be addressed

- *Delineating Pathology*: Careful examination of the disease is crucial in the acute stage. What may appear as a full-thickness scar on slit-lamp examination may only involve the superficial layers of the cornea. Anterior segment optical coherence tomography (AS-OCT) is useful for determining the depth and layers of corneal involvement, aiding the decision between lamellar and full-thickness keratoplasty [15]. For instance, superficial scarred dendrites typically do not require surgical intervention, whereas deep stromal scars may necessitate deep anterior lamellar keratoplasty (DALK). It can also aid in distinguishing corneal endotheliitis from other pathologies by detecting previous keratic precipitates and corneal thickening, in contrast to the corneal thinning typically observed in normal cases, along with identifying guttate changes and widening of the Descemet membrane double layer (Fig. 26.11a, b).
- *Reducing Inflammation and Vascularisation*: Preoperative treatment focuses on reducing inflammation and vascularisation especially in those patients presenting with atypical features such as sub-tarsal fibrosis in dry eyes mimicking cicatrizing diseases and the quite rare herpetic sclerokeratitis. What initially appears as a scar with vascularisation may, upon staining, reveal fluorescent stippling of the epithelium, indicative of either residual healing dendrites or surface irregularities overlying the scar. In cases of deep vascularisation, especially in more than two quadrants, the risk of graft failure is high. Fine needle diathermy (FND) is often used to regress deep corneal vessels in high-risk grafts of healed viral keratitis, lipid keratopathy and failed graft with stromal vessels [14].
  Monopolar cautery is applied using a parallelly positioned needle to larger vessels and perpendicular to tufts of smaller vessels, with careful attention to depth. This technique coagulates corneal collagen, effectively occluding small vessels, which can occur rapidly over an existing scar which is observed as stromal whitening, intracorneal haemorrhages and striae of the corneal tissue. Keratoplasty should be scheduled within 3–4 months after FND to avoid vessel recanalisation [14] (Fig. 26.12a, b).
- *Antiviral Cover*: The indications for oral antivirals can be either for treatment of active viral disease or for prophylaxis against recurrence. Patients undergoing penetrating keratoplasty (PK) for visual loss due to HSV keratitis are at high risk for recurrence of active infection in the graft. HSV endotheliitis in the post-PK patient can closely resemble allograft rejection, complicating the diagnosis and confusing the clinician. To mitigate the risk of recurrence, Antiviral prophylaxis with acyclo-

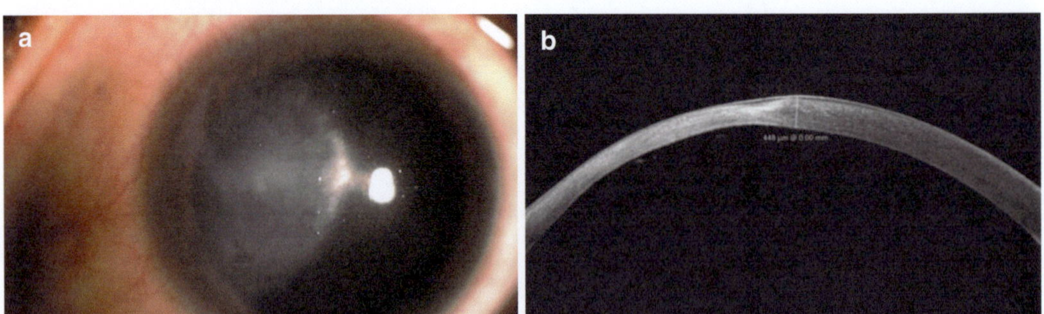

Fig. 26.11 (**a**) Diffuse slit-lamp photo delineating a healed stromal herpetic keratitis. (**b**) Its corresponding AS-OCT image

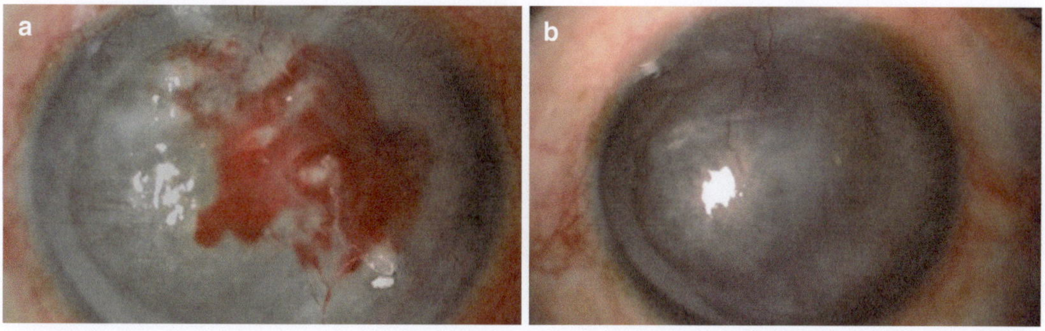

Fig. 26.12 Slit-lamp images. (**a**) Pre-FND showing deep stromal vascularisation. (**b**) Post-FND showing regression of deep vessels

vir or valacyclovir is essential [16, 17]. Acyclovir is a widely used oral antiviral drug and is considered safe and well-tolerated. It acts by inhibiting DNA replication, thereby reducing the risk of latent HSV reactivation in the trigeminal ganglion and preventing recurrence. Topical antivirals act only locally on the cornea and do not contribute to improved overall graft survival [18]. Valacyclovir, being a prodrug has improved bioavailability, thereby reducing frequency of administration and better patient adherence. While some literature suggests a one-year course of antivirals in renal-competent patients, indefinite antiviral cover is preferred due to the lifelong latency of HSV [19].

26.5 Intraoperative Considerations

Careless trephination and suturing are of paramount importance to avoid wound leaks in areas of variable thickness, especially in those corneas with extreme thinning [20].

Although HSV keratitis is primarily diagnosed clinically, surgeons should utilise this opportunity to obtain samples of both corneal tissue and aqueous humour for microbiological confirmation, including PCR analysis, which may add value to the diagnosis [21].

Chronic use of topical antivirals can lead to impaired corneal innervation and reduced tear secretion, which can negatively affect graft function. In case of severe neurotrophic corneal grafts, tarsorrhaphy is an effective treatment option. In these cases of neurotrophic keratitis and severe dry eye, the corneal graft is at a high risk of further damage due to lack of tear production and corneal innervation. Preoperatively, there should be a complete assessment of the patients tear function before deciding on the procedure. A temporary tarsorrhaphy, which can last up to 3 months, may be achieved with Botox injections to provide short-term relief. However, for more significant and long-term graft protection, a surgical tarsorrhaphy is more effective, as it ensures complete lid coverage of the graft defect area, aiding in epithelialisation and preventing further complications. Punctal cautery, for the same reason, can also be a very effective treatment in post-herpetic keratoplasty. It promotes tear retention, thereby aiding epithelisation and faster healing of the graft.

In grafts with multiple recurrences, extensive scarring with vascularisation, there is a high probability of developing limbal stem cell deficiency (Fig. 26.13). HSV keratitis can lead to severe damage to the ocular surface along with corneal scarring leading to significant decrease in vision. Patients with LSCD face significant challenges in re-epithelializing the corneal graft following keratoplasty. The absence of sufficient stem cells to regenerate the corneal epithelium can impede healing, leading to prolonged recovery times, increased risk of graft rejection, and persistent epithelial defects or infection. This slow re-epithelialisation process is a common

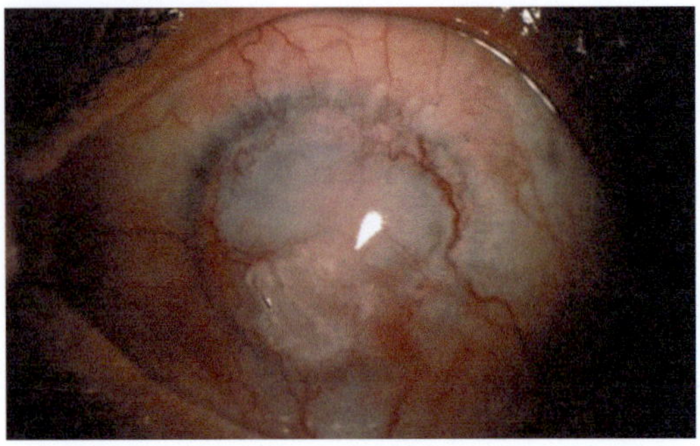

Fig. 26.13 Failed corneal graft post multiple recurrences of HSV keratitis with florid vascularisation

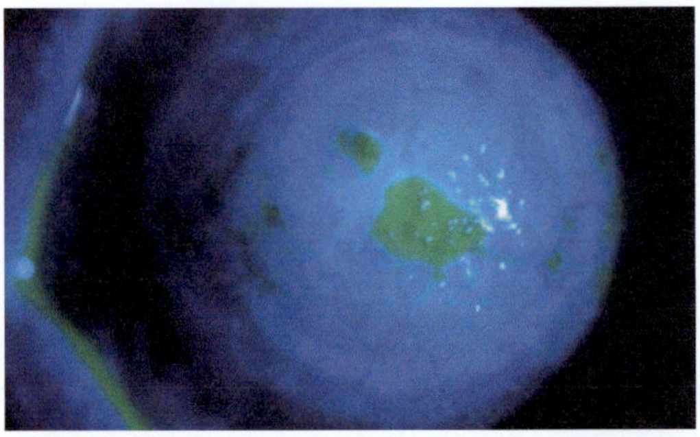

Fig. 26.14 Recurrence of geographic epithelial keratitis post keratoplasty

obstacle in LSCD cases, even after successful keratoplasty, as the underlying stem cell deficiency hinders the ability to restore the normal epithelial barrier effectively. Surgeons in this case should consider allo-SLET (allo-simple limbal epithelial transplantation) from the same donor eye being used for keratoplasty, coupled with postoperative immunosuppressive therapy [22]. Allo SLET can restore the corneal epithelium and has the potential to improve the ocular surface and enhance visual outcomes.

Preoperatively, both the surgeon and patient must be prepared for additional procedures, as well as potential complications, to ensure optimal outcomes. This includes proper diagnosis and clear expectations regarding recovery and healing.

26.6 Postoperative Considerations

Postoperatively, the most common concern is the recurrence of HSV keratitis, mainly epithelial dendrites. It is important to note that epithelial dendrites that appear soon after surgery are usually unlikely to be HSV-related, as the corneal nerves, which carry the virus, must regenerate before reactivation occurs [23]. Another useful tip to remember is that, the position of the epithelial defect across the graft–host junction, especially staining with rose Bengal, should arouse suspicion of recurrent dendritic keratitis [24]. In a postoperative scenario, it is important to note that epithelial recurrence has the potential to extend into the stroma which is not very common prior to surgery (Fig. 26.14).

Other postoperative concerns include graft rejection, particularly in high-risk grafts. Signs of rejection include inflammation at the graft–host junction, presence of pigments and keratic precipitates and recurrent dendritic keratitis. Graft rejection is an immune-mediated reaction which involves the activation of T lymphocytes and production of antibodies against the donor tissue antigen. Graft failure on the other hand is non-immunological and can be due to various factors such as graft rejection, mishandling of corneal tissue intraoperatively and recurrence of keratitis.

After an initial infection, HSV can remain dormant in the trigeminal ganglion. Surgical procedures such as cataract surgery, LASIK or Collagen cross-linking can be a trigger for reactivation of the virus due to the insult to the corneal tissue during these procedures [25–27]. Any ocular procedure requires continued antiviral prophylaxis to prevent reactivation of the virus. Conservative approach would be to avoid these procedures.

26.7 Conclusion

The management of HSV keratitis, particularly in its advanced stages, requires careful clinical judgement, precise surgical planning and long-term antiviral therapy. It entails distinct set of challenges faced by surgeons and steps that can be taken to prevent and manage those cases of healed HSV keratitis that would require a keratoplasty. Differentiating between HSV and other similar corneal diseases is essential for effective treatment. In cases requiring keratoplasty, preoperative and postoperative considerations, including vascular management and antiviral prophylaxis, play a critical role in improving surgical outcomes. Long-term vigilance is necessary to prevent recurrence and ensure the health of the transplanted cornea.

Key Points

1. Corneal grafts in healed HSV keratitis are high risk grafts and face high rejection and failure risk.
2. HSV keratitis can present as epithelial, stromal or endotheliitis or present with atypical features making clinical diagnosis very important.
3. Clinical evaluation, viral culture, PCR and immunologic tests help confirm HSV keratitis.
4. AS-OCT helps delineate the scars and aid us in recognizing those cases which require keratoplasty.
5. Oral antivirals (acyclovir/valacyclovir) are essential for prophylaxis to prevent recurrence post-surgery.
6. Severe scarring with vascularisation often necessitates fine needle diathermy (FND) used to regress corneal vessels preoperatively.
7. Intraoperatively, precise trephination and suturing are crucial to avoid complications.
8. Allo-SLET, tarsorrhaphy and punctal cautery can aid in protecting neurotrophic grafts and improving epithelial healing.

References

1. Lomholt JA, Baggesen K, Ehlers N. Recurrence and rejection rates following corneal transplantation for herpes simplex keratitis. Acta Ophthalmol Scand. 1995;73:29–32.
2. Ahmad B, Gurnani B, Patel BC. Herpes simplex keratitis. [Updated 2024 Mar 10]. In: StatPearls [Internet]. Treasure Island: StatPearls Publishing; 2025. Available from: https://www.ncbi.nlm.nih.gov/books/NBK545278/.
3. Cohen EJ, Laibson PR, Arentsen JJ. Corneal transplantation for herpes simplex keratitis. Am J Ophthalmol. 1983;95(5):645–50. https://doi.org/10.1016/0002-9394(83)90384-7. PMID: 6342400.
4. Kowalski RP, Gordon YJ. Evaluation of immunologic tests for the detection of ocular herpes simplex virus. Ophthalmology. 1989;96(11):1583–6. https://doi.org/10.1016/s0161-6420(89)32683-2. PMID: 2559384.
5. Seitzman GD, Strauss EC, Margolis TP. "Steel wool keratopathy": a clinical sign of chronic inflammation. Cornea. 2006;25(6):742–4.
6. Bialasiewicz A. Adenoviral keratoconjunctivitis. Sultan Qaboos Univ Med J. 2007;7(1):15–23. PMID: 21654940; PMCID: PMC3086413.
7. Jayamanne DGR, Dayan M, Jenkins D, Porter R. The role of staphylococcal superantigens in the pathogenesis of marginal keratitis. Eye. 1997;11(5):618–21. https://doi.org/10.1038/eye.1997.165.
8. Smolin G, Okumoto M. Staphylococcal blepharitis. Arch Ophthalmol. 1977;95:812–6.
9. Sibley D, Larkin DFP. Update on Herpes simplex keratitis management. Eye (Lond). 2020;34(12):2219–26.
10. Valerio GS, Lin CC. Ocular manifestations of herpes simplex virus. Curr Opin Ophthalmol. 2019;30(6):525–31.
11. Ambrósio R, Periman LM, Netto MV, Wilson SE. Bilateral marginal sterile infiltrates and diffuse lamellar keratitis after laser in situ keratomileusis. J Refract Surg. 2003;19(2):154–8.
12. Epstein RJ, Seedor JA, Dreizen NG, et al. Penetrating kerato-plasty for herpes simplex keratitis and keratoconus. Allograft rejection and survival. Ophthalmology. 1987;94:935–44.
13. Al-Yousuf N, Mavrikakis I, Mavrikakis E, Daya SM. Penetrating keratoplasty: indications over a 10-year period. Br J Ophthalmol. 2004;88:998–1001.
14. Ravichandran S, Natarajan R. Fine-needle diathermy for corneal vascularisation. Indian J Ophthalmol. 2022;70(5):1868.
15. Sridhar MS, Martin R. Anterior segment optical coherence tomography for evaluation of cornea and ocular surface. Indian J Ophthalmol. 2018;66(3):367–72.

16. Foster CS, Barney NP. Systemic acyclovir and penetrating keratoplasty for herpes simplex keratitis. Doc Ophthalmol. 1992;80:363–9.
17. Akova YA, Onat M, Duman S. Efficacy of low-dose and long-term oral acyclovir therapy after penetrating keratoplasty for herpes simplex keratitis. Ocul Immunol Inflamm. 1999;7:51–60.
18. Moyes AL, Sugar A, Musch DC, Barnes RD. Antiviral therapy after penetrating keratoplasty for herpes simplex keratitis. Arch Ophthalmol. 1994;112:601–7.
19. Dias C, Nashed Y, Atluri H, Mitra A. Ocular penetration of acyclovir and its peptide prodrugs valacyclovir and val-valacyclovir following systemic administration in rabbits: an evaluation using ocular microdialysis and LC-MS. Curr Eye Res. 2002;25(4):243–52. [PubMed: 12658558].
20. Speakman JS, Jones JD. Corneal trephining for penetrating keratoplasty. Br J Ophthalmol. 1956;40(4):216–21.
21. Espy MJ, Ross TK, Teo R, Svien KA, Wold AD, Uhl JR, et al. Evaluation of LightCycler PCR for implementation of laboratory diagnosis of herpes simplex virus infections. J Clin Microbiol. 2000;38(8):3116–8.
22. Riedl JC, Musayeva A, Wasielica-Poslednik J, Pfeiffer N, Gericke A. Allogenic simple limbal epithelial transplantation (alloSLET) from cadaveric donor eyes in patients with persistent corneal epithelial defects. Br J Ophthalmol. 2021;105(2):180–5.
23. Azher TN, Yin XT, Tajfirouz D, Huang AJ, Stuart PM. Herpes simplex keratitis: challenges in diagnosis and clinical management. Clin Ophthalmol. 2017;11:185–91.
24. Beyer CF, Byrd TJ, Hill JM, Kaufman HE. Herpes simplex virus and persistent epithelial defects after penetrating keratoplasty. Am J Ophthalmol. 1990;109:95–6.
25. Jhanji V, Ferdinands M, Sheorey H, et al. Unusual clinical presentations of new-onset herpetic eye disease after ocular surgery. Acta Ophthalmol. 2012;90:514.
26. de Rojas Silva MV, Díez-Feijóo E, Javaloy J, Sánchez-Salorio M. Prophylactic perioperative antiviral therapy for LASIK in patients with inactive herpetic keratitis. J Refract Surg. 2006;22(4):404–6. https://doi.org/10.3928/1081-597X-20060401-19. PMID: 16629075.
27. Abbouda A, Abicca I, Alió JL. Infectious keratitis following corneal crosslinking: a systematic review of reported cases: management, visual outcome, and treatment proposed. Semin Ophthalmol. 2016;31(5):485.

Corneal Transplantation in Viral Keratitis

27

Abhishek Kumar, Brindha Periasamy, Bhavana Sharma, and Radhika Tandon

Abstract

Viral keratitis is a significant cause of corneal blindness worldwide, with herpes simplex virus (HSV) and varicella-zoster virus (VZV) being the most common etiologic agents. These infections can cause recurrent inflammation, leading to corneal scarring, neovascularization, and endothelial dysfunction. In cases with significant impairment of visual acuity with limited options available in terms of medical management, corneal transplantation is considered the treatment of choice. This chapter provides an overview of types of transplants, indications, surgical techniques, postoperative care, and outcomes associated with corneal transplantation in cases of viral keratitis.

Keywords

Corneal transplantation · Recurrence · Graft failure · Graft rejection

A. Kumar · R. Tandon (✉)
RP Centre, AIIMS New Delhi, New Delhi, India

B. Periasamy · B. Sharma
AIIMS Bhopal, Bhopal, Madhya Pradesh, India

27.1 Introduction

Viral keratitis is a common cause of corneal blindness, particularly in developed countries. The most common manifestation of recurrent ocular HSV infection is HSV keratitis. Herpetic Eye Disease Study reported recurrence as epithelial keratitis in 47% of cases, while HSV stromal keratitis accounted for 16% [1]. Epithelial keratitis involves direct infection of corneal epithelial cells, while the pathogenesis of HSV stromal keratitis is mainly immunologic. Thus, epithelial keratitis is treated primarily by antiviral medications, whereas HSV stromal keratitis necessitates surgical intervention in addition to medical management.

Although HSV affects all layers of the cornea, stromal keratitis is the primary cause of permanent loss of corneal transparency, necessitating full-thickness corneal transplantation. In some instances, keratoplasty might be needed for maintenance of the globe's integrity. However, there are specific risks associated with corneal transplantation in viral keratitis, including a higher chance of graft rejection, viral recurrence, and challenges with long-term immunosuppressive treatment. Corneal grafts have better survival rates in the presence of inactive corneal scarring compared to active keratitis [2]. Despite these challenges, the graft survival rate has increased with the systemic antiviral prophylaxis and advanced surgical procedures. Patient compli-

B. Sharma et al. (eds.), *Viral Keratitis*, https://doi.org/10.1007/978-981-95-3148-6_27

ance and vigilant post op monitoring are essential for a successful corneal transplant in viral keratitis patients.

27.2 Pathophysiology

Viral keratitis poses significant challenges in the context of corneal transplantation. HSV and VZV have latency in the trigeminal ganglion due to neurotropism, which is responsible for periodic shedding of the virus and multiple recurrences. Keratoplasty and the post-transplant immunosuppression are the stressors of viral reactivation. The underlying pathophysiology involves both direct viral cytopathic effects and immune-mediated tissue damage, which can compromise graft survival and function. Also, the chronic inflammation due to multiple episodes makes the cornea hypoxic, and so the vascularization. This results in a loss of immune privilege, increasing the risk of graft rejection. The pathophysiology of viral keratitis in corneal transplantation is explained in Flowchart 27.1.

27.3 Indications for Corneal Transplantation

Viral infections have a greater propensity for recurrences and prolonged inflammation, which remain important hallmarks of the disease process and increase the patient's risk of developing corneal scarring, neovascularization, and consequent blindness (Fig. 27.1a, b). Corneal scarring, neovascularization, thinning, necrosis, and perforation are the main indications for corneal transplantation in HSV keratitis [3, 4].

Initial management of viral keratitis is medical, involving topical and systemic antivirals (e.g., acyclovir, ganciclovir) and the judicious use of corticosteroids, particularly in cases of stromal disease. Surgery is considered when there is dense stromal scarring affecting the visual axis, the globe integrity is at risk, or the disease is progressing despite the maximum medical therapy. The corneal transplantation in viral keratitis can be

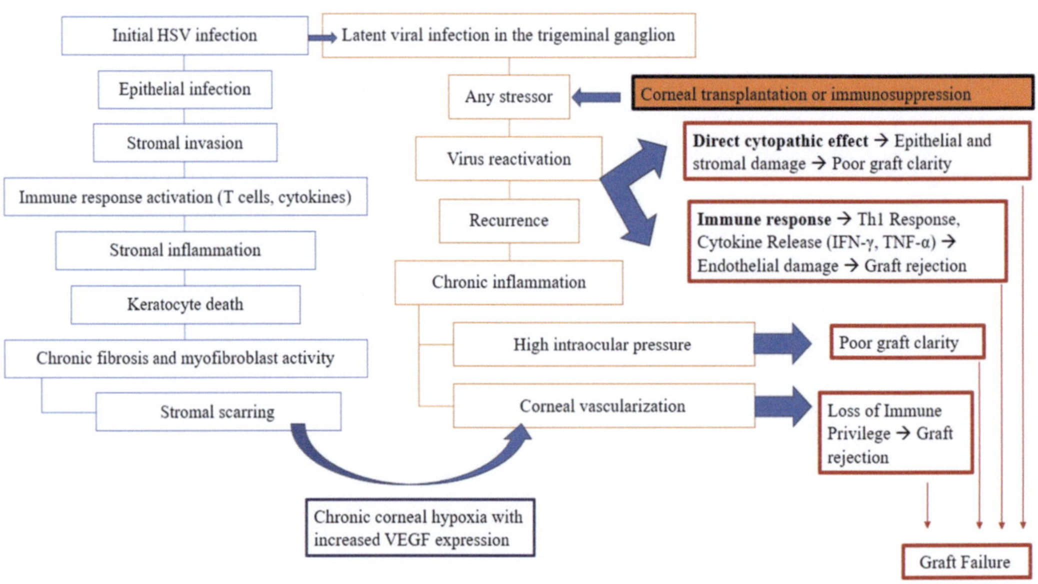

Flowchart 27.1 Pathophysiology of viral keratitis in corneal transplantation

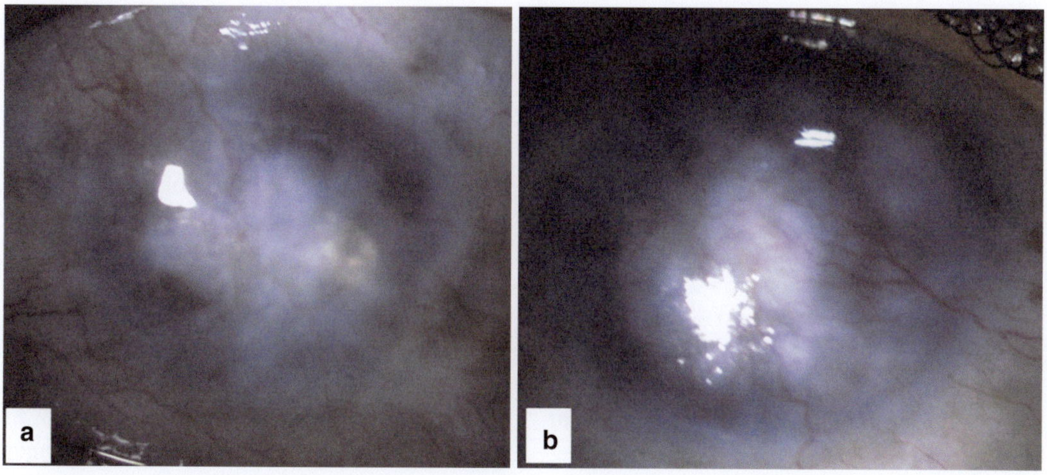

Fig. 27.1 (**a**, **b**) Bilateral vascularized leukomatous corneal opacity following recurrent viral stromal keratitis

A. *Optical*: Visual rehabilitation due to central scarring or irregular astigmatism
B. *Tectonic*: To preserve globe integrity in cases of thinning or perforation
C. *Therapeutic*: To remove active infectious foci in resistant cases

Table 27.1 illustrates various indications for corneal transplantation in cases of viral keratitis.

Table 27.1 Indications for corneal transplantation in viral keratitis

Indications	Type of corneal transplantation
Central corneal opacification or stromal scarring	Optical PK/DALK (based on depth of opacity)
Corneal decompensation following viral endothelitis	Optical PK/DSEK/DMEK (based on severity)
Recurrent episodes of immune-mediated keratitis	Therapeutic PK
Cases refractory to medical therapy	Therapeutic PK
Severe stromal keratitis with stromal melting/perforation	Tectonic PK
Corneal perforation secondary to persistent epithelial defect with little or no active stromal inflammation (that cannot be treated with other modalities)	Tectonic PK

PK penetrating keratoplasty, *DALK* deep anterior lamellar keratoplasty, *DSEK* descemet's stripping endothelial keratoplasty, *DMEK* descemet membrane endothelial keratoplasty

27.4 Types of Corneal Transplants

Corneal transplantation in viral keratitis can be full-thickness or lamellar keratoplasty. The indications may vary depending on the size and depth of involvement. Thus, detailed assessment is necessary for surgical planning. The following are the surgical techniques that are employed.

Penetrating Keratoplasty (PK)

PK is a procedure that replaces the diseased corneal tissue with a full-thickness donor graft. It is suitable for eyes with extensive stromal involvement and endothelial compromise, in severe HSV/VZV keratitis with central dense scarring. PK is also indicated in frank perforation or severe progressive keratitis refractory to medical therapy. However, patients with active inflammation, active ulceration, perforation, or extensive neovascularization secondary to HSV keratitis have shown to have poorer outcomes [5].

Prolonged inflammation may lead to stromal thinning, corneal irregularity, and consequent visual impairment. In such corneas of high irregularity and peripheral asymmetry, peripheral intrastromal hydration with balanced salt solution in areas of relative thinning can be used to facilitate optimal trephination [4, 6].

There is a significant recurrence rate of HSV keratitis in patients who undergo PK without antiviral prophylaxis [7]. Whereas preoperative oral antiviral treatment has been found to reduce the risk of graft failure [8]. Patients receiving oral antivirals are less likely to have a failed graft at 5 years postoperatively compared with those on no antiviral medication [8]. In a study by Wu et al., patients who received oral acyclovir 200 mg five times daily in the first 3 months, tapered to 400 mg twice daily for 12–18 months, recurrence was 21% while the immune rejection rate was 41%, and 22% of patients developed graft failure over 4–6 years. The causes for graft failure included immune rejection as most common, followed by recurrence of HSV keratitis [9].

Deep Anterior Lamellar Keratoplasty (DALK)

DALK selectively uses the anterior donor lamella to restore the damaged corneal stroma. It is preferred in high-risk cases like extensive inflammation and vascularization with healthy endothelium. Advantages include reduced risk of recurrence, rejection, and graft failure with better long-term graft survival, owing to retained host corneal endothelium, which is not amenable to immune rejection [10, 11]. Furthermore incidence of steroid-induced glaucoma and cataract is significantly lower as compared to PK [12].

The big-bubble technique is most widely used; however, it may be difficult to employ when the post-herpetic corneal opacities have residual Descemet's scarring. In such cases, manual dissection is preferred, though visual outcome may be limited by residual deep stromal layer.

Stromal rejection is considered to be a rare complication of DALK surgery, particularly with long-term antiviral prophylaxis, acyclovir 400 mg five times daily for 1 month, tapered to 400 mg twice daily for another 12–36 months [13, 14]. Antiviral prophylaxis may minimize the risk; however, it does not eliminate the recurrence of HSV keratitis after DALK. Thus, it is important to achieve a quiet anterior segment before the surgical intervention. Recurrence rates of HSV keratitis have been reported to be double of DALK, while rejection rates upto 41% in PK as compared to no rejection in the DALK group [15].

Mushroom Keratoplasty

It is a subtype of penetrating keratoplasty to preserve maximum host endothelium, if healthy. It involves transplantation of a large 9 mm diameter anterior lamella and a smaller 6 mm diameter posterior lamella. It is a hybrid of PK and DALK and carries the advantage of DALK while performing PK. Postoperative outcomes for 2-piece MK compare favourably with the results of PK in eyes both at low- and high-risk for immunologic rejection [16]. Main advantage of MK is to retain the recipient's healthy endothelium, thereby minimizing immunologic rejection due to lower antigen-presenting cells and a greater distance from limbal vessels in addition to its use of a large-diameter anterior lamellar graft with better postoperative refractive outcomes [17].

Endothelial Keratoplasty

Endothelial keratoplasty is preferred in endothelial dysfunctions following viral endothelitis. Both Descemet's membrane endothelial keratoplasty (DMEK) and Descemet's Stripping Automated Endothelial Keratoplasty (DSAEK) can be done, with the advantage of faster recovery, fewer suture-related complications, noncompromised wound strength, less post-surgery astigmatism, and early visual rehabilitation. Additionally, lower incidence of allograft rejection following DSAEK is a major advantage [18]. Post-DSAEK allograft rejection has been reported in 0.6% of patients with HSV [19]. Few cases of viral endothelitis that underwent DMEK developed HSV recurrence in 20% of cases [20, 21]. In the postoperative period, it is important to differentiate allograft rejection from recurrent viral endotheliitis as the treatment is different in both entities. Presenting features are visual deterioration, corneal oedema, DM folds, variable-sized KPs with variable AC reaction. Immunological rejection necessitates increasing the frequency of topical steroids supplemented with systemic steroids or intravenous methyl prednisolone 1 g daily for 3 days as per the clinical condition. Whereas recurrence of disease is to be treated by systemic antivirals in therapeutic doses of Acyclovir 400 mg five times over 2 weeks, followed by a maintenance dose of

Table 27.2 Differences between post-keratoplasty graft rejection and viral reactivation

Characteristics	Graft rejection	Viral reactivation
Time of presentation	Any time after transplantation	Usually, after 12 months of transplantation
Epithelial changes	Epithelial rejection line	Dendritic/geographic ulcer/atypical ulcer patterns
Inflammation	Confined only to the donor cornea	Both the host and donor cornea are involved
Keratic precipitates (KPs)	Seen on donor endothelium	Seen on both host and donor endothelium
Khodadoust line on endothelium	Present	Absent
Treatment	Topical steroids with IVMP (Intravenous Methylprednisolone) followed by oral steroids on a tapering dose	Oral acyclovir 400 mg five times over 2 weeks, followed by a maintenance dose of 400 mg three times over 6–12 months and 400 mg twice a day lifelong

400 mg three times over 6–12 months. Differentiating features of post-keratoplasty graft rejection and viral reactivation are explained in Table 27.2 below.

27.5 Challenges in Corneal Transplantation

Keratoplasty in a case of herpetic eye disease poses significant challenges. Stromal vascularization is more common following viral keratitis, which increases the risk of graft rejection. Even in an inactive eye, surgical stress and postoperative corticosteroids increase the risk of recurrence. Herpetic recurrence-induced inflammation can further augment the rejection episode. Graft rejection and herpetic recurrence are the most common causes of graft failure in these cases, and it is also difficult to differentiate them. The main differentiating feature remains the timing of presentation. While immunologic rejection may present any time during the postoperative period as opposed to recurrence of disease which is mainly seen after 12 months which is not before regeneration of severed corneal nerves.

27.6 Surgical Considerations

A. *Preoperative*:

Keratoplasty in eyes with viral keratitis is considered to confer a high risk of graft failure [22]. Reactivation of latent infection, increases the risk of immunologic rejection; however, advancements in surgical techniques along with pre and postoperative antiviral prophylaxis have significantly improved the success rates of keratoplasty [23].

Preoperative evaluation Must include ocular surface stability, absence of active inflammation, and systemic antiviral coverage. Patients should undergo thorough slit-lamp examination to look for red flag signs such as significant stromal vascularization (>3 clock hours), active inflammation, active ulceration, or perforation. Cases with these signs secondary to HSV keratitis have been shown to have poor success rates following keratoplasty.

Inflammation control Due to its recurrence and chronicity, viral keratitis is associated with inflammation. Inflammation per se is a risk factor for graft failure. It also induces vascularization and increased intraocular pressure, making the graft prone to rejection and failure. In cases of severe active inflammation, it is necessary to start on high-frequency topical steroids (every hour) under antiviral cover and then taper slowly, to improve the graft survival.

Intraocular pressure (IOP) control Due to corneal scarring, accurate IOP measurement is not reliable in all cases. With the Goldmann applanation tonometer (GAT), readings are not reproducible because the irregular corneal surface causes pooling of the fluorescein dye and irregular images of the circles, in addition to altered biomechanics of scarred vascularized corneas. Further, the scarred corneas may lead to artificially high-pressure readings. Tono-Pen, a small, handheld applanation device, similar to the Mackay Marg working principle, may be useful in such cases. It is important to take the measurement in an area that is normal and clear. However, an off-centre measurement may result in overestimation, since the peripheral cornea is thicker than the central cornea. Thus, the optimal site of measurement with maximum advantage through the remaining normal cornea should be aimed. Other procedures which can be performed in such cases are 'I care' tonometer, Schiotz tonometer, or digital tonometry.

If IOP is increased, topical antiglaucoma medications can be started, and based on the response, treatment can be modified. Prostaglandin analogues should be avoided as they are prone to increase inflammation and reactivate the latent HSV virus. In refractory cases or cases with secondary glaucoma, plan for augmented trabeculectomy with mitomycin-C (0.02% for 2 minutes or 0.04% for 4 minutes). Trabeculectomy can be combined with keratoplasty or two-staged. Adequate IOP control is essential for the graft clarity.

Corneal vascularization Deep stromal vascularization (>3 clock hours) is associated with graft rejection than the superficial type. However, both should be considered as high risk for keratoplasty as they breach the immune-privileged status of the cornea. Topical steroids suppress the inflammation-induced vascularization (Fig. 27.2a, b). As the hypoxic cornea expresses more VEGF (Vascular Endothelial Growth Factor) molecules, the off-label use of subconjunctival anti-VEGF injections (Bevacizumab/Ranibizumab) shows promising results in limiting angiogenesis. The dose of subconjunctival Bevacizumab is 2.5 mg/0.1 ml [24]. The injection can be given on the day of keratoplasty at the quadrant with dense vascularization 1 mm poste-

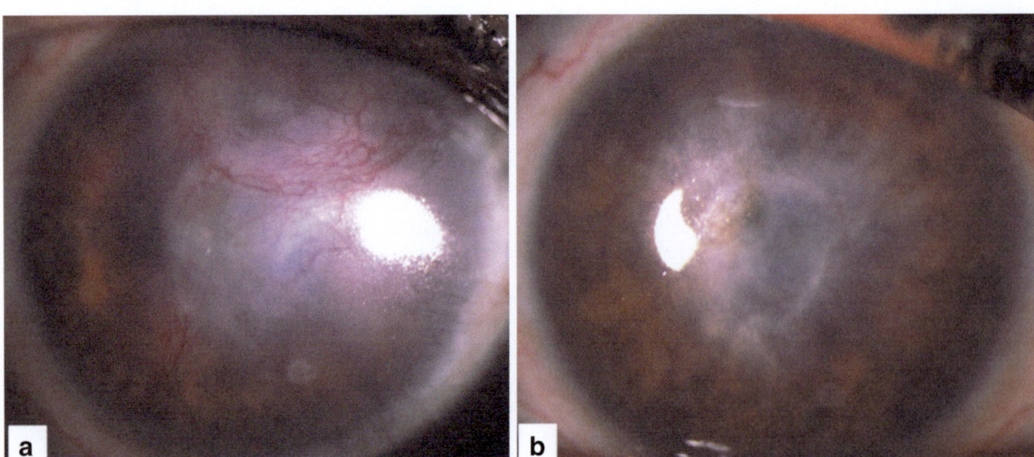

Fig. 27.2 (**a**) Healed HSV stromal keratitis with deep stromal vascularization, and (**b**) shows resolution of vascularization following topical Loteprednol 0.1% for 2 months

rior to the sclerocorneal junction. Some studies have reported topical bevacizumab (10 mg/mL) four times daily for 1 month post-keratoplasty, then tapering over 6 months. Complications include epitheliopathy and progression of stromal thinning [25]. Furthermore, corneal neo vessels can be obliterated by fine-needle diathermy or argon laser photocoagulation, but the latter carries the risk of virus reactivation.

Assessment of depth of corneal scarring Anterior Segment OCT (ASOCT) can be performed to measure the depth of corneal scarring and to decide upon the plan of surgery, whether penetrating keratoplasty or DALK, or endothelial keratoplasty.

Documentation of corneal sensations Corneal hypoesthesia is more prominent in VZV keratitis than HSV. Still, it should be documented in all cases of viral keratitis, and the patients should be monitored for epithelial integrity or development of neurotrophic ulcer following keratoplasty.

Perioperative antiviral prophylaxis Antiviral prophylaxis remains the most important therapeutic measure for preventing recurrence and consequently reducing failure of corneal grafts performed for herpetic scars. Systemic antivirals reduce the risk of HSV recurrence, prolong the recurrence-free interval, and duration of herpetic disease. Systemic antiviral medications are started preoperatively and continued for at least 1 year of post keratoplasty. Oral acyclovir 400 mg twice daily or oral valacyclovir 500 mg OD should be started preoperatively. This regimen prevents reactivation of latent HSV and reduces the risk of allograft rejection in vascularized corneas through downregulation of viral shedding and HSV-associated inflammation [26]. The Herpetic Eye Disease Study (HEDS) demonstrated the effectiveness of long-term oral acyclovir prophylaxis in preventing herpetic recurrence [1].

Timing of surgery A quiescent eye (disease-free for at least 6–12 months) is preferred before elective surgeries like optical PK or endothelial keratoplasty.

B. *Intraoperative*:

Donor selection Young healthy donors with good endothelial cell density should be preferred, as there is a risk of pronounced inflammation and high IOP following keratoplasty in viral keratitis. As the corneal sensation is compromised in the recipients, opt for an excellent or good grade donor cornea with intact epithelium and short preservation time.

Graft preparation Larger grafts are to be avoided as the limbal proximity increases the risk of rejection and also carries a high chance of PAS formation and glaucoma. Slightly oversized grafts may be used in tectonic cases.

Recipient bed preparation Careful dissection to avoid perforation in cases of lamellar keratoplasty. In therapeutic cases, at least 1 mm of healthy rim is to be excised.

Suturing Interrupted sutures are preferred as the opacified and vascularized corneas heal asymmetrically. Longer bites are advised in edematous corneas.

In cases with visually significant cataract, triple procedure with keratoplasty, cataract extraction, and Intraocular lens implantation can be done.

27.7 Postoperative Management

Oral acyclovir 400 mg five times daily for the first 3 months, followed by 400 mg twice daily or oral valacyclovir 500 mg OD for 1 year for the next 12 months, has been found to improve the outcomes of PK. The American Academy of Ophthalmology strongly recommends using high-dose oral acyclovir (800 mg three times daily for at least 1 year) as antiviral prophylaxis after keratoplasty [26].

High-risk cases with a history of multiple recurrences and immunosuppression might require lifelong treatment. Topical corticosteroids should be started with high frequency and later tailored as per the degree of inflammation. Patients should be vigilantly monitored for recurrence and rejection. Long-term follow-up is mandatory for keratoplasty in herpetic keratitis.

Herpetic reactivation can be triggered immunologically by local trauma during surgery, which is a significant cause of corneal graft failure [27]. Therefore, the same acyclovir dosage used in the HEDS trials is likely not suitable for eyes undergoing keratoplasty for herpetic scars.

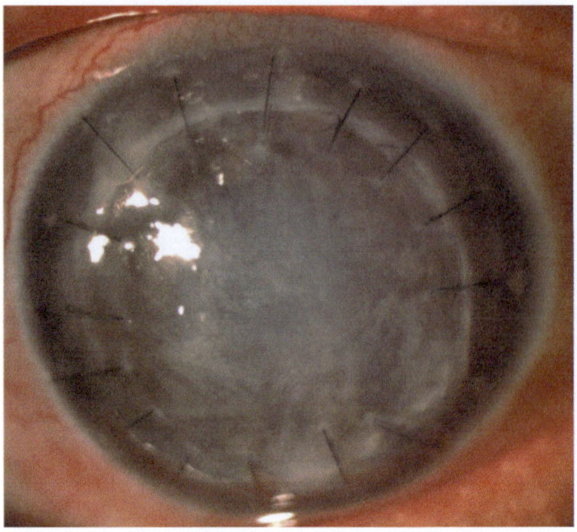

Fig. 27.3 Irreversible endothelial rejection post-penetrating keratoplasty done for healed viral keratitis. (Image courtesy: Dr. Rakhi Kusumesh, Professor, Indira Gandhi Institute of Medical Science, Patna)

27.8 Complications

Major complications after corneal transplantation done for viral keratitis comprise:

1. *Graft Rejection*:
   Graft survival is generally lower in viral keratitis compared to non-infectious indications due to higher immune rejection rates, viral recurrence, and preexisting ocular surface disease. Visual outcomes depend on the extent of preexisting damage and prompt management of complications. Despite advances in techniques, use of topical steroids and antiviral prophylaxis, allograft rejection remains an important cause of graft failure following PK for herpetic keratitis. Immune rejection and endothelial graft failure, often resulting from significant endothelial cell loss, continue to be the primary reasons for graft failure (Fig. 27.3) [12, 28].
   Graft failure in PK for herpetic keratitis is most commonly attributed to allograft rejection rather than viral recurrence [2]. However, in the absence of pathognomonic signs such as a dendritic or geographic ulcer, it can be clinically challenging to differentiate between rejection and viral recurrence, which may sometimes coexist.
2. *Recurrence of Viral Disease*:
   HSV recurrence in epithelium or stroma, post corneal transplantation, is usually seen after 12 months till the regeneration of severed corneal nerves is completed (Figs. 27.4 and 27.5). The incidence of recurrent HSV illness is 12–19% when PK is used to treat corneal scarring [29–32].
   This is attributed to virus migration, which starts from the peripheral host cornea to involve the graft lenticule in a retrograde fashion along the corneal nerves.
   The primary approach to treatment involves the use of antiviral medications, which can be administered orally as acyclovir 800 mg five times, valacyclovir 1000 mg BD, or famciclovir 500 mg TDS for 2–4 weeks. Additionally, topical ganciclovir 0.15%, or acyclovir 3% five times a day, is administered until the keratitis heals, after which the frequency is tapered to three times a day for an additional week. Trifluridine 1% can be prescribed eight to nine times a day. However, caution should be exercised to timely discontinue the use of antiviral drops given the potential for corneal toxicity.

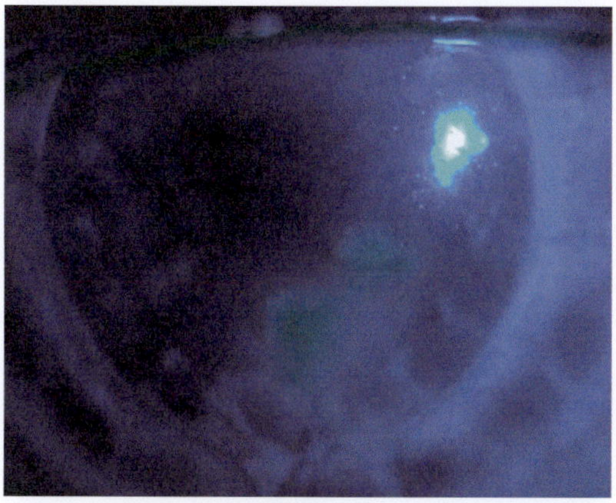

Fig. 27.4 Viral epithelial recurrence in post-penetrating keratoplasty. (Image courtesy: Dr. Rakhi Kusumesh, Professor, Indira Gandhi Institute of Medical Science, Patna)

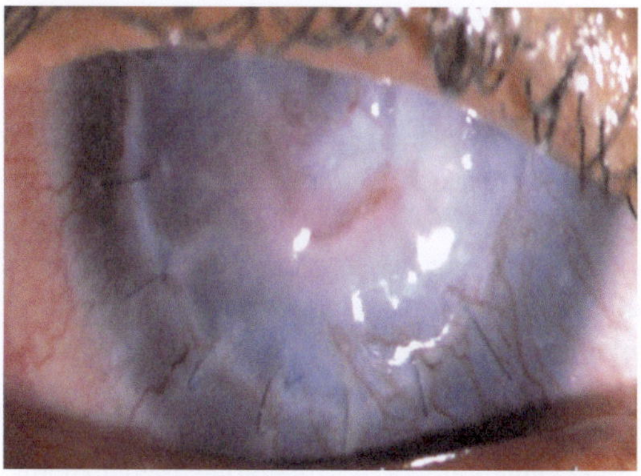

Fig. 27.5 HSV recurrence at 6 months following DALK done for healed viral keratitis

3. *Secondary Glaucoma*:
   Post-keratoplasty glaucoma is associated with poor graft survival. Herpetic keratitis and keratouveitis are frequently associated with high intraocular pressures due to inflammation and trabeculitis. Hence viral keratitis cases are high-risk candidates for secondary glaucoma in the post operative period. Other risk factors include large graft, eccentric graft, adherent leukoma, and regrafting. Postoperatively, all cases should have an IOP check during each follow-up. Sudden IOP spike episodes, which are common in herpetic keratitis, are more deleterious than constant high IOP, resulting in graft rejection.

   High IOP following keratoplasty can be with open or closed angles. Mechanisms include inflammatory debris in the angle, trabeculitis, chronic inflammation, steroid use, angle distortion in large grafts, and progressive peripheral anterior synechiae causing synechial angle closure.

   Iridoplasty and iridectomy can be performed as prophylactic measures to prevent synechiae formation. If patients present with post op high IOP, proper evaluation of the cause and appropriate management should be advised. Medical management can be initiated with aqueous suppressants. In case of pupillary block, laser peripheral iridotomy is to be performed under the cover of systemic antiviral as the laser carries risk of HSV recurrence. In cases of inflammatory glaucoma, short course of topical corticosteroids can be given. Cases refractory to medical therapy, surgical management should be performed. Synechial angle closure might require synechiolysis.

27.9 Special Scenarios

(a) *Pediatric viral keratitis*: If amblyopia is not a concern, surgery can be postponed until adulthood to avoid complications of pediatric keratoplasty. Following corneal transplant, amblyopia management is as important as the post-op follow-up and antiviral prophylaxis.
(b) *Immunocompromised patients*: Carry a higher risk of recurrence and poor wound healing. Lifelong antivirals and regular follow-ups are mandatory.
(c) *Refractory cases*: May require repeat grafts, amniotic membrane transplantation, or keratoprosthesis in selected cases.

27.10 Outcomes

Usually, a corneal transplant in viral keratitis carries a guarded prognosis. But with perioperative systemic antiviral cover, surgical advances, and

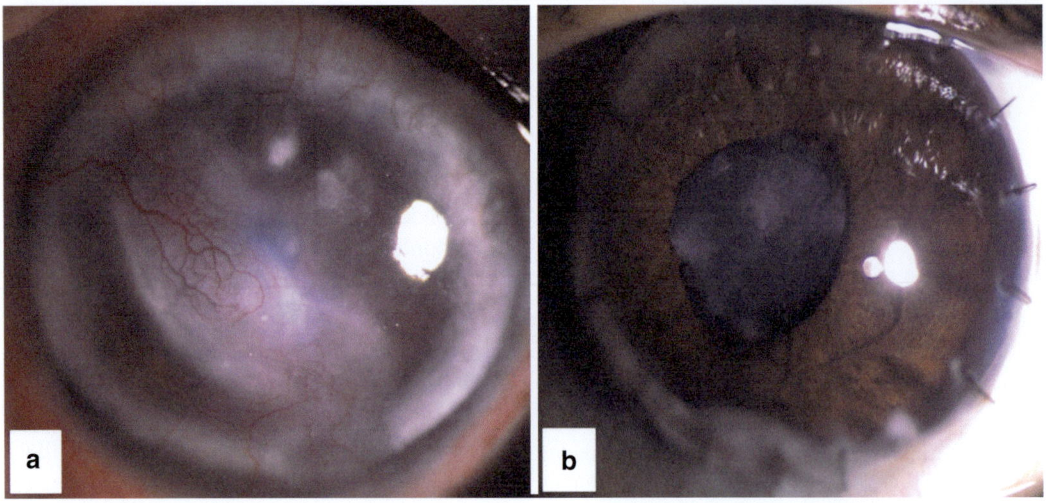

Fig. 27.6 Slit-lamp image showing (**a**) healed viral stromal keratitis with vascularized corneal opacity, (**b**) clear graft post-penetrating keratoplasty on 6-month follow-up

meticulous post-op follow-up, the outcomes have been reported to be improved (Fig. 27.6a, b).

27.11 Future Directions

Advances in molecular diagnostics, antiviral therapies, and tissue engineering hold promise. Recent development of sustained antiviral ocular drug delivery systems like nanocarriers, nanoemulsions, liposomes, and in situ gels helps to increase the ocular bioavailability, and so the treatment effectiveness [33].

Aganirsen eye drops are studied for suppressing the corneal vascularization. It is an antisense oligonucleotide, which limits the mRNA expression of Insulin Receptor Substrate (IRS-1) involved in the pathway of corneal neovascularization [34]. Newer anti-VEGFs like Aflibercept show promising results in limiting the corneal vascularization in cases that are poorly tolerating bevacizumab [25].

Bioengineered corneas and regenerative approaches may eventually reduce reliance on donor tissue. Gene therapy targeting latent viral reservoirs is an area of ongoing research.

27.12 Conclusion

Corneal transplantation in the setting of viral keratitis presents a complex clinical challenge. While keratoplasty can offer significant visual rehabilitation in cases with stromal scarring or corneal decompensation, the risk of graft failure is high due to the recurrent nature of herpetic infections and associated immune responses. Preoperative planning, meticulous surgical technique, and vigilant postoperative management, including long-term antiviral prophylaxis and balanced immunosuppression, are critical for graft survival.

Key Points

- Corneal transplantation is a vital intervention in advanced viral keratitis.
- Optimal timing (quiescent phase) and surgical planning improve outcome.
- DALK is preferable when the endothelium is intact; PK is needed in full-thickness disease.
- Long-term and rarely life-long antiviral prophylaxis is necessary to prevent recurrences.
- Multidisciplinary care and patient education enhance long-term success.

References

1. Herpetic Eye Disease Study Group. Oral acyclovir for herpes simplex virus eye disease: effect on prevention of epithelial keratitis and stromal keratitis. Arch Ophthalmol. 2000;118:1030–6.
2. Ficker LA, Kirkness CM, Rice NS, Steele AD. Longterm prognosis for corneal grafting in herpes simplex keratitis. Eye Lond Engl. 1988;2(Pt 4):400–8.
3. Azher TN, Yin XT, Tajfirouz D, Huang AJ, Stuart PM. Herpes simplex keratitis: challenges in diagnosis and clinical management. Clin Ophthalmol Auckl NZ. 2017;11:185–91.
4. Wilhelmus KR, Sugar J, Hyndiuk RA, Stulting RD. Corneal thickness changes during herpes simplex virus disciform keratitis. Cornea. 2004;23:154–7.
5. Foster CS, Duncan J. Penetrating keratoplasty for herpes simplex keratitis. Am J Ophthalmol. 1981;92:336–43.
6. Bovone C, Myerscough J, Friehmann A, Elkadim M, Parmeggiani F, Busin M. Peripheral intrastromal hydration facilitates safe, deep trephination in corneas of irregular thickness. Cornea. 2020;39:207–9.
7. Lomholt JA, Baggesen K, Ehlers N. Recurrence and rejection rates following corneal transplantation for herpes simplex keratitis. Acta Ophthalmol Scand. 1995;73:29–32.
8. Goodfellow JFB, Nabili S, Jones MNA, Nguyen DQ, Armitage WJ, Cook SD, et al. Antiviral treatment following penetrating keratoplasty for herpetic keratitis. Eye Lond Engl. 2011;25:470–4.
9. Wu SQ, Zhou P, Zhang B, Qiu WY, Yao YF. Long-term comparison of full-bed deep lamellar keratoplasty with penetrating keratoplasty in treating corneal leucoma caused by herpes simplex keratitis. Am J Ophthalmol. 2012;153:291–299.e2.
10. Watson SL, Ramsay A, Dart JKG, Bunce C, Craig E. Comparison of deep lamellar keratoplasty and penetrating keratoplasty in patients with keratoconus. Ophthalmology. 2004;111:1676–82.
11. Noble BA, Agrawal A, Collins C, Saldana M, Brogden PR, Zuberbuhler B. Deep Anterior Lamellar Keratoplasty (DALK): visual outcome and complications for a heterogeneous group of corneal pathologies. Cornea. 2007;26:59–64.
12. Anshu A, Li L, Htoon HM, de Benito-Llopis L, Shuang LS, Singh MJ, et al. Long-term review of penetrating keratoplasty: a 20-year review in Asian eyes. Am J Ophthalmol. 2021;224:254–66.
13. Leccisotti A. Air-assisted manual deep anterior lamellar keratoplasty for treatment of herpetic corneal scars. Cornea. 2009;28:728–31.
14. Li J, Ma H, Zhao Z, Hou C, Shao Y, Waller S, et al. Deep anterior lamellar keratoplasty using precut anterior lamellar cap for herpes simplex keratitis: a long-term follow-up study. Br J Ophthalmol. 2014;98:448–53.
15. Reinhart WJ, Musch DC, Jacobs DS, Lee WB, Kaufman SC, Shtein RM. Deep anterior lamellar keratoplasty as an alternative to penetrating keratoplasty a report by the American Academy of Ophthalmology. Ophthalmology. 2011;118:209–18.
16. Yu AC, Spena R, Fusco F, Dondi R, Myerscough J, Fabbri F, et al. Long-term outcomes of two-piece mushroom keratoplasty for traumatic corneal scars. Am J Ophthalmol. 2022;236:20–31.
17. Yu AC, Friehmann A, Myerscough J, Socea S, Furiosi L, Giannaccare G, et al. Initial high-dose prophylaxis and extended taper for mushroom keratoplasty in vascularized herpetic scars. Am J Ophthalmol. 2020;217:212–23.
18. Price MO, Gorovoy M, Price FW, Benetz BA, Menegay HJ, Lass JH. Descemet's stripping automated endothelial keratoplasty: three-year graft and endothelial cell survival compared with penetrating keratoplasty. Ophthalmology. 2013;120:246–51.
19. Yin D, Huang A, Warrow D, Ritterband DC, Seedor JA, McCormick SA, et al. Detection of herpes simplex virus type 1 in failed descemet stripping automated endothelial keratoplasty grafts. Cornea. 2013;32:1189–92.
20. Basak SK, Basak S. Descemet membrane endothelial keratoplasty in irreversible corneal edema due to herpes simplex virus endotheliitis. Cornea. 2020;39:8–12.
21. Basak SK, Basak S. Recurrence of herpes simplex virus endotheliitis in a Descemet membrane endothelial keratoplasty graft: mimicking fungal interface infection. BMJ Case Rep CP. 2019;12:e229441.
22. The Collaborative Corneal Transplantation Studies (CCTS). Effectiveness of histocompatibility matching in high-risk corneal transplantation. The Collaborative Corneal Transplantation Studies Research Group. Arch Ophthalmol Chic Ill. 1960;1992(110):1392–403.
23. Pellegrini M, Yu AC, Spena R, Bovone C, Zauli G, Busin M. Outcomes of large-diameter deep anterior lamellar keratoplasty and converted two-piece mushroom penetrating keratoplasty for herpetic corneal scars. Eye Lond Engl. 2024;38:614–9.
24. Dohlman TH, Singh RB, Amparo F, Carreno-Galeano T, Dastjerdi M, Coco G, et al. Suppression of neovascularization by topical and subconjunctival bevacizumab after high-risk corneal transplantation. Ophthalmol Sci. 2024;4:100492.
25. Al-Debasi T, Al-Bekairy A, Al-Katheri A, Al Harbi S, Mansour M. Topical versus subconjunctival anti-vascular endothelial growth factor therapy (Bevacizumab, Ranibizumab and Aflibercept) for treatment of corneal neovascularization. Saudi J Ophthalmol. 2017;31:99–105.
26. White ML, Chodosh J. Herpes simplex virus keratitis: a treatment guideline. Hoskins Cent Qual Eye Care Am Acad Ophthalmol Website. 2014:1–69.
27. Nicholls SM, Shimeld C, Easty DL, Hill TJ. Recurrent herpes simplex after corneal transplantation in rats. Invest Ophthalmol Vis Sci. 1996;37:425–35.

28. Park CY, Lee JK, Gore PK, Lim CY, Chuck RS. Keratoplasty in the United States: a 10-year review from 2005 through 2014. Ophthalmology. 2015;122:2432–42.
29. Langston RH, Pavan-Langston D. Penetrating keratoplasty for herpetic keratitis: decision-making and management. Int Ophthalmol Clin. 1975;15:125–40.
30. Cohen EJ, Laibson PR, Arentsen JJ. Corneal transplantation for herpes simplex keratitis. Am J Ophthalmol. 1983;95:645–50.
31. Fine M, Cignetti FE. Penetrating keratoplasty in herpes simplex keratitis. Recurrence in grafts. Arch Ophthalmol Chic Ill. 1960;1977(95):613–6.
32. Ficker LA, Kirkness CM, Rice NS, Steele AD. The changing management and improved prognosis for corneal grafting in herpes simplex keratitis. Ophthalmology. 1989;96:1587–96.
33. Pandey M, Choudhury H, Abdul-Aziz A, Bhattamisra SK, Gorain B, Su JST, et al. Advancement on sustained antiviral ocular drug delivery for herpes simplex virus keratitis: recent update on potential investigation. Pharmaceutics. 2020;13:1.
34. Cursiefen C, Viaud E, Bock F, Geudelin B, Ferry A, Kadlecová P, et al. Aganirsen antisense oligonucleotide eye drops inhibit keratitis-induced corneal neovascularization and reduce need for transplantation: the I-CAN study. Ophthalmology. 2014;121:1683–92.

Ancillary Procedures

28

Manu Muraleekrishna, Noopur Gupta, Neiwete Lomi, M. Vanathi, and Radhika Tandon

Abstract

Management of viral keratitis comprises a variety of approaches, ranging from topical antiviral therapy to full-thickness corneal transplantation, depending on the clinical presentation. Typically, medical management is the primary treatment option, while cases with corneal opacification and/or perforation/corneal thinning may necessitate penetrating/lamellar keratoplasty. However, the limited availability of corneal tissues and the poor outcomes in certain clinical scenarios pose challenges for performing corneal transplantation. Several alternative surgical options have been proposed to address this gap between medical management and penetrating keratoplasty including their use in emergency situations such as amniotic membrane transplantation, tissue adhesives combined with bandage contact lenses, SMILE-derived lenticule patch grafts, Tenon's patch grafts, corneal patch grafts, conjunctival flap procedures, corneal neurotization, and tarsorrhaphy. These procedures utilize biological tissues from the patient, such as Tenon's capsule, conjunctiva, and corneal lamellar patch, or easily accessible synthetic materials, such as tissue adhesives and bandage contact lenses. While these alternatives benefit small perforations, they generally provide only temporary tectonic support and limited visual gain. In this chapter, we explore the various surgical options available for managing viral keratitis, along with their indications, advantages, and drawbacks.

Keywords

Viral keratitis · AMG · Patch graft · Conjunctival flap · Corneal neurotization · Tarsorrhaphy

28.1 Introduction

Medical treatment is the primary approach for treating viral keratitis. Topical and systemic antiviral drugs are generally used to treat infectious viral keratitis, whereas topical steroids are the primary treatment options for immune-mediated stromal and endothelial keratitis. Antiviral agents such as Acyclovir and Ganciclovir have effectively reduced viral replication and improved clinical outcomes. Additionally, adjunctive measures such as lubrication, corticosteroids, nonsteroidal anti-inflammatory, and immunomodulatory agents alleviate symptoms by reducing ocular surface inflammation and promoting tissue repair. Despite timely intervention with antiviral agents, some cases of viral keratitis may progress to severe forms, leading to corneal ectasia and thinning, perforation, anterior staphyloma, total cor-

M. Muraleekrishna · N. Gupta (✉) · N. Lomi · M. Vanathi · R. Tandon
RP Centre, AIIMS Delhi, New Delhi, India

B. Sharma et al. (eds.), *Viral Keratitis*, https://doi.org/10.1007/978-981-95-3148-6_28

neal opacity, or advanced neovascular secondary glaucoma. These include mainly aggressive infection, resistance to topical medications, and advanced stages of disease at presentation. In such cases, surgical intervention is necessary to restore corneal integrity and visual function. This chapter provides an overview of the current perspectives and surgical interventions other than full-thickness keratoplasties in managing viral keratitis.

Surgical management may be needed in up to 30–40% of infectious keratitis cases, depending on the severity of the infection [1]. It is usually required in patients with necrotizing viral keratitis, where progressive corneal melting and perforation can occur, and chronic neurotrophic keratopathies, which can cause persistent epithelial defects and stromal lysis. The different surgical modalities mainly aim to:

1. Provide temporary or permanent tectonic support to the globe in an impending or acute perforation.
2. Provide mediators to decrease inflammation and enhance healing, such as amniotic membrane graft.

Visual gain is not a primary goal and late-stage surgical procedures may be required after the complete resolution of infection and inflammation. The preferred modalities for surgical management depend on size and site of the perforation, and also the underlying aetiology. Commonly practiced surgical methods include amniotic membrane grafting, glue with bandage contact lens, Tenon's patch grafting, corneal patch graft, conjunctival flap, corneal neurotization, and tarsorrhaphy.

28.2 Amniotic Membrane Graft (AMG)

The human amniotic membrane (AM) is the innermost layer of the placenta and consists of three basic layers: an epithelial monolayer, a thick basement membrane, and an avascular hypocellular stromal layer [2, 3]. Transplantation of the amniotic membrane in the setting of corneal ulceration and persistent epithelial defect (PED), promotes epithelial wound healing, decreases inflammation, and promotes anti-scarring and anti-angiogenic effects on the ocular surface [4]. The structural integrity, transparency, and elasticity of the amniotic basement membrane make it a widely accepted tissue replacement material for ocular surface reconstruction procedures. It promotes epithelial cell adhesion, migration, and differentiation. It also supports the growth of epithelial progenitor cells by prolonging their lifespan, maintaining normal morphology, and preventing epithelial cell apoptosis [5]. This helps AMG to facilitate epithelialization in cases of persistent epithelial defects in neurotrophic keratopathies, which is a common complication of recurrent viral keratitis [6].

Corneal denervation and desensitization in cases of viral keratitis leads to recurrent epithelial defects, persistent epithelial defects, and neurotrophic ulcerations with a risk of corneal stromal exposure to multiple inflammatory mediators and can result in stromal lysis and perforation, including secondary bacterial/fungal infection. Amniotic membrane transplantation (AMT) promotes healing by releasing neuro-epitheliotrophic factors and anti-inflammatory mediators, along with mechanically covering the defect, which blocks the access of inflammatory mediators to the exposed bare stroma. This mechanical support also helps to reduce pain and discomfort in severely symptomatic patients.

28.2.1 Surgical Technique

Different surgical techniques have been described for AMT depending on the size, location, and the cause of corneal perforation. The three basic principles are (1) the inlay or graft technique, (2) the overlay or patch technique, and (3) filling or multi-layered application. The inlay technique is commonly used for persistent epithelial defects, where the AM is trimmed to the size of the defect with the epithelial side up and sutured to the edges with 10-0 monofilament nylon and then covered temporarily with a bandage contact lens [6]. The membrane acts as a scaffold for migrating surrounding healthy epithelial cells.

An overlay or patch technique is required on an inflamed surface where AM acts as a protective barrier to the underlying healing epithelium from the surface inflammatory mediators. Here, the larger membrane should cover the entire affected cornea with the stromal side up and sutured to the perilimbal conjunctiva using absorbable 8-0 vicryl sutures (Fig. 28.1). In this technique, AM acts as a biological contact lens.

The multi-layered technique is used in cases of deep ulcers, the stromal defect is filled with multiple pieces of AM as an inlay, and then a large AM is used to cover the entire surface as an onlay technique. Beguiga et al. described this technique as suturing a large overlay AM followed by filling the underlying stromal defect by sliding the pieces beneath it [7].

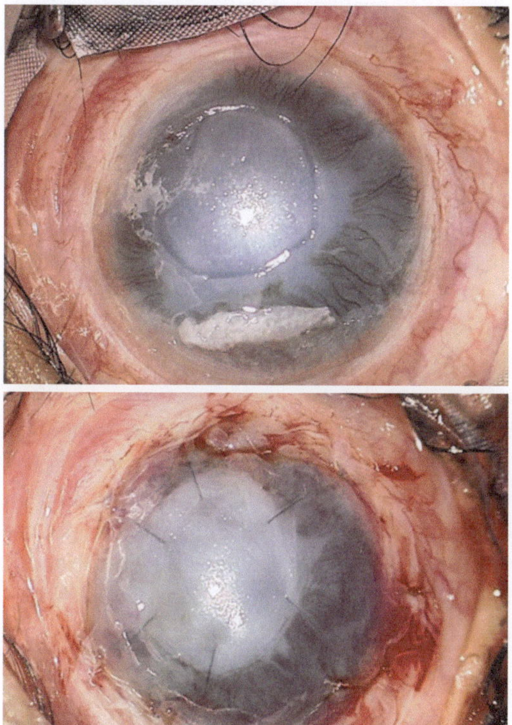

Fig. 28.1 Preoperative and postoperative images of amniotic membrane grafting in a case of persistent epithelial defect

28.2.2 Complications

Although it is a safe procedure, few complications and disadvantages such as suture site granuloma and hypopyon have been reported after this technique [8]. Infections with gram-positive organisms after freshly prepared amniotic membrane transplants are not uncommon. The reported incidence of microbial infection following freshly prepared AM is 8% and that of the preserved form is 1.6% [9, 10].

28.3 Tissue Adhesives

The purpose of using tissue adhesives for corneal gluing in viral keratitis is to provide tectonic support to the globe in cases of impending perforations, descemetocele, or small perforations of less than 3 mm. Two commonly used tissue adhesives compounds are: (1) synthetic tissue adhesives, mainly based on cyanoacrylates and other polymers, and (2) tissue adhesives based on naturally derived polymers, such as polysaccharides and proteins [11].

The main advantages of synthetic tissue adhesives are their low cost, high purity, and ease of availability. The most commercially available and widely used form is cyanoacrylate glue. Naturally derived tissue adhesives are mainly protein-based and include fibrin, collagen, and albumin. Fibrin-based adhesives are the most commonly used and FDA-approved form for ophthalmic use.

28.3.1 Surgical Technique

Various surgical techniques have been described for tissue-adhesive applications for different ophthalmic indications. The basic steps to be followed in all cases include strict aseptic surgical environment, adequate anaesthesia, maintenance of a dry surface before application, removal of necrotic tissue from the base of the ulcer or stromal defect, debridement of 1–2 mm of epithelium surrounding the area of application, and controlled use of minimum required glue to avoid excess spillage over the unaffected tissue [12]. The release of iris tissue from the defect and maintenance of a well-formed anterior chamber before application of glue are also important to avoid contact of glue with the iris tissue and severe post-operative inflammation.

28.3.1.1 Techniques of Application of Cyanoacrylate Glue

(a) A simple method is the direct application of glue over the dry surface using a 1 ml syringe and 26G needle in a controlled fashion and allowing it to polymerize for 20–30 seconds before application of a bandage contact lens to cover the rough surface [13]. This is possible if there is an impending perforation or micro-perforation without significant tissue loss and uveal tissue plugging (Fig. 28.2).

(b) A drape-and-patch technique has been described for small corneal perforations where a 3 mm trimmed disc of the non-adhesive part of a surgical drape is used to plug the defect along with cyanoacrylate glue [14]. This helps to avoid dislodgement of the glue and better sealing. Gandhewar et al. modified this technique using a double drape and patch method to avoid glue leakage into the anterior chamber and contact with uveal tissue, especially in larger perforations with iris incarceration [15].

(c) Sykakis et al. described the contact lens sandwich technique for glue application, where a BCL patch was used instead of a surgical drape and then covered with a complete BCL application [16]. The shape of BCL resembles that of a normal corneal contour. For perforations of more than 3 mm in size, Moschos et al. used a suture reticulum with 10-0 nylon to act as a scaffold for glue application [17].

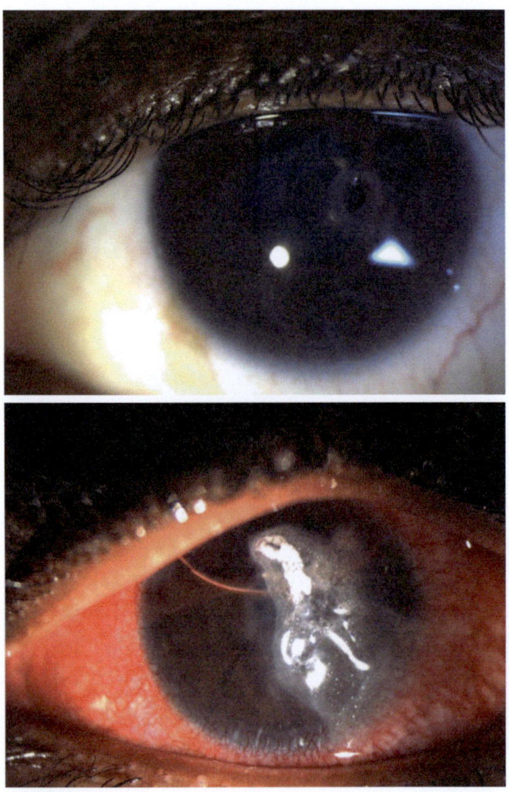

Fig. 28.2 Preoperative and postoperative images of corneal gluing with bandage contact lens for small corneal perforation

The success rate of corneal gluing depends on the stage of the ulcer, severity, size of the perforation, and etiological agent. It varies from 37% to 75% in overall microbial keratitis [18–20]. In a retrospective case series analysis, Moorthy et al. studied the role of cyanoacrylate glue (direct application or patch technique) in corneal perforation secondary to active herpetic keratitis. This study included 46 eyes and reported that complete healing with corneal scarring was achieved in 37% (17 eyes) of eyes, and the remaining 53% (26 eyes) had to undergo therapeutic keratoplasty. They concluded that this method is not useful for complete healing in cases of herpetic keratitis-associated perforation. Compared to cyanoacrylate glue, a better success rate of 78–81% has been documented with the use of fibrin glue in overall microbial keratitis [21, 22]. However, the outcomes of herpetic keratitis and perforations larger than 2 mm are poorer than those of bacterial keratitis.

Tissue adhesives are commonly used surgical techniques for impending perforations and small perforations, with different modifications. It provides an option to avoid full-thickness keratoplasty in these patients and avoids all risks associated with an open-sky procedure.

Moreover, this simple procedure does not require any eye banking facility or surgical expertise. Another important advantage of cyanoacrylate glue is its bacteriostatic and antifungal properties, which help to control disease activity along with providing tectonic support to the globe [23].

28.4 Tenon's Patch Graft

Tenon's patch graft (TPG) is a technique used to seal small corneal perforations and descemetocele using the Tenon's tissue retrieved from the patient. Tenon's capsule can produce autologous fibroblasts and promote healing when incorporated into corneal tissues [24]. This property of Tenon's tissue, along with their vascularity and elasticity, has made them an alternative option to corneal patch grafting or cyanoacrylate glue application to seal small corneal perforations. The main advantage of TPG is the ease of harvesting tissue from the same patient and the lack of an immunological reaction to this autologous tissue.

28.4.1 Surgical Technique

Tenon's tissue of adequate size, preferably 1 mm larger than the corneal perforation, is harvested from the same eye of the patient after a localized peritomy and separating the overlying conjunctiva. The corneal ulcer needs to be debrided to remove necrotic tissue and unhealthy epithelium for better graft attachment (Fig. 28.3). The anterior chamber should be maintained with air after releasing the iris tissue if it is plugged into the defect [25, 26]. A temporary BCL application is recommended for the initial 2 weeks until the graft tissue is smoothly taken up by the new environment.

For perforations less than 3 mm in size, TPG secured with cyanoacrylate glue has also been described instead of nylon sutures [27]. This procedure is easier to perform and avoids suture-related complications, including suture cutting through the Tenon's graft and graft dislodgement during the postoperative period. Another method is tuck-in a Tenon's patch graft, where a stromal pocket is created around the margin of the corneal defect and the donor Tenon's graft is tucked into the pocket [28]. This provides better tissue adhesion with less chances of graft dislodgement.

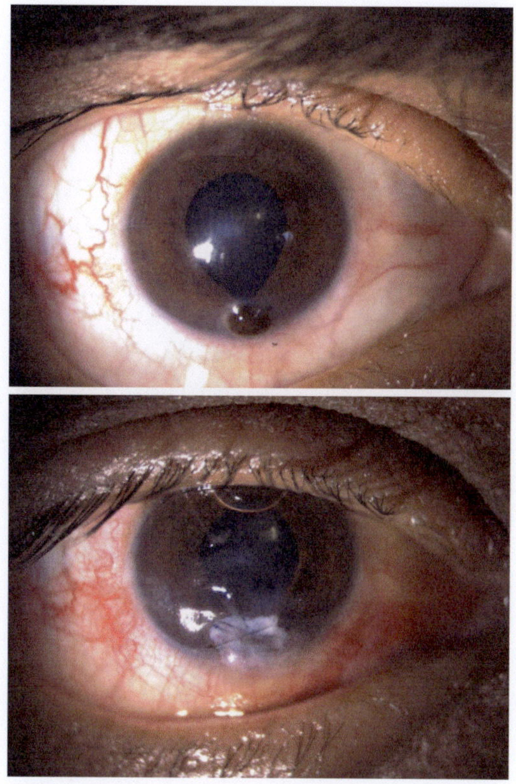

Fig. 28.3 Preoperative and postoperative image of Tenon's patch graft in a patient with peripheral corneal perforation

28.4.2 Complications

The major disadvantage of TPG is the opaque nature of the graft, which causes obscuration of the visual axis and can only provide tectonic support to the globe. This becomes a major concern when dealing with central corneal perforations, for which a corneal patch graft may be preferred over TPG. Post-operative wound leakage, graft retraction, dislodgement, graft thinning, and staphyloma formation are possible complications associated with this procedure [25, 28].

28.5 SMILE-Derived Lenticule Patch Graft

Introduction of Small Incision Lenticule Extraction (SMILE, Carl Zeiss Meditec AG), a kerato-refractive lenticule extraction (KLEx) procedure added the option of using the extracted corneal stromal lenticule for patching the defect in cases of perforated corneal ulcers. The corneal stromal lenticule is a by-product of all KLEx procedures with variable thickness, depending on the refractive error of the treated patient. The use of a freshly extracted or cryo-preserved lenticule can be utilized for corneal patching as it provides tectonic support without the backup of eye banking facilities. This provides temporary support to the affected surface until full-thickness corneal tissue is available for optical keratoplasty, particularly in developing countries.

28.5.1 Surgical Technique

The surgical procedure for host bed preparation is similar to that used for TPG. The retrieved lenticule can be transferred to the thinned-out or perforated site and sutured with 10-0 MFN sutures or adhesive fibrin glue (Fig. 28.4). A moderately myopic patient lenticule can add a thickness of 50–100 microns to the stromal bed. Multiple lenticules can be sutured together if thinning is severe or if there is a descemetocele with an impending perforation. An amniotic membrane can be used as an overlay to accelerate healing in some cases [29].

Fang Wu and co-workers introduced the use of SMILE lenticule patch as a surgical alternative to close wounds in corneal perforation [30]. They achieved a 100% success rate in closing the wound, and 50% of their patients had improved best-corrected visual acuity postoperatively. Successive studies on this technique have also shown successful wound sealing with an increase in visual acuity in perforated corneal ulcers [31, 32].

The major advantage of the SMILE lenticule patch graft is the use of a transparent graft of adequate thickness, which can provide tectonic support with visual gain simultaneously and can even avoid subsequent surgical procedures for visual rehabilitation in many cases. Since the grafted tissue is also a corneal stromal layer, it is easily taken up by the host bed with better graft survival. However, the lack of this refractive surgical facility and cryopreservation of the lenticule limits the use of this technique in many centres.

28.6 Corneal Patch Graft

Small perforations can be effectively managed using the aforementioned surgical techniques. However, perforations greater than 3 mm in size and involving the peripheral cornea may require small lamellar or full-thickness corneal patch

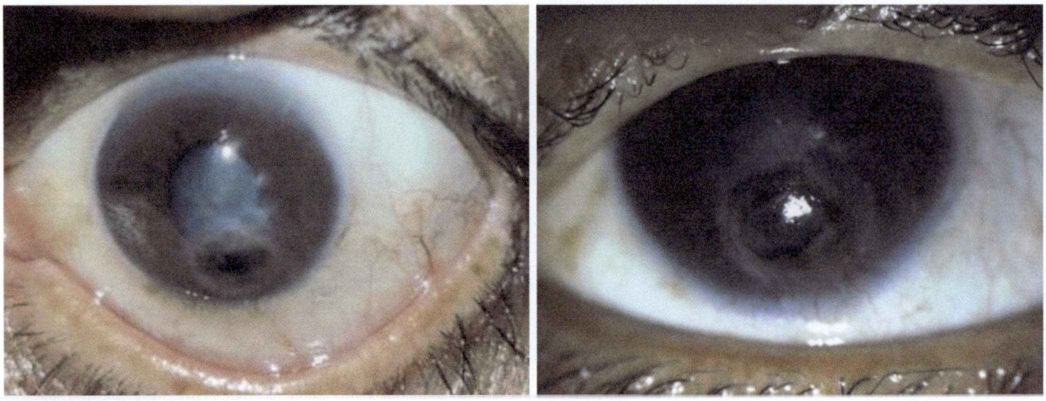

Fig. 28.4 SMILE (Small Incision lenticule extraction)-lenticule assisted patch graft in a patient with viral keratitis

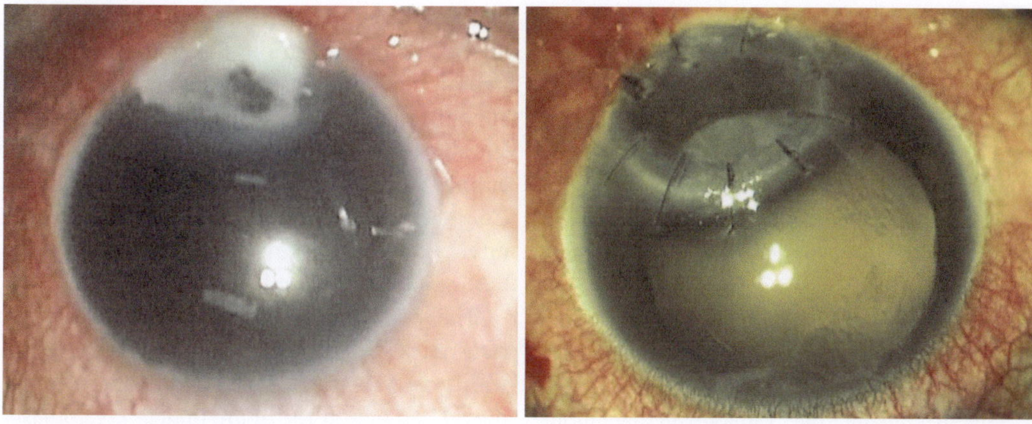

Fig. 28.5 Preoperative and postoperative images in a patient treated with sutured corneal patch graft for viral keratitis with secondary bacterial infection and corneal perforation

grafts. These larger perforations necessitate more substantial support, and adhesive glue, bandage contact lenses, and Tenon's patch grafts alone may be insufficient. A lamellar patch graft has the advantage of reducing the risk of an open-sky procedure and is a preferred option for impending perforations and descemetoceles. Nevertheless, a full-thickness patch graft is necessary for perforated ulcers. For peripheral perforations, a corneal patch graft should be considered, as the suture does not interfere with the visual axis. Non-optical grade tissue can also be used for corneal patch grafting, providing temporary tectonic support to the globe and buying time for future optical keratoplasty, if necessary, for visual rehabilitation.

28.6.1 Surgical Technique

The surgical methodology for this procedure is akin to full-thickness keratoplasty. The dimensions of the donor tissue are contingent upon the size and location of the perforation. Subsequent to releasing the uveal tissue from the wound and thoroughly dissecting the infected tissue, the graft of equal dimensions can be obtained utilizing a dermatome punch. In cases where perforations are imminent, or descemetoceles are present, lamellar grafts that have been manually dissected can also be employed. The corneal patch graft may be secured with 10-0 monofilament nylon sutures (Fig. 28.5) or fibrin glue. Gupta N et al. have reported a case series of sutureless full-thickness and lamellar corneal patch grafts in perforations ranging in size from 3 to 5 mm, utilizing fibrin glue [33].

Long-term functional and anatomical outcomes of corneal patch grafts have demonstrated encouraging results in cases of peripheral corneal melts resulting from various causes. In a retrospective analysis of 49 patients conducted by Sharma et al., it was found that 60% of the cases had both anatomical and functional success with penetrating and lamellar corneal patch grafts [34].

28.7 Conjunctival Flap

Conjunctival flap procedure can be considered for neurotrophic keratopathy and progressive corneal thinning following recurrent herpetic keratitis. However, it is not an option for active ongoing viral keratitis or frank corneal perforation. A mobilized conjunctival flap helps the blood vessels reach the ulcer area and enhance the healing process. It has been described as an effective management option for corneal thinning due to infective keratitis [35–37].

28.7.1 Surgical Technique

The two major techniques for conjunctival flap surgery are the Gundersen and partial pedicle flaps:

(a) The conjunctival flap technique for the treatment of corneal disease was first described by Gundersen [38], later popularized as the Gundersen flap technique. Here, the entire cornea is covered with conjunctival tissue. Complete coverage of the cornea by the conjunctiva using the Gundersen technique makes it difficult for surgeons to assess the progression of the underlying disease and detailed anterior segment examination.
(b) The partial pedicle flap technique uses a part of the conjunctival pedicle with vasculature to cover only the affected part of the cornea rather than the complete cornea (Fig. 28.6). Localized peritomy and conjunctival dissection are performed from the quadrant nearer to the affected area, mobilized, and sutured with non-absorbable sutures. It avoids complete conjunctivalization of the cornea and allows assessment of the rest of the anterior segment structures and better visual outcome for non-central ulcers. This technique has almost replaced the Gundersen flap technique owing to these added advantages.

The major advantage of the conjunctival flap procedure is the use of autologous tissue, which is readily available and simple procedure that can be performed even in a basic ophthalmic care centre without any eye bank support. This provides temporary mechanical support to the thinning cornea, which can otherwise lead to perforation at any time. Conjunctival flaps with blood vessels provide direct access to serum mediators, thereby, promoting faster healing [38].

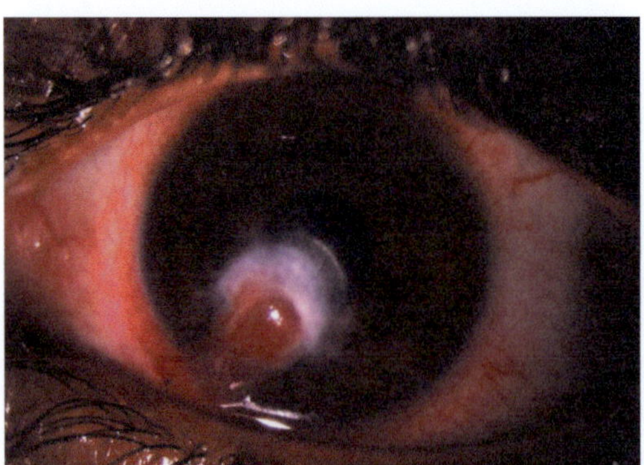

Fig. 28.6 Clinical picture of a patient with peripheral corneal perforation treated with conjunctival pedicle graft

The conjunctival flap procedure is usually reserved as a late resort for non-healing ulcers with poor visual prognosis because it does not provide an option for future optical keratoplasty or reduces the chance of survival of a future graft due to vascularization of the host bed.

28.8 Corneal Neurotization

Corneal neurotization is a relatively novel technique for the treatment of post-viral neurotrophic keratopathy. This aims to provide sensory reinnervation to an anaesthetic or hypoaesthetic cornea and nerve-derived epithelial growth factors to enhance the healing process [39].

28.8.1 Surgical Technique

Two methods of corneal neurotization have been described:

(a) Direct neurotization- Transposition of the supraorbital or supratrochlear nerve to the cornea [39, 40] and Indirect neurotization- Transposition of the sural nerve graft [41]. In the direct technique, a healthy contralateral supraorbital or supratrochlear nerve is retrieved by a coronal incision and transferred to the affected cornea through a tunnel incision crossing the nasal bridge and reaching the limbal area. In cases of corneal anaesthesia due to localized ciliary nerve damage, the ipsilateral supraorbital nerve can also be transposed.
(b) Indirect technique- Sural nerve graft is anastomosed with the contralateral healthy supratrochlear nerve and transpositioned subcutaneously to cross the nasal bridge, and

then subconjunctivally to reach the perilimbal area of the affected eye [42]. Temporary tarsorrhaphy can also be performed to allow for complete nerve regeneration.

An average duration of 3–6 months is required to regain corneal sensations after successful neurotization [43]. The outcome of the procedure can be assessed by direct visualization of regenerated nerve fibres using confocal microscopy or corneal sensations assessment using a Cochet-Bonnet esthesiometer.

28.9 Tarsorrhaphy

Tarsorrhaphy is not recommended for active viral keratitis, which can affect antiviral therapy and does not allow the treating surgeon to assess the underlying disease progression completely. However, a temporary tarsorrhaphy can provide external support to the severely affected globe until an emergency therapeutic keratoplasty can be undertaken.

Lateral permanent tarsorrhaphy is preferred in cases of persistent epithelial defects and neurotrophic keratopathy resulting from long-standing herpetic viral keratitis (Fig. 28.7a, b). It helps in corneal healing by decreasing corneal exposure, maintaining the tear film layer, and decreasing constant rubbing by the lids over newly formed epithelium, especially on a poor ocular surface. It is often used as an adjunct to other procedures, such as amniotic membrane grafting in non-healing neurotrophic viral keratitis. Cosar et al. reported a 90% success rate in healing epithelial defects after permanent tarsorrhaphy [44].

The major disadvantage of this procedure is the cosmesis related to the patient. However, the major concern with the treating doctor is the underlying disease activity, poor drug penetration, and retention of tear inflammatory mediators, including collagenolytic enzymes, over the exposed stroma, which can further damage the surface and lead to perforation. Proper case selection and timing of the procedure are important to avoid such complications.

28.10 Conclusion

Timely and appropriate surgical intervention can significantly improve patient outcomes and preserve visual function in viral keratitis; the management of which often mandates surgical intervention in cases refractory to medical therapy. Various techniques, including amniotic membrane grafting, tissue adhesives, Tenon's

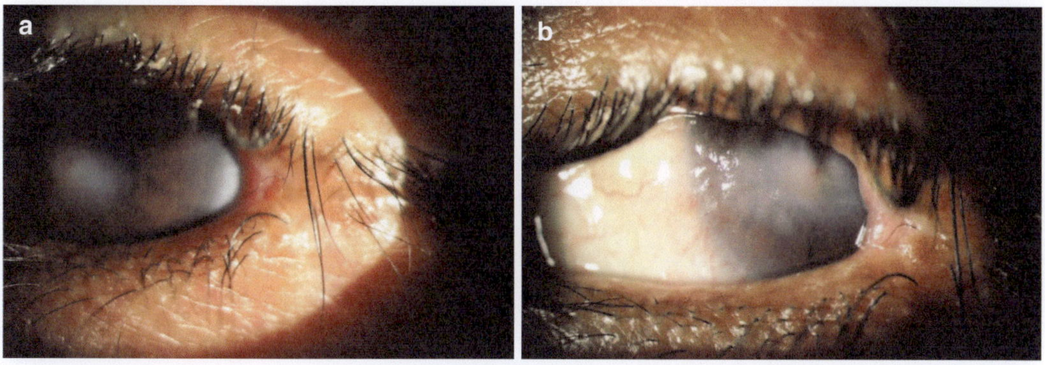

Fig. 28.7 (**a**, **b**) Patient with neurotrophic keratopathy shows complete healing of corneal pathology following lateral tarsorrhaphy

patch grafts, and corneal patch grafts, provide effective options for addressing corneal perforations and promoting healing with each method having its own unique advantages and potential complications. Emerging techniques, such as corneal neurotization and the use of SMILE-derived lenticules, offer promising alternatives for enhancing corneal repair and sensory function.

Key Points

- Management of viral keratitis often necessitates surgical intervention, including penetrating keratoplasty.
- Different ancillary procedures with minor variations in surgical techniques can serve as alternative options to a full-thickness keratoplasty, especially in cases of small corneal perforations and non-healing ulcers.
- While these procedures are cost-effective and simple to perform, the visual outcome is not typically favourable.
- Tenon's patch graft and conjunctival flap surgeries can lead to corneal vascularization, which may have an adverse impact on the success rate of future corneal transplant procedures.
- Various methods for transplanting amniotic membrane have demonstrated optimal clinical outcomes in treating non-healing corneal ulcers. However, the cost and accessibility of this technique are significant factors affecting their universal usage.
- Corneal neurotization is a relatively new procedure that holds promise for improving outcomes in patients with neurotrophic keratopathies.

References

1. Said DG, Rallis KI, Al-Aqaba MA, Ting DSJ, Dua HS. Surgical management of infectious keratitis. Ocul Surf. 2023;28:401–12.
2. Sangwan VS, Burman S, Tejwani S, Mahesh SP, Murthy R. Amniotic membrane transplantation: a review of current indications in the management of ophthalmic disorders. Indian J Ophthalmol. 2007;55(4):251.
3. Tuli S, Gray M. Surgical management of corneal infections. Curr Opin Ophthalmol. 2016;27(4):340–7.
4. Tseng SCG, Espana EM, Kawakita T, Di Pascuale MA, Li W, He H, et al. How does amniotic membrane work? Ocul Surf. 2004;2(3):177–87.
5. Grueterich M, Tseng SCG. Human limbal progenitor cells expanded on intact amniotic membrane ex vivo. Arch Ophthalmol. 2002;120(6):783–90.
6. Lee SH, Tseng SC. Amniotic membrane transplantation for persistent epithelial defects with ulceration. Am J Ophthalmol. 1997;123(3):303–12.
7. Berguiga M, Mameletzi E, Nicolas M, Rivier D, Majo F. Long-term follow-up of multilayer amniotic membrane transplantation (MLAMT) for non-traumatic corneal perforations or deep ulcers with descemetocele. Klin Monatsbl Augenheilkd. 2013;230(4):413–8.
8. Gabler B, Lohmann CP. Hypopyon after repeated transplantation of human amniotic membrane onto the corneal surface. Ophthalmology. 2000;107(7):1344–6.
9. Khokhar S, Sharma N, Kumar H, Soni A. Infection after use of nonpreserved human amniotic membrane for the reconstruction of the ocular surface. Cornea. 2001;20(7):773–4.
10. Marangon FB, Alfonso EC, Miller D, Remonda NM, Muallem MS, Tseng SCG. Incidence of microbial infection after amniotic membrane transplantation. Cornea. 2004;23(3):264–9.
11. Trujillo-de Santiago G, Sharifi R, Yue K, Sani ES, Kashaf SS, Alvarez MM, et al. Ocular adhesives: design, chemistry, crosslinking mechanisms, and applications. Biomaterials. 2019;197:345–67.
12. Rana M, Savant V. A brief review of techniques used to seal corneal perforation using cyanoacrylate tissue adhesive. Cont Lens Anterior Eye. 2013;36(4):156–8.
13. Fogle JA, Kenyon KR, Foster CS. Tissue adhesive arrests stromal melting in the human cornea. Am J Ophthalmol. 1980;89(6):795–802.
14. Jhanji V, Young AL, Mehta JS, Sharma N, Agarwal T, Vajpayee RB. Management of corneal perforation. Surv Ophthalmol. 2011;56(6):522–38.
15. Gandhewar J, Savant V, Prydal J, Dua H. Double drape tectonic patch with cyanoacrylate glue in the management of corneal perforation with iris incarceration. Cornea. 2013;32(5):e137–8.
16. Sykakis E, Parmar DN. Management of non traumatic corneal perforations with cyanoacrylate tissue adhesive: the 'contact lens sandwich' technique. Cont Lens Anterior Eye. 2014;37(2):121.
17. Moschos M, Droutsas D, Boussalis P, Tsioulias G. Clinical experience with cyanoacrylate tissue adhesive. Doc Ophthalmol. 1997;93(3):237–45.
18. Yin J, Singh RB, Al Karmi R, Yung A, Yu M, Dana R. Outcomes of cyanoacrylate tissue adhesive application in corneal thinning and perforation. Cornea. 2019;38(6):668–73.
19. Garg P, Gopinathan U, Nutheti R, Rao GN. Clinical experience with N-butyl cyanoacrylate tissue adhesive in fungal keratitis. Cornea. 2003;22(5):405–8.

20. Moorthy S, Jhanji V, Constantinou M, Beltz J, Graue-Hernandez EO, Vajpayee RB. Clinical experience with N-butyl cyanoacrylate tissue adhesive in corneal perforations secondary to herpetic keratitis. Cornea. 2010;29(9):971–5.
21. Siatiri H, Moghimi S, Malihi M, Khodabande A. Use of sealant (HFG) in corneal perforations. Cornea. 2008;27(9):988–91.
22. Sharma A, Kaur R, Kumar S, Gupta P, Pandav S, Patnaik B, et al. Fibrin glue versus N-butyl-2-cyanoacrylate in corneal perforations. Ophthalmology. 2003;110(2):291–8.
23. Dogan C, Aygun G, Bahar-Tokman H, Yazgan Z, Mergen B, Ozdamar A, et al. In vitro antifungal effect of acrylic corneal glue (N-butyl-2-cyanoacrylate). Cornea. 2019;38(12):1563–7.
24. Kakizaki H, Takahashi Y, Nakano T, Asamoto K, Ikeda H, Ichinose A, et al. Anatomy of Tenon's capsule. Clin Experiment Ophthalmol. 2012;40(6):611–6.
25. Singhal D, Sahay P, Maharana PK, Amar SP, Titiyal JS, Sharma N. Clinical presentation and management of corneal fistula. Br J Ophthalmol. 2019;103(4):530–3.
26. Maharana PK, Singhal D, Sahay P, Titiyal JS. Tenon patch graft for corneal fistula: a rare entity treated by a simple technique. BMJ Case Rep. 2017;2017:bcr2017222790. https://doi.org/10.1136/bcr-2017-222790.
27. Korah S, Selvin SST, Pradhan ZS, Jacob P, Kuriakose T. Tenon's patch graft in the management of large corneal perforations. Cornea. 2016;35(5):696–9.
28. Sharma N, Singhal D, Maharana PK, Vajpayee RB. Tuck-in tenon patch graft in corneal perforation. Cornea. 2019;38(8):951–4.
29. Baum J. Thygeson lecture. Amniotic membrane transplantation: why is it effective? Cornea. 2002;21(4):339–41.
30. Wu F, Jin X, Xu Y, Yang Y. Treatment of corneal perforation with lenticules from small incision lenticule extraction surgery: a preliminary study of 6 patients. Cornea. 2015;34(6):658–63.
31. Bhandari V, Ganesh S, Brar S, Pandey R. Application of the SMILE-derived glued lenticule patch graft in microperforations and partial-thickness corneal defects. Cornea. 2016;35(3):408–12.
32. Jiang Y, Li Y, Liu XW, Xu J. A novel tectonic keratoplasty with femtosecond laser intrastromal lenticule for corneal ulcer and perforation. Chin Med J (Engl). 2016;129(15):1817–21.
33. Gupta N, Sachdev R, Tandon R. Sutureless patch graft for sterile corneal melts. Cornea. 2010;29(8):921–3.
34. Sharma S, Rathi A, Murthy SI, Trivedi M, Patel C, Mohamed A, et al. Outcomes of penetrating and lamellar corneal patch grafts. Cornea. 2021;40(5):618–23.
35. Sun GH, Li SX, Gao H, Zhang WB, Zhang MA, Shi WY. Clinical observation of removal of the necrotic corneal tissue combined with conjunctival flap covering surgery under the guidance of the AS-OCT in treatment of fungal keratitis. Int J Ophthalmol. 2012;5(1):88–91.
36. Khodadoust A, Quinter AP. Microsurgical approach to the conjunctival flap. Arch Ophthalmol. 2003;121(8):1189–93.
37. Nizeyimana H, Zhou DD, Liu XF, Pan XT, Liu C, Lu CW, et al. Clinical efficacy of conjunctival flap surgery in the treatment of refractory fungal keratitis. Exp Ther Med. 2017;14(2):1109–13.
38. Gundersen T. Conjunctival flaps in the treatment of corneal disease with reference to a new technique of application. AMA Arch Ophthalmol. 1958;60(5):880–8.
39. Terzis JK, Dryer MM, Bodner BI. Corneal neurotization: a novel solution to neurotrophic keratopathy. Plast Reconstr Surg. 2009;123(1):112–20.
40. Allevi F, Fogagnolo P, Rossetti L, Biglioli F. Eyelid reanimation, neurotisation, and transplantation of the cornea in a patient with facial palsy. BMJ Case Rep. 2014;2014:bcr2014205372.
41. Elbaz U, Bains R, Zuker RM, Borschel GH, Ali A. Restoration of corneal sensation with regional nerve transfers and nerve grafts: a new approach to a difficult problem. JAMA Ophthalmol. 2014;132(11):1289–95.
42. Bains RD, Elbaz U, Zuker RM, Ali A, Borschel GH. Corneal neurotization from the supratrochlear nerve with sural nerve grafts: a minimally invasive approach. Plast Reconstr Surg. 2015;135(2):397e–400e.
43. Tuli S, Gray M, Shah A. Surgical management of herpetic keratitis. Curr Opin Ophthalmol. 2018;29(4):347–54.
44. Cosar CB, Cohen EJ, Rapuano CJ, Maus M, Penne RP, Flanagan JC, et al. Tarsorrhaphy: clinical experience from a cornea practice. Cornea. 2001;20(8):787–91.

Correction to: Disciform Keratitis

Purvasha Narang, Bhavana Sharma, Snehal Nimje,
and Aviral Vasudeo

Correction to:
Chapter 12 in: B. Sharma et al. (eds.), *Viral Keratitis*, https://doi.org/10.1007/978-981-95-3148-6_12

The first name of Snehal Nimje was unfortunately published with an error. The initially published version has now been corrected.

The updated version of this chapter can be found at
https://doi.org/10.1007/978-981-95-3148-6_12

B. Sharma et al. (eds.), *Viral Keratitis*, https://doi.org/10.1007/978-981-95-3148-6_29

Editorial Note

This essential resource offers a detailed description of viral keratitis, covering the spectrum of causative agents including Herpes Simplex Virus (HSV), Varicella-Zoster Virus (VZV), Adenovirus, and other significant viral pathogens. Structured across 28 comprehensive chapters over five sections, this book provides a thorough understanding of the pathogenesis, clinical manifestations, diagnosis, and management of viral keratitis, making it invaluable for ophthalmologists, residents, and researchers alike. It provides clear guidance on epidemiology for understanding the disease spread and risk factors for early identification, in addition to practical insights into current treatment modalities, and actionable prevention strategies. This book shall serve to be an indispensable tool for eye care professionals seeking a practical and thorough understanding of viral keratitis management.

HAPPY READING

B. Sharma et al. (eds.), *Viral Keratitis*, https://doi.org/10.1007/978-981-95-3148-6

MIX
Papier aus verantwortungsvollen Quellen
Paper from responsible sources
FSC® C105338

If you have any concerns about our products,
you can contact us on
ProductSafety@springernature.com

In case Publisher is established outside the EU,
the EU authorized representative is:
Springer Nature Customer Service Center GmbH
Europaplatz 3, 69115 Heidelberg, Germany

Printed by Libri Plureos GmbH
in Hamburg, Germany